Shoulder Instability

Editors

JONATHAN F. DICKENS
BRIAN C. LAU

CLINICS IN
SPORTS MEDICINE

www.sportsmed.theclinics.com

Consulting Editor
F. WINSTON GWATHMEY

October 2024 • Volume 43 • Number 4

ELSEVIER

1600 John F. Kennedy Boulevard ● Suite 1800 ● Philadelphia, Pennsylvania, 19103-2899

http://www.theclinics.com

CLINICS IN SPORTS MEDICINE Volume 43, Number 4
October 2024 ISSN 0278-5919, ISBN-13: 978-0-443-12873-8

Editor: Megan Ashdown
Developmental Editor: Malvika Shah

Clinics in Sports Medicine (ISSN 0278-5919) is published quarterly by Elsevier Inc., 360 Park Avenue South, New York, NY 10010-1710. Months of issue are January, April, July, and October. Business and Editorial Offices: 1600 John F. Kennedy Blvd., Ste. 1800, Philadelphia, PA 19103-2899. Customer Service Office: 3251 Riverport Lane, Maryland Heights, MO 63043. Periodicals postage paid at New York, NY and additional mailing offices. Subscription prices are $390.00 per year (US individuals), $100.00 per year (US students), $430.00 per year (Canadian individuals), $100.00 (Canadian students), $504.00 per year (foreign individuals), and $235.00 per year (foreign students). For institutional access pricing please contact Customer Service via the contact information below. Foreign air speed delivery is included in all *Clinics* subscription prices. All prices are subject to change without notice. Orders, claims, and journal inquiries: Please visit our Support Hub page https://service.elsevier.com for assistance.

Reprints. For copies of 100 or more of articles in this publication, please contact the Commercial Reprints Department, Elsevier Inc., 360 Park Avenue South, New York, NY 10010-1710. Tel.: 212-633-3874; Fax: 212-633-3820; E-mail: reprints@elsevier.com.

Clinics in Sports Medicine is covered in *MEDLINE/PubMed (Index Medicus) Current Contents/Clinical Medicine, Excerpta Medica,* and *ISI/Biomed.*

Contributors

CONSULTING EDITOR

F. WINSTON GWATHMEY, MD
Associate Professor of Orthopaedic Surgery, University of Virginia Health System, Charlottesville, Virginia, USA; Vice Chair for Orthopaedic Education and Residency Program Director, Team Physician, UVA and JMU Athletics, Charlottesville, Virginia, USA

EDITORS

JONATHAN F. DICKENS, MD, COL, MC, USAR
Professor and Fellowship Director, Department of Orthopaedics, Duke Sports Medicine, Duke University, Durham, North Carolina, USA; Department of Orthopaedic Surgery, Walter Reed National Military Medical Center Uniformed Services, University of Health Sciences, Bethesda, Maryland, USA; Department of Orthopaedics, Institute of Clinical Sciences, Sahlgrenska Academy, Gothenburg University, Gothenburg, Sweden

BRIAN C. LAU, MD
Assistant Professor, Department of Orthopaedic Surgery, Duke University School of Medicine, Durham, North Carolina, USA; Department of Orthopaedic Surgery, Walter Reed National Military Medical Center Uniformed Services, University of Health Sciences, Bethesda, Maryland, USA

AUTHORS

MARCO ADRIANI, MD
Resident, Department of Medical and Surgical Specialties, Radiological Sciences, and Public Health, University of Brescia, Brescia, Italy; Steadman Philippon Research Institute, Vail, Colorado, USA

ROBERT A. ARCIERO, MD
Professor, Department of Orthopaedic Surgery, University of Connecticut Health Center, University of Connecticut Health Musculoskeletal Institute, Farmington, Connecticut, USA

JUSTIN W. ARNER, MD
Clinical Assistant Professor, Department of Orthopaedic Surgery, University of Pittsburgh Medical Center, Pittsburgh, Pennsylvania, USA; Sports Medicine Orthopaedic Surgery, Burke and Bradley, Pittsburgh, Pennsylvania, USA

ANNA E. BOZZONE, BA
Orthopaedic Surgery Research Assistant, Medical College of Georgia at Augusta University, Augusta, Georgia, USA

JAMES P. BRADLEY, MD
Professor, Department of Orthopaedic Surgery, University of Pittsburgh Medical Center, Burke and Bradley Orthopedics, Pittsburgh, Pennsylvania, USA

JOSEPH C. BRINKMAN, MD
Resident, Department of Orthopedic Surgery, Mayo Clinic, Phoenix, Arizona, USA

GARRETT S. BULLOCK, DPT, DPhil
Assistant Professor, Department of Orthopaedic Surgery and Rehabilitation, Wake Forest University School of Medicine, Winston-Salem, North Carolina, USA

GARRETT V. CHRISTENSEN, MD
Resident Physician, Department of Orthopedics and Rehabilitation, University of Iowa Hospitals and Clinics, Iowa City, Iowa, USA

ELIZABETH DAMITIO
Undergraduate Research Assistant, Institute of Protein Design, University of Washington, Seattle, Washington, USA

MIKALYN T. DEFOOR, MD
Orthopaedic Surgery Resident, San Antonio Military Medical Center, San Antonio, Texas, USA

GIOVANNI DI GIACOMO, MD
Orthopaedic Surgeon, Orthopedics and Traumatology Unit, Concordia Hospital, Rome, Italy

ALEX FAILS, DPT
Postdoctoral Researcher, Department of Orthopaedic Surgery, UPMC Freddie Fu Sports Medicine Center, Pittsburgh, Pennsylvania, USA

ANTHONY P. FIEGEN, MD
Fellow, Department of Orthopaedic Surgery and Rehabilitation, Wake Forest University School of Medicine, Winston-Salem, North Carolina, USA

JOSEPH W. GALVIN, DO
Associate Professor of Surgery USUHS, Orthopaedic Surgery, Madigan Army Medical Center, Tacoma, Washington, USA

PHOB GANOKROJ, MD
Faculty of Medicine Siriraj Hospital, Department of Orthopaedic Surgery, Mahidol University, Bangkok, Thailand; Steadman Philippon Research Institute, Vail, Colorado, USA

MARK A. GLOVER, BS
Medical Student, Wake Forest University School of Medicine, Winston Salem, North Carolina, USA

BRANUM GAGE GRISWOLD, MD
Orthopaedic Shoulder and Elbow Fellow, Denver Shoulder, Western Orthopaedics, Denver, Colorado, USA

JEFFREY D. HASSEBROCK, MD
Assistant Professor, Department of Orthopedic Surgery, Mayo Clinic, Phoenix, Arizona, USA

ELAINE HE, BA
Student, Department of Orthopedics, The Warren Alpert Medical School of Brown University, Providence, Rhode Island, USA

ZACHARY J. HERMAN, MD
Resident, Department of Orthopaedic Surgery, UPMC Freddie Fu Sports Medicine
Center, Pittsburgh, Pennsylvania, USA

CRAIG M. JOHNSON, DO
Orthopaedic Surgery Resident, Madigan Army Medical Center, Tacoma, Washington,
USA

GRANT JONES, MD
Orthopedic Surgeon, Department of Orthopaedics, Sports Medicine Research Institute,
Wexner Medical Center, The Ohio State University, Columbus, Ohio, USA

JILLIAN KARPYSHYN, MD, FRCSC
Resident, Division of Orthopaedics, Department of Surgery, Dalhousie University, Halifax,
Nova Scotia, Canada

AYUB KARWANDYAR, MD
Resident, Department of Orthopaedic Surgery, Vanderbilt University Medical Center,
Nashville, Tennessee, USA

MICHAEL J. KUTSCHKE, MD
Resident, Department of Orthopedics, The Warren Alpert Medical School of Brown
University, Providence, Rhode Island, USA

ALBERT LIN, MD
Professor, Department of Orthopaedic Surgery, UPMC Freddie Fu Sports Medicine
Center, Pittsburgh, Pennsylvania, USA

JIE MA, MES
Division of Orthopaedics, Department of Surgery, Dalhousie University, Halifax, Nova
Scotia, Canada

MICHAEL R. MANCINI, MD
Resident, Department of Orthopaedic Surgery, University of Connecticut Health Center,
University of Connecticut Health Musculoskeletal Institute, Farmington, Connecticut,
USA

GIANMARCO MARCELLO, MD
Resident Doctor in Orthopaedics and Traumatology, Orthopedics and Traumatology Unit,
Campus Bio-Medico University, Rome, Italy

ERIC C. McCARTY, MD
Professor, Chief of Sports Medicine and Shoulder Surgery, Department of Orthopedic
Surgery, University of Colorado School of Medicine, Aurora, Colorado, USA

KRISTEN F. NICHOLSON, PhD
Assistant Professor, Department of Orthopaedic Surgery and Rehabilitation, Wake Forest
University School of Medicine, Winston-Salem, North Carolina, USA

LANCE E. LeCLERE, MD
Associate Professor, Department of Orthopaedic Surgery, Vanderbilt University Medical
Center, Nashville, Tennessee, USA

OLIVIA C. O'REILLY, MD
Resident Physician, Department of Orthopedics and Rehabilitation, University of Iowa
Hospitals and Clinics, Iowa City, Iowa, USA

BRETT D. OWENS, MD
Professor, Department of Orthopedics, The Warren Alpert Medical School of Brown University, Providence, Rhode Island, USA

STEPHEN A. PARADA, MD
Director of Shoulder Surgery, Professor, Orthopaedic Surgery, Vice-Chair, Orthopaedic Research, Medical College of Georgia at Augusta University, Augusta, Georgia, USA

LUIGI PISCITELLI, MD
Orthopaedic Surgeon, Orthopedics and Traumatology Unit, Concordia Hospital, Rome, Italy

ADAM POPCHAK, PT, PhD
Associate Professor, Department of Orthopaedic Surgery, UPMC Freddie Fu Sports Medicine Center, Pittsburgh, Pennsylvania, USA

Capt MATTHEW T. PROVENCHER, MD, MBA, CAPT MC USNR (Ret.)
Professor of Surgery and Orthopaedics, The Steadman Clinic, Steadman Philippon Research Institute, Vail, Colorado, USA

CHARLES QIN, MD
Orthopedic Surgeon, Department of Orthopaedics, Sports Medicine Research Institute, Wexner Medical Center, The Ohio State University, Columbus, Ohio, USA

RAJIV P. REDDY, BS
MD Candidate, Department of Orthopaedic Surgery, UPMC Freddie Fu Sports Medicine Center, Pittsburgh, Pennsylvania, USA

BENJAMIN B. ROTHRAUFF, MD, PhD
Orthopaedic Surgery Resident, Department of Orthopaedic Surgery, University of Pittsburgh Medical Center, Pittsburgh, Pennsylvania, USA

ANNA E. SUMPTER, BA
Research Fellow, School of Medicine, Vanderbilt University, Nashville, Tennessee, USA

EDWARD J. TESTA, MD
Resident, Department of Orthopedics, The Warren Alpert Medical School of Brown University, Providence, Rhode Island, USA

JOHN M. TOKISH, MD
Consultant, Department of Orthopedic Surgery Sports Medicine, Mayo Clinic, Phoenix, Arizona, USA

NICHOLAS A. TRASOLINI, MD
Assistant Professor, Department of Orthopaedic Surgery and Rehabilitation, Wake Forest University School of Medicine, Winston-Salem, North Carolina, USA

BRIAN R. WATERMAN, MD
Professor, Department of Orthopaedic Surgery and Rehabilitation, Wake Forest University School of Medicine, Winston-Salem, North Carolina, USA

RYAN J. WHALEN, BS, CSCS
Research Coordinator, Steadman Philippon Research Institute, Vail, Colorado, USA

BRIAN R. WOLF, MD, MS
Professor and Vice-Chairman of Finance and Academic Affairs, Department of Orthopaedics and Rehabilitation, Kim and John Callaghan Endowed Chair, Director, Sports Medicine, University of Iowa Hospitals and Clinics, Iowa City, Iowa, USA

IVAN WONG, MD, FRCSC, MAcM, Dip Sports Med, FAANA
Professor, Division of Orthopaedics, Department of Surgery, Dalhousie University, Halifax, Nova Scotia, Canada

Contents

The glenohumeral joint is the least congruent and least constrained joint with a complex relationship of static and dynamic stabilizers to balance its native mobility with functional stability. In the young athlete, anterior shoulder instability is multifactorial and can be a challenge to treat, requiring a patient-specific treatment approach. Surgical decision-making must consider patient-specific factors such as age, sport activity and level, underlying ligamentous laxity, and goals for return to activity, in addition to careful scrutiny of the underlying pathology to include humeral and glenoid bone loss and surrounding scapular bone morphology.

Shoulder glenohumeral joint dislocations and subluxations are a relatively common injury among athletic populations. Evaluating the patient both on the field initially and through early recovery helps to determine the best treatment strategies and predict the natural history of each unique injury.

In the evaluation of shoulder instability, recognition of relevant pathology on imaging is critical to planning a surgical treatment that minimizes the risk for recurrent instability. The purpose of this review is to (1) discuss the use of radiography, computed tomography, and MRI in evaluating shoulder instability and (2) demonstrate how various imaging modalities are useful in identifying critical pathologies in the shoulder that are relevant for treatment.

In-season management of anterior shoulder instability in athletes is a complex problem. Athletes often wish to play through their current season, though recurrent instability rates are high, particularly in contact sports.

Utilizing fresh distal tibia allograft in anterior glenoid reconstruction has emerged as a highly advantageous approach in addressing instances of failed anterior shoulder stabilization with glenoid bone loss. This procedure offers several benefits, including the absence of donor-site morbidity, restoration of significant glenoid defects, reestablishment of joint congruity with the humeral head, restoration of glenoid biomechanics, and the addition of cartilage to the glenoid. Furthermore, it provides a robust and reliable alternative for managing failed stabilization procedures, leading to improved clinical outcomes and a high graft healing rate, while maintaining a low occurrence of recurrent instability.

The indications for bone block augmentation of the glenoid following recurrent anterior shoulder instability are expanding. Arthroscopic anatomic glenoid reconstruction (AAGR) is an evolving technique with similar clinical results to the Latarjet procedure and other open bone block procedures. Multiple types of bone grafts and fixation techniques have been described, with varying results on bony integration, resorption, articular congruity, and recurrence rates. This review focuses on biomechanics, patient workup, indications, current evidence, and the authors' preferred surgical technique for AAGR.

Overhead athletes with anterior, posterior, and multidirectional shoulder instability present with a wide range of symptoms, especially considering the injury mechanism and affected supportive structures. As such, the management of shoulder instability is widely variable and relies on rehabilitation, operative management, and sport-specific considerations, such as positional and seasonal demands on the athlete. Biomechanical analysis may further aid in the recovery process or serve as a predictive tool to identify an increased risk for injury.

There has been growing interest in the rehabilitation process and timing of returning an athlete to sport following the management options for anterior shoulder instability. The purpose of this article is to review the current rehabilitation and return to sport (RTS) protocols for various nonoperative and operative management strategies following anterior shoulder instability events. When appropriate in the rehabilitation protocol, RTS testing should be criteria based, rather than time based, with a special focus given to psychological readiness in order to promote successful return to athletics and prevention of recurrent instability episodes in the future.

Posterior glenohumeral instability represents a wide spectrum of pathoanatomic processes. A key consideration is the interplay between the posterior capsulolabral complex and the osseous anatomy of the glenoid and humeral head. Stability is dependent upon both the presence of soft tissue pathology (eg, tears to the posteroinferior labrum or posterior band of the inferior glenohumeral ligament, glenoid bone loss, reverse Hill Sachs lesions, and pathologic glenoid retroversion or dysplasia) and dynamic stabilizing forces. This review highlights unique pathoanatomic features of posterior shoulder instability and associated biomechanics that may exist in patients with posterior glenohumeral instability.

Posterior shoulder instability is a distinct subcategory of shoulder instability with an incidence higher than previously reported. Pain is typically the primary complaint, with pathology due to repetitive microtrauma being more common that a specific traumatic event. If nonoperative treatment fails, arthroscopic posterior capsulolabral repair has been shown to result in excellent outcomes and return to sport, with American football players having the best outcomes and throwers being slightly less predictable. Risk factors for surgical failure include decreased glenoid bone width, rotator cuff injury, female gender, and the use of less than 3 anchors.

Recurrent posterior shoulder instability after primary repair is uncommon, but presents a challenging clinical scenario. Most revisions in failed labral repair were associated with glenoid bone morphology related to critical bone loss, retroversion, or dysplasia. A variety of treatment options exist which include revision labral repair with or without capsular plication, glenoid osteotomy, humeral rotational osteotomy, or glenoid bone augmentation. No single technique has been shown to be superior and each technique has strengths and limitations. Therefore, thoughtful evaluation and planning is critical to address each patient's individual pathology to maximize success after revision surgery.

CLINICS IN SPORTS MEDICINE

SERIES OF RELATED INTERESTED

Orthopedic Clinics
https://www.orthopedic.theclinics.com/
Foot and Ankle Clinics
https://www.foot.theclinics.com/
Hand Clinics
https://www.hand.theclinics.com/
Physical Medicine and Rehabilitation Clinics
https://www.pmr.theclinics.com/

THE CLINICS ARE AVAILABLE ONLINE!
Access your subscription at:
www.theclinics.com

CLINICS IN SPORTS MEDICINE

FORTHCOMING ISSUES

January 2025
Building a Sports Medicine Practice Guide
to Navigating the First Five Years
James R. Carroll, Editor

April 2025
The Baseball Athlete
Steven Cohen, Editor

July 2025
Cartilage
Sandra A. Ross, Editor

RECENT ISSUES

July 2024
Pediatric ACL Reconstruction
Vehar Musahl and Gino Osgood
Action

April 2024
Ethnicity, Diversity, and Inclusion in Sports
Medicine
Constance Chu, Brea Taylor and Joel Boyd,
Editors

January 2024
Renal Health Considerations in the
Athlete
Siobhan ...

SERIES OF RELATED INTEREST

Orthopedic Clinics
https://www.orthopedic.theclinics.com/
Foot and Ankle Clinics
https://www.foot.theclinics.com/
Hand Clinics
https://www.hand.theclinics.com/
Physical Medicine and Rehabilitation Clinics
https://www.pmr.theclinics.com/

Foreword
Shoulder Instability

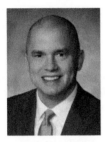

F. Winston Gwathmey, MD
Consulting Editor

The athlete relies on the power and precision of a well-functioning shoulder to perform at the highest level. The extraordinary functional anatomy of the glenohumeral joint, which allows for this power and precision through the extremes of motion in all planes, also contributes to the unique pathophysiology of the unstable shoulder. The shoulder is particularly vulnerable to the stresses and potential injuries of sport. Once the intricate stabilizing mechanisms of the glenohumeral joint are compromised, restoring stability while maintaining function presents significant treatment challenges with potential pitfalls. The delicate balance between mobility and stability is often at odds when considering surgical treatment options in the athlete, and the ramifications of a persistently stiff or unstable shoulder can be devastating.

Addressing the underlying etiology of the unstable shoulder is essential to preventing recurrent instability and further shoulder damage. The failed shoulder stabilization generates further difficulty and often requires complex procedures. In this issue of *Clinics in Sports Medicine*, guest editors Drs Jonathan F. Dickens, and Brian C. Lau explore the entire spectrum of shoulder function and dysfunction in the athlete. Starting with a review of the functional anatomy and biomechanics of the shoulder, this issue takes the reader through the evaluation and treatment of the unstable shoulder from the field to the clinic to the operating room and through the recovery. This issue also addresses failed surgery and revision shoulder stabilization. Treatment of anterior and posterior instability, including arthroscopic and open techniques, is described in detail.

Clin Sports Med 43 (2024) xv–xvi
https://doi.org/10.1016/j.csm.2024.04.003
0278-5919/24/© 2024 Elsevier Inc. All rights are reserved, including those for text and data mining, AI training, and similar technologies.

sportsmed.theclinics.com

Restoring stability and mobility is essential to returning an injured shoulder to high function in an athlete. This issue delineates how to effectively navigate that delicate balance.

Sincerely,

F. Winston Gwathmey, MD
Associate Professor of Orthopaedic Surgery
University of Virginia Health System
Charlottesville, Virginia, USA

Vice Chair for Orthopaedic Education and Residency
Program Director, Team Physician
UVA and JMU Athletics
Charlottesville, Virginia, USA

E-mail address:
FWG7D@uvahealth.org

Preface

The Athlete's Shoulder

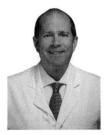
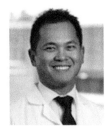

Jonathan F. Dickens, MD, COL, MC, USAR   Brian C. Lau, MD
Editors

Shoulder instability in the athlete stands as a critical and often high-stakes aspect of sports medicine, encompassing nuances in diagnosis, treatment, and rehabilitation that resonate deeply with the athletes and practitioners involved. The human shoulder joint empowers athletes to perform feats that push the limits of physical capability—whether it's a pitcher propelling a fastball at 95 miles per hour, a gymnast executing a rings routine, or a linebacker making a crucial tackle. Yet, amidst the glory of athletic prowess, the presence of shoulder instability jeopardizes an athlete's foundational trust in their shoulder, inevitably impacting performance.

From the inception of shoulder surgery to the present day, the intricate complexities of shoulder instability have captivated the attention of team physicians and shoulder surgeons. In this context, we embarked on the journey to create a comprehensive and up-to-date review dedicated to the unstable shoulder in athletes.

Throughout our careers in orthopedic surgery, and particularly in our exploration of shoulder instability, we have been profoundly fortunate to benefit from the guidance of remarkable friends and mentors—true giants in the field. It is through their generosity that we have had the privilege of assembling this issue. We extend our eternal gratitude for the opportunity to bring together a consortium of world-renowned experts on shoulder instability, with the shared aspiration of offering clearer guidance to surgeons dedicated to the care of athletes. The field of shoulder instability is evolving rapidly, and our aim has been to document the current state of scientific knowledge in this dynamic domain.

Clin Sports Med 43 (2024) xvii–xviii
https://doi.org/10.1016/j.csm.2024.02.003
0278-5919/24/© 2024 Published by Elsevier Inc.

sportsmed.theclinics.com

In presenting this *Clinics in Sports Medicine* dedicated to Shoulder Instability, we hope to offer a valuable updated reference for the care of athletes.

Sincerely,

Jonathan F. Dickens, MD, COL, MC, USAR
Department of Orthopaedic Surgery
James R. Urbaniak Sports Sciences Institute
3475 Erwin Road
Durham, NC 27705, USA

Brian C. Lau, MD
Department of Orthopaedic Surgery
James R. Urbaniak Sports Sciences Institute
3475 Erwin Road
Durham, NC 27705, USA

E-mail addresses:
jonathan.f.dickens@duke.edu (J.F. Dickens)
brian.lau@duke.edu (B.C. Lau)

Functional Anatomy and Biomechanics of Shoulder Instability

Craig M. Johnson, DO[a], Mikalyn T. DeFoor, MD[b],
Branum Gage Griswold, MD[c], Anna E. Bozzone, BA[d],
Joseph W. Galvin, DO[e], Stephen A. Parada, MD[f],*

KEYWORDS

- Glenohumeral joint • Stability • Biomechanics • Functional anatomy

KEY POINTS

- The glenohumeral joint is composed of static and dynamic stabilizers that allow the humeral head to remain centered on the glenoid.
- Glenoid bone loss can be measured with a variety of methods and should be addressed with a bony reconstruction procedure when bone loss reaches a critical value.
- Humeral bone loss is present in nearly all patients with recurrent dislocations and can be addressed with capsulotenodesis of the posterior cuff (remplissage).

INTRODUCTION

Anterior shoulder instability is a common diagnosis in young athletes. Shoulder stability is the result of a complex interplay between the static and dynamic stabilizers of the glenohumeral joint. Static stabilizers include the articular anatomy, negative intra-articular pressure, fibrocartilaginous labrum, and the glenohumeral ligaments. The dynamic stabilizers of the shoulder include the rotator cuff muscles and the scapulothoracic stabilizers. With increased utilization of advanced imaging and computed tomographic (CT) scans with 3 dimensional (3D) reconstructions, there is an improved understanding of the importance of bipolar bone loss on the outcomes following shoulder stabilization surgery. Herein, we provide a comprehensive review of the

[a] Madigan Army Medical Center, 9040 Jackson Avenue, Tacoma, WA 98431, USA; [b] San Antonio Military Medical Center, 3551 Roger Brooke Drive, San Antonio, TX 78234, USA; [c] Denver Shoulder/Western Orthopaedics, 1830 Franklin Street, Denver, CO 80218, USA; [d] Medical College of Georgia at Augusta University, 1120 15th Street, Augusta, GA 30912, USA; [e] Orthopaedic Surgery, Madigan Army Medical Center, 9040 Jackson Avenue, Tacoma, WA 98431, USA; [f] Orthopaedic Research, Medical College of Georgia at Augusta University, 1120 15th Street, Augusta, GA 30912, USA
* Corresponding author. Medical College of Georgia at Augusta University, 1120 15th Street, Augusta, GA 30912.
E-mail address: sparada@augusta.edu

Clin Sports Med 43 (2024) 547–565
https://doi.org/10.1016/j.csm.2024.03.016
sportsmed.theclinics.com
0278-5919/24/© 2024 Elsevier Inc. All rights reserved.

functional anatomy of the glenohumeral joint with a focus on scapular morphology and glenoid and humeral bone loss.

STATIC AND DYNAMIC STABILIZERS OF THE GLENOHUMERAL JOINT

The glenohumeral joint is composed of both static and dynamic stabilizers, which allow the humeral head to remain stable and centered on the relatively flat glenoid socket through a large range of shoulder motion. The static stabilizers of the glenohumeral joint include the articular anatomy of the glenoid and humeral head, the fibrocartilaginous labrum, the negative intra-articular pressure and the superior, middle, and inferior glenohumeral ligaments (superior glenohumeral ligament [SGHL], middle glenohumeral ligament [MGHL], and inferior glenohumeral ligament [IGHL]). The dynamic stabilizers of the shoulder joint include the rotator cuff muscles of the supraspinatus, infraspinatus, subscapularis, and the teres minor. With anterior instability, the subscapularis is particularly important in providing a dynamic restraint to anterior humeral translation. If the horizontal force couple is disrupted, this can lead to recurrent anterior instability (**Fig. 1**). The scapulothoracic stabilizer muscles are also a key dynamic stabilizer of the glenohumeral joint.

Understanding glenoid morphology plays an important role in evaluating the stability of the shoulder joint. The normal glenoid diameter measures 26.2 mm in women and 30.3 mm in men. The normal glenoid version ranges from $-4°$ of retroversion to $7°$ of anteversion. The amount of inclination varies from $0°$ to $10°$ of inclination.[1-4] **Fig. 2** demonstrates a 3D CT reconstruction of the glenoid denoting the clock-face orientation often used when describing glenoid and labral morphology.

Cadaveric studies have demonstrated that the human anterior inferior glenoid labrum is a fibrous rounded structure, which is confluent with the hyaline cartilage of the glenoid articular surface.[5] Histologically, there is a narrow fibrocartilaginous transition zone between the glenoid hyaline cartilage and the fibrous labral tissue. This narrow transition zone is composed of numerous collagen bundles in a woven pattern within the hyaline cartilage.

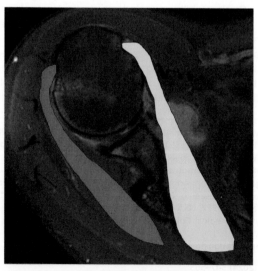

Fig. 1. Axial proton dense fat saturation image on an MRI that demonstrates the subscapularis (green) and the infraspinatus (red), which act as a force couple to balance the shoulder.

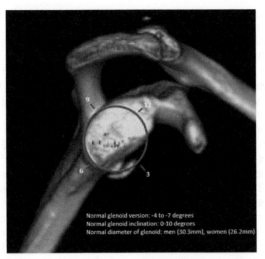

Normal glenoid version: -4 to -7 degrees
Normal glenoid inclination: 0-10 degrees
Normal diameter of glenoid: men (30.3mm), women (26.2mm)

Fig. 2. Three-dimensional CT reconstruction of the glenoid and scapula demonstrating the clock-face orientation used for describing glenoid morphology.

The glenoid labrum provides depth to the glenoid and a bumper to prevent anterior inferior dislocation. Vaswani and colleagues performed a retrospective case–control study of patients undergoing primary anterior arthroscopic shoulder stabilization and matched those who sustained a failure of Bankart repair to those who did not. They found that a diffusely small labral morphology was a significant risk factor for sustaining a postoperative redislocation.[6]

The anterior inferior and posterior inferior glenoid labrum also serve as an important attachment site for the anterior and posterior bands of the inferior glenohumeral ligament (anterior-inferior glenohumeral ligament [AIGHL], posterior-inferior glenohumeral ligament [PIGHL]) that serve as a "hammock-like" structure to statically stabilize the shoulder.[7] The AIGHL and PIGHL undergo reciprocal shortening and lengthening in 90° of glenohumeral abduction and serve as a "check rein" to anterior and posterior translation.[8] Plastic deformation of the AIGHL with an associated Bankart is the classic pathologic lesion that occurs following anterior inferior glenohumeral dislocation. In addition to tearing of the anterior inferior labrum from the glenoid (Bankart lesion), the AIGHL can also tear at its attachment on the humerus, the so-called humeral avulsion of the glenohumeral ligament lesion.[9] Finally, the AIGHL can also rupture from both the labrum and the humerus, the "floating AIGHL."[10]

GLENOID BONE LOSS

The pathologic lesion of an anterior glenohumeral dislocation is an anterior inferior glenoid labral tear and a posterior humeral head impaction fracture (Hill–Sachs [HS] lesion).[11] However, commonly with recurrent anterior shoulder instability, patients develop anterior glenoid bone loss. Attritional glenoid bone loss has been well defined as a risk factor for failure of an arthroscopic soft tissue repair (Bankart).[12] Wiesel and colleagues[13] reported glenoid bone loss as the most common cause for failure of a primary arthroscopic soft-tissue stabilization procedure resulting in increased morbidity and cost.

Glenoid rim defects can be identified as glenoid rim fractures or attritional bone loss. Bigliani and colleagues[12] described a classification system for glenoid bone lesions with 3 different types. Type I is a displaced avulsion fracture with attached capsule. Type II is a medially displaced fragment malunited to the glenoid rim. Type III can be defined as erosion of the glenoid rim with less than 25% (Type IIIA) or greater than 25% (Type IIIB) deficiency (**Fig. 3**).

In a prospective cohort study, Dickens and colleagues evaluated the degree of glenoid bone loss after initial and recurrent instability events. Glenoid bone loss after a first-time instability event was noted to be 6.8%, which increased to 22.8% in the setting of recurrent instability.[14] Milano and colleagues[15] analyzed a cohort of 161 patients with recurrent shoulder instability, glenoid bone defects were identified in 72% of patients with an average size of 6.9%. In a separate cohort of 218 patients, 71% of cases were noted to have bone loss with a mean size of 10.8%.[16] Shaha and colleagues[17] investigated the amount of glenoid bone loss in a young active-duty population noting 89.2% of their patients had bone loss with a mean of 14.5%. In comparison of these studies, it can be identified that the military population is a high-risk group for glenoid bone loss, which typically constitutes large defects.[14,17,18] Early stabilization is often recommended after an initial instability event in a young, active patient due to the risk of recurrent instability and increasing bone loss.

Initial assessment involves radiographs including anteroposterior (AP), Grashey, Axillary, and Scapular Y views. The West Point view and the Bernageau view can be obtained to assess for glenoid defects.[19,20] These radiographs can assist in identifying glenoid defects but are noted to have a reduced sensitivity compared to advanced imaging including CT and MRI.[21]

A CT scan with 3D reconstruction and humeral head subtraction allows for the identification and assessment of the size of the glenoid lesion through an en face view. In a cadaveric study, Huysman and colleagues[22] identified the inferior glenoid as a true circle and the bare spot as a means for identifying the center of that circle. A best-fit circle technique can be used to quantify the amount of bone loss within the area of circle that does not overlap bone as percentage of bone loss. There are several other methods of quantifying bone loss including the Pico method, circle line method, linear measurement percentage (LMP) method, and glenoid arc angle method (**Table 1**).[21,23–26] All these methods begin with the assumption that a best-fit circle can be placed on the inferior glenoid (**Fig. 4**).

There is evidence that supports these methods can be reliably performed on MRI as well; however, experts recommend 3D CT as the most current accurate study to assess bone loss.[27] Huijsmans and colleagues[28] performed a cadaveric study

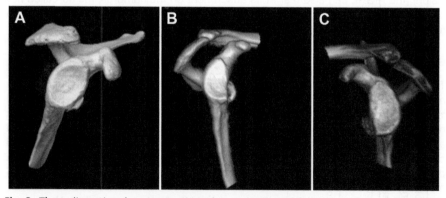

Fig. 3. Three-dimensional reconstructions demonstrating Bigliani glenoid rim defects with (A) type I, (B) type II, and (C) type III (B) lesions.

Table 1
Various methods of quantifying glenoid bone loss

Measurement Technique	Description	Equation
Best-fit circle method	True circle is centered on the inferior two-thirds of the glenoid, and the diameter of the circle and AP diameter of glenoid are measured at the same level	% GBL = (A − B)/A × 100% A = surface area of best-fit circle B = surface area of glenoid
Pico method	Circumference of the unaffected inferior glenoid based on a true circle is obtained, and then transferred to the affected glenoid; the glenoid defect is manually traced out in the affected shoulder to calculate surface area of bone loss	% GBL = (A − B)/A × 100% A = surface area of unaffected glenoid B = surface area of affected glenoid
Circle-line method	Best-fit circle is drawn as a line from center to the edge and compared with center to the bone defect; uses chord length to calculate area of a circular segment (ie, area of bone loss) and percent bone loss	Chord length = 2r sin (C/2) Area of bone loss (A) = $r^2/2$ (π/180C − sin C) % GBL = A/B × 100% A = area of bone loss B = total area of circle C = central angle r = radius of glenoid
LMP technique	Linear, ratio-based technique to measure the expected diameter of the glenoid based on a best-fit circle with a line drawn from center of circle to edge and compared with center to glenoid defect	% GBL = w/D × 100% D = best-fit circle diameter w = width of bone defect
Glenoid arc angle method	Center of the circle and central angle is defined by lines drawn to the upper and lower aspects of the glenoid defect; superior and inferior points at which the glenoid defect intersects the perimeter of the circle represents the central angle toward the center point of the circle	% GBL = [(α-sin α)/2 π] × 100% α = glenoid arc angle
Griffith's index	AP width measurements made perpendicular to a line through the vertical access of the glenoid from the supra-infra glenoid tubercle, which is compared between the affected and unaffected side to determined percent width loss	% GBL = B/A × 100% A = AP glenoid width of unaffected shoulder B = AP glenoid width of affected shoulder
Glenoid index (width) method	Using a best-fit circle, compare affected glenoid radius to unaffected native glenoid radius to give percentage bone loss, similar to arthroscopic bare spot technique	(R − r)/(2R) × 100% r = affected glenoid radius R = unaffected glenoid radius

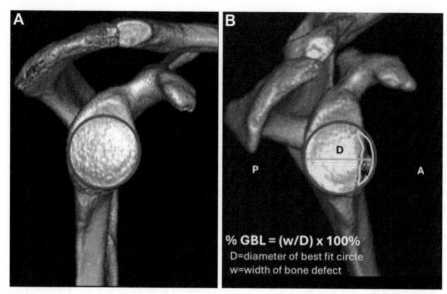

Fig. 4. A CT reconstruction with 3D reformat en face view of the glenoid demonstrating a best-fit circle drawn along the inferior portion of the glenoid shown on an intact glenoid without bone loss (*A*) as well as on a glenoid with attritional bone loss and medialized bone on the glenoid neck (*B*). A, anterior; P, posterior.

quantifying the amount of bone loss with the circle method and found no statistical differences between 3D CT and MRI. Magnetic resonance arthrography can allow for the assessment of soft-tissue injuries in addition to bone loss and has been found to have strong interobserver and intraobserver correlation of bone loss measurement compared to CT.[29]

Glenoid bone loss has been associated with failure of soft-tissue stabilization procedures resulting in worse clinical outcomes. Hettrich and colleagues prospectively followed 892 patients to assess predictors for bone loss in anterior shoulder instability. Anterior glenoid bone loss was identified in 20.7% of patients and was associated with an increased number of dislocations, increasing age, male sex, non-White race, and contact sports participation.[18] Milano and colleagues[15] evaluated a cohort of 161 patients with anterior shoulder instability and noted that the most significant predictors of bone loss were number of dislocations and age at first dislocation. It is important to identify bone loss because the failure rate of performing an arthroscopic Bankart repair alone in the setting of significant bone loss leads to increased failure rates.[30,31]

Boileau and colleagues[31] noted that glenoid bone loss greater than 25% was a risk factor for recurrent instability after arthroscopic stabilization. There have been several studies that analyze the amount of bone loss that indicates risk for recurrence of instability as well as the morphology of these glenoid rim lesions. Historically, glenoid defects have been classified as "critical" and necessitating bony augmentation procedures anywhere from 20% to 25%.[12,32–34] Itoi and colleagues performed a classic cadaveric study to assess the effect of different sizes of glenoid defects on stability and range of motion after Bankart repair. Their study demonstrated that an osseous defect of 21% may cause instability and limit range of motion.[35]

Further studies have evaluated "subcritical" amounts of bone loss. Shaha and colleagues analyzed a cohort of 72 anterior instability patients in a military population. In their patient population, bone loss of greater than 13.5% yielded clinically significant differences in outcome scores even in the setting of patients that did not have recurrent instability.[17] Yamamoto and colleagues performed a follow-up study to Shaha and colleagues analyzing the amount of bone loss that led to worse outcome scores and recurrent rates in a cohort of 43 patients. This study demonstrated that a bone loss of greater than 17% was associated with worse Western Ontario Shoulder Instability Index (WOSI) scores especially in male patients that participated in sporting activities.[36] These studies indicate that the critical size necessitating bony augmentation procedures may be lower than the often cited threshold of 20% to 25%.[17,35,36]

Anterior instability and the morphology of glenoid defects has a characteristic pattern that is different from other forms of instability. Sugaya and colleagues performed a 3D CT study evaluating the glenoid rim morphology in 100 patients with recurrent instability. 90% had a glenoid rim defect with 50% being true bony Bankart lesions and 40% with loss of the normal circular configuration of the inferior glenoid.[37] The location of these lesions in anterior glenoid instability has been identified ranging from 12 to 6 o'clock on the glenoid clock face with the majority of lesions ranging between 2:30 and 4:20.[38]

Defects associated with anterior instability are vastly different than those associated with posterior instability. Ernat and colleagues quantitatively compared the anatomic and morphologic differences between anterior and posterior shoulder instability patients with the use of CT. Anterior glenohumeral instability was associated with anterior glenoid lesions that have a steeper slope, higher percentage of bone loss, and greater superior-inferior defect height. Posterior glenohumeral instability was primarily associated with a greater degree of retroversion rather than bone loss and occurs in the posterior inferior quadrant of the glenoid.[39]

As previously discussed, the amount of glenoid bone loss necessitating bony reconstruction surgery has been described as the "critical" amount of bone loss. Recent publications by Moroder and colleagues have challenged the concept of a specific threshold of bone loss that may necessitate these procedures. In a case–control study, Moroder and colleagues evaluated 96 shoulders with CT images to evaluate the bony glenoid concavity and the bony shoulder stability ratio (BSSR). The mean BSSR as depicted in the equation shown in **Fig. 5** was used to determine the stability between anterior shoulder instability and a control group.

In this cohort of patients, anterior shoulder instability was associated with a flattening of the normal glenoid concavity, which led to a significantly decreased BSSR.[40] In a more recent publication, Moroder and colleagues evaluated the capability of glenoid bone loss measurements to accurately depict the biomechanical effect of glenoid defects. Their study determined that conventional measurements with CT are unable to accurately estimate the biomechanical effect of glenoid defects due to the nonlinear relation between defect size and biomechanical effect as well as

$$BSSR = \frac{\sqrt{1 - (\frac{r-d}{r})^2}}{\frac{r-d}{r}}$$

Fig. 5. BSSR equation which is a mathematical equation depicting the stability of the shoulder joint based on CT measurements of the glenoid concavity. (*From:* Moroder P, Ernstbrunner L, Pomwenger W, Oberhauser F, Hitzl W, Tauber M, et al. Anterior Shoulder Instability Is Associated With an Underlying Deficiency of the Bony Glenoid Concavity. Arthrosc J Arthrosc Relat Surg Off Publ Arthrosc Assoc N Am Int Arthrosc Assoc. 2015 Jul;31(7):1223–31.)

the inability to assess the glenoid concavity shape differences. This study indicates that a "critical" threshold for bone loss does not accurately depict who may need a bony augmentation procedure and that glenoid bone restoration involves restoring both the width and concavity of the glenoid.[41]

HUMERAL BONE LOSS

An HS lesion, present in 70% of first-time dislocators and over 90% in recurrent dislocations, is defined by an impaction fracture of the posterior-superior humeral head against the anterior glenoid rim.[42] Although humeral bone defects have traditionally been considered less important than glenoid bone defects, there is increasing attention toward defects of the humeral head as a significant contributor to recurrent anterior shoulder instability.[23,43,44]

CT, especially with 3D reconstructions, is the gold standard for quantifying humeral bone defects,[45,46] and methods for measuring humeral bone loss continue to evolve over time. The first method used for quantifying HS lesions was performed on plain radiographs as a percentage of bone loss involvement in a 180° arc on the surface of the humeral head.[47] In this quantitative method, the HS depth index is calculated based on the ratio of the maximum depth of the notch defect (p) in internal rotation and the radius of the humeral head (R; **Fig. 6**).[48] This method has since been extrapolated to CT and MRI studies and was further expanded by Rowe and colleagues[49] to account for both the depth and width of bone loss to develop a grading scheme based on clinical severity. This classification system ranges from mild (<0.5 cm deep and <2 cm long), moderate (0.5–1 cm deep and 2–4 cm long) and severe (>1 cm deep and >4 cm long). The depth and width of humeral bone loss can be divided by the diameter of the humeral head and quantified as percentage of the humeral head diameter measured on both axial and coronal CT images, with bone loss greater than 40% being clinically significant.[50–52]

Increasing evidence suggests that the location and orientation of the HS lesion, extending from 0 mm to 24 mm from the top of the humeral head, in addition to the size, can affect clinical outcomes and provide prognostic value in predicting recurrent instability.[23] Twenty-five percent of humeral bone loss has been suggested as the critical threshold to recommend surgical intervention, mostly from studies that have

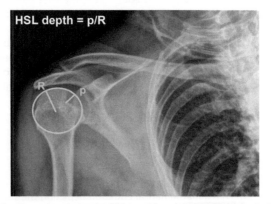

Fig. 6. An AP plain film of a right shoulder with a large Hill–Sachs lesion (HSL) demonstrating a quantitative method for measuring the HSL depth index, based on the ratio of the maximum depth of the notch defect (p) in internal rotation and the radius of the humeral head (R).

shown biomechanical alterations and clinical failure leading to instability at this threshold of humeral head volume loss.[43,44,53,54] In addition to volume of humeral head bone loss, the extent of bone loss in relation to the glenoid should also be considered, as studies support that humeral bone loss greater than 21% of the superior-inferior length of the glenoid or greater than 25% of the glenoid depth also leads to instability.[54] In recurrent instability, the posterolateral notch of the HS lesion increases in depth and the overall volume of humeral head bone loss increases.[35] Peebles and colleagues[45] additionally noted that glenoid bone loss was directly related to the characteristics of an HS lesion, and patients with smaller glenoid defects had narrower and deeper HS lesions with less humeral head surface area loss, while greater glenoid bone loss was associated with wider and shallower HS lesions.

The risk of an HS lesion engaging with the anterior rim of the glenoid is greatest at the end-range of abduction, external rotation, and horizontal extension because this is the position that the glenoid overrides the HS lesion.[35] The concept of glenoid track (GT) was introduced to describe the relationship of engagement of the glenoid and humeral head articular surfaces during movement at varying positions of abduction and external rotation.[36] This concept suggests that the location of the HS lesion is a significant contributing risk factor to recurrent instability, demonstrating that there is risk of engagement if the lesion extends beyond the medial margin of the zone of contact between the articular surfaces of the glenoid and humeral head.[36] In an on-track lesion, the HS defect stays within the GT and no engagement or dislocation occurs. Conversely, if the HS defect falls outside of the GT, termed an off-track lesion, the anterior rim of the glenoid may engage with the HS, leading to a recurrent dislocation.[55]

Glenoid bone loss has a high occurrence up to 100% in the presence of an HS lesion, described as a bipolar lesion.[43,55] In a bipolar lesion, the GT area is smaller and, therefore, the medial margin draws closer to the footprint, increasing the risk of engagement.[43,56] Nakagawa and colleagues[57] found one-third of all shoulders with primary instability had bipolar lesions, as did 60% of shoulders with recurrent instability, with a significant difference in recurrent instability noted in the setting of HS lesions and the inverted pear-shaped glenoid lesions.[58]

Three-dimensional CT scans are used in daily practice to measure on-track versus off-track lesions, using en face views of both the glenoid and posterior aspect of the humeral head (**Fig. 7**A).[45,59] This estimation is performed by a formula proposed by Di Giacomo and colleagues[59] and validated in several subsequent studies[35,55,60,61] (**Box 1**). The location of the medial margin of the GT is 83% of the entire glenoid width with the arm in 90° of abduction in normal shoulders.[62] As a result, the width of the GT in the setting of bone loss is defined as 0.83(D) – d, where D is the diameter of the inferior glenoid (**Fig. 7**B) and d is the width of the anterior glenoid bone loss (**Fig. 7**C). The GT width is applied to the posterior aspect of the humeral head. The Hill–Sachs interval (HSI) is subsequently measured as the distance from the rotator cuff attachment to the medial rim of the HS lesion, which is equal to the width of the HS lesion and the width of the intact bone bridge (BB) between the rotator cuff and the HS lesion. If the HSI is greater than the GT width, the medial rim of the HS extends past the glenoid rim with no bony support adjacent to the HS, identifying an off-track or engaging lesion. Contrarily, if the HSI is less than the GT width, there is bony support adjacent to the HS lesion and the medial rim of the HS is contained within the glenoid rim, identifying an on-track or nonengaging lesion. The effect of on-track and off-track lesions may potentially guide surgical decision-making in terms of arthroscopic soft tissue repair with or without the addition of humeral-sided procedures (ie, humeral head bone graft or remplissage).[46,63,64]

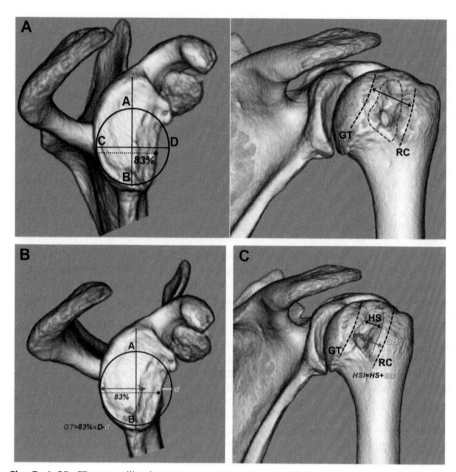

Fig. 7. A 3D CT scan utilized to measure GT in the presence of an HS lesion. (*A*) Three-dimensional CT scan with en face views of a left shoulder with glenoid bone loss (left) and posterior humeral head with a medium HS lesion (right). Line A–B represents the long axis of the glenoid, and the perpendicular line C–D is the diameter of the inferior glenoid. The width of a normal GT is defined as 83% of the inferior glenoid width (*dotted line*). Dotted line GT indicates the medial margin of the GT; dotted line RC indicates the medial margin of the posterior rotator cuff attachments. The boundary of the HS lesion is outlined in the red-dotted circle. (*B*) Three-dimensional CT scan with en face view of a left shoulder glenoid with bone loss of width d (*yellow line*). With glenoid bone loss, GT = 0.83 × D – d. D represents the inferior glenoid width of a normal glenoid without bone loss; line A–B is the long axis of the glenoid. The width of a normal GT without bone loss is defined as 83% of the inferior glenoid width (*dotted line*). (*C*) Three-dimensional CT scan with en face view of a left posterior humeral head with an HS lesion. The HSI is defined as the width of the HS lesion (boundary outlined in the red-dotted circle) plus the width of the intact BB between the HS and the posterior rotator cuff (RC) attachments. Dotted line GT indicates the medial margin of the GT; dotted line RC indicates the medial margin of the posterior RC attachments.

Historically, on-track and off-track lesions have been thought of as a binary variable, yet more recent studies describe this paradigm as a spectrum of risk of recurrent instability, introducing the term near-track lesions.[65–67] More specifically, on-track lesions with a small distance-to-dislocation (DTD) value, in which the medial edge of the

---

Box 1
Measurement of on-track versus off-track Hill–Sachs lesion

1. Obtain 3D CT scan with en face view of the glenoid (with humeral head subtraction) and the posterior view of the humeral head

2. Measure the diameter (D) of the inferior glenoid (perpendicular line to the long axis of the glenoid)

3. Measure the width of the anterior glenoid bone loss (d)

4. Calculate the width of the GT:
   GT = 0.83 × D–d

5. Measure the width of the HS lesion

6. Measure the width of the remaining BB between the posterior rotator cuff attachment and lateral aspect of the HS lesion

7. Calculate the width of the HSI:
   HSI = HS + BB

8. If HSI > GT, HS lesion is off-track (engaging); if HSI < GT, HS lesion is on-track (nonengaging)

From: Di Giacomo G, Itoi E, Burkhart SS. Evolving concept of bipolar bone loss and the Hill-Sachs lesion: from "engaging/non-engaging" lesion to "on-track/off-track" lesion. Arthrosc J Arthrosc Relat Surg Off Publ Arthrosc Assoc N Am Int Arthrosc Assoc. 2014 Jan;30(1):90–8.

HS lesion is still within but in close proximity to the medial edge of the GT are still at a higher risk of failure and recurrent dislocation. The DTD is defined as the distance between the edge of the anterior aspect of the glenoid and the medial border of the HS lesion.[66] As the GT narrows and HS size increases, on-track lesions demonstrate a smaller DTD value and subsequently fall into the continuum of a near-track lesion.

The term near-track lesions suggests that not all on-track lesions are the same and the clinical implications of the DTD value require further investigation. Li and colleagues[66] demonstrated that a DTD of less than 8 mm in a near-track lesion is a risk factor for failure after arthroscopic Bankart repair, especially in patients aged 20 years or older, suggesting that the DTD value is a continuous marker to predict the risk of failure. Similarly, Barrow and colleagues[65] found that as the DTD approached 0 mm (the threshold for an off-track lesion), the risk of recurrent dislocation after arthroscopic Bankart repair increased. Furthermore, the authors demonstrated that a DTD of less than 10 mm was associated with an exponentially higher risk of failure, with a higher risk of recurrence for collision athletes at even higher DTD values compared to noncollision athletes. However, in a retrospective study of a Dutch military population by Verweij and colleagues,[67] there was no relationship demonstrated between a smaller DTD in predicting recurrent anterior instability, which may be due to the high-demand population or mid-range instability.

INFLUENCE OF SCAPULAR MORPHOLOGY

Variations in glenoid, coracoid, and acromial morphology have implications in anterior shoulder instability. Anterior instability is associated with a flattened AP radius of curvature of the glenoid, larger height to width index ratio, shallower cavity with loss of sphericity, and more anteversion and inferior inclination of the glenoid.[68–72] Glenoid version is thought to have a linear effect on the force required for dislocation. In a cadaveric study by Eichinger and colleagues,[73] increased glenoid anteversion of 10° resulted in spontaneous dislocation in 25% of specimens. A shallow glenoid in conjunction with a large humeral head may also predispose patients to recurrent dislocation after arthroscopic Bankart repair.[74] Vaswani and colleagues[74] demonstrated patients with a shallow glenoid morphology (radius of curvature $\geq$24.5 mm) and a larger humeral head volume ($\geq$80 mm^3) had a 4 fold increased odds of postoperative dislocation. As understanding improves upon the relationship of glenohumeral instability and variations in glenoid morphology, there is increasing awareness that soft tissue stabilization procedures alone do not address the pathologic bony anatomy and may contribute to a patient's baseline predisposition to recurrent anterior instability.[74,75]

The sagittal morphology of the coracoacromial arch plays an increasingly recognized role in the pathogenesis of anterior instability. Owens and colleagues[69] identified the coracohumeral distance as an independent risk factor for traumatic anterior instability, noting a 20% increased risk of instability for every 1 mm increase in coracohumeral distance. Patients with anterior instability have been shown to have a more obtuse coracoacromial arch (decreased shoulder arch angle), in addition to a shorter coracoid with a superomedial offset and larger anterior coracoid tilt.[75] Altered contact between the conjoint tendon and the subscapularis as a result of altered coracoid morphology may lead to an altered line of force through the subscapularis, limiting the restraint to anterior humeral head translation during anterior shoulder dislocation.[76]

The acromion exhibits the highest variance of all periarticular scapular anatomic structures in relation to the glenoid.[76] An acromion with a more posterior origin of the scapular spine and more vertical orientation contributes to traumatic anterior shoulder instability.[76] Additionally, a flatter acromial roof and less containment of the humeral head can further contribute to traumatic instability.[68,75] A more vertical orientation of the acromion likely results in a greater percentage of the deltoid posterior to the center of the glenoid, providing less resistance to anterior translation. Increased posterior acromial coverage and posterior acromial tilt are described protective factors against recurrent anterior instability, suggesting that the anatomy of the entire arch, including both anterior and posterior elements, is important in anterior stability.[69,75]

CONTRIBUTION FROM THE LONG HEAD OF THE BICEPS TENDON

The long head of the biceps tendon (LHBT) is a dynamic stabilizer of the glenohumeral joint, with variable contribution to anterior shoulder instability.[77] While some studies have suggested that the LHBT plays a negligible role in dynamic stability of the shoulder, there is some evidence that the tendon offers some contribution to static stabilization of the shoulder as a humeral head depressor depending on the position of shoulder elevation in overhead activity.[78–80] As forward elevation of the shoulder stresses the posterior aspect of the unconstrained glenohumeral joint, biomechanical loading of the LHBT in cadaveric specimens demonstrated resistance to posterior translation of the humeral head during forward elevation, suggesting its role as a posterior stabilizer specifically at 60° of glenohumeral forward elevation.[81]

A recent review of 214 articles examining the contribution of the LHBT in shoulder stability found a minimal role of the LHB in glenohumeral stability in healthy controls.[82] However, hyperactivity of the LHB detected by electromyography in patients with rotator cuff failure or absent LHBT suggested a more significant role in shoulder stability and potential compensatory function in pathologic shoulders and instability. Ten studies evaluated the role of the proximal biceps in joint stability with variable results. One study of 20 asymptomatic volunteers noted a dynamic role of the LHBT in shoulder stability during low angles of shoulder elevation (<30°),[83] while another study of 5 patients undergoing LGBT tenodesis demonstrated no change in joint position or activity compared to healthy controls.[84] In addition to rotator cuff failure, there is increasing awareness for potential LHBT lesions in acute traumatic dislocations, particularly in patients aged over 45 years. Feuerriegel and colleagues[85] noted 52% of patients with traumatic dislocations demonstrated pathology of the biceps pulley system, all of which showed associated partial tear of the rotator cuff. Furthermore, patients with recurrent anterior shoulder instability with greater than 5 dislocation have demonstrated increasing rates of associated biceps pathology requiring treatment at the time of surgical stabilization.[86]

BIOMECHANICS

Glenohumeral instability is a pathologic condition in which the humeral head is unable to maintain its position in the center of the glenoid fossa due to damage of 1 of more of these stabilizers.[87]

When considering glenoid reconstruction for anterior glenoid bone loss, it is important to understand the different reconstruction options and their effect on the glenohumeral biomechanics. Rauck and colleagues sought to evaluate the proportion of the glenoid width restoration necessary to restore glenohumeral stability after Latarjet. The authors measured anterior humeral heading translation and force distribution on the coracoid graft. They found that restoration of native glenoid width restored anterior stability while preventing coracoid graft overload and that restoration of 100% of native glenoid width should be the minimum goal when performing anterior glenoid reconstruction.[81] Distal tibial allograft (DTA) is a reasonable option for large glenoid reconstruction, as it offers a graft with a cartilaginous surface to reconstruct the joint (**Fig. 8**). Rodrigueza and colleagues evaluated DTA versus Latarjet for glenoid

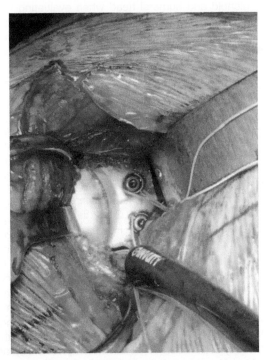

Fig. 8. Intraoperative photograph of right shoulder anterior glenoid reconstruction with distal tibia allograft demonstrating anatomic reconstruction of cartilaginous surface.

reconstruction with respect to joint kinematics and cartilage pressure mapping in shoulders undergoing 25% anterior glenoid-defect reconstruction. The authors concluded that Latarjet and DTA reconstructions exhibit similar glenohumeral kinematics regarding glenohumeral joint stability. However, joint compression load and articular contact pressure distribution may favor DTA reconstruction.[88] Also, when considering the biomechanics of anterior instability, the presence of a humeral head lesion must also be taken into consideration. Patel and colleagues designed a study to investigate the effects of Latarjet only reconstruction and the presence of varying humeral head defects. The authors found that anterior glenoid augmentation with a bone block can provide increased translation to dislocation in the presence of humeral defect sizes of 19% to 31% of the humeral head. However, Latarjet was not sufficient in defects greater than 31% and would require humeral augmentation.[89] Soft-tissue repair may be a valuable treatment option for patients with minimal bone loss; however, one must account for the negative and additive effect of humeral lesions. Arciero and colleagues evaluated the biomechanical efficacy of a Bankart repair in the setting of bipolar bone defects. The authors found that bipolar defects have an additive and negative effect on glenohumeral stability. As little as a 2 mm glenoid defect with a medium-sized HS lesion demonstrated a compromise in soft-tissue Bankart repair, while a small-sized HS lesion showed compromise of soft-tissue repair with 4 mm or more glenoid bone loss.[63]

SUMMARY

Shoulder stability is the result of a complex interplay between the static and dynamic stabilizers of the glenohumeral joint. It is important to understand the bipolar nature of bone loss from the glenoid and humeral head when evaluating the stability of the shoulder joint. While there are several cutoffs and treatment algorithms detailing options for treatment of bone loss, it is important to utilize a thorough history, physical examination, and evaluate the entirety of the glenohumeral joint stabilizers including the surrounding soft tissue structures as well as the morphology of the scapula.

DISCLOSURE

Dr S.A. Parada serves as a consultant to Arthrex, Inc and Exactech, Inc and receives research support from Exactech, Inc.

REFERENCES

1. Serrano N, Kissling M, Krafft H, et al. CT-based and morphological comparison of glenoid inclination and version angles and mineralisation distribution in human body donors. BMC Muscoskel Disord 2021;22:849.
2. Cyprien JM, Vasey HM, Burdet A, et al. Humeral retrotorsion and glenohumeral relationship in the normal shoulder and in recurrent anterior dislocation (scapulometry). Clin Orthop 1983;175:8–17.
3. Randelli M, Gambrioli PL. Glenohumeral osteometry by computed tomography in normal and unstable shoulders. Clin Orthop 1986;208:151–6.
4. Mathews S, Burkhard M, Serrano N, et al. Glenoid morphology in light of anatomical and reverse total shoulder arthroplasty: a dissection- and 3D-CT-based study in male and female body donors. BMC Muscoskel Disord 2017;18:9.
5. Cooper DE, Arnoczky SP, O'Brien SJ, et al. Anatomy, histology, and vascularity of the glenoid labrum. An anatomical study. J Bone Joint Surg Am 1992;74(1):46–52.

6. Vaswani R, Gasbarro G, Como C, et al. Labral Morphology and Number of Pre-operative Dislocations Are Associated With Recurrent Instability After Arthro-scopic Bankart Repair. Arthrosc J Arthrosc Relat Surg 2020;36(4):993–9.
7. O'Brien SJ, Neves MC, Arnoczky SP, et al. The anatomy and histology of the infe-rior glenohumeral ligament complex of the shoulder. Am J Sports Med 1990; 18(5):449–56.
8. Warner JJ, Caborn DN, Berger R, et al. Dynamic capsuloligamentous anatomy of the glenohumeral joint. J Shoulder Elbow Surg 1993;2(3):115–33.
9. Arner JW, Peebles LA, Bradley JP, et al. Anterior Shoulder Instability Manage-ment: Indications, Techniques, and Outcomes. Arthrosc J Arthrosc Relat Surg 2020;36(11):2791–3.
10. Homan BM, Gittins ME, Herzog RJ. Preoperative magnetic resonance imaging diagnosis of the floating anterior inferior glenohumeral ligament. Arthrosc J Ar-throsc Relat Surg 2002;18(5):542–6.
11. Owens BD, Nelson BJ, Duffey ML, et al. Pathoanatomy of First-Time, Traumatic, Anterior Glenohumeral Subluxation Events. JBJS 2010;92(7). Available at: https://journals.lww.com/jbjsjournal/fulltext/2010/07070/pathoanatomy_of_first_time,_traumatic,_anterior.5.aspx.
12. Bigliani LU, Newton PM, Steinmann SP, et al. Glenoid rim lesions associated with recurrent anterior dislocation of the shoulder. Am J Sports Med 1998;26(1):41–5.
13. Wiesel BB, Gartsman GM, Press CM, et al. What Went Wrong and What Was Done About It: Pitfalls in the Treatment of Common Shoulder Surgery. JBJS 2013;95(22):2061. Available at: https://journals.lww.com/jbjsjournal/citation/2013/11200/what_went_wrong_and_what_was_done_about_it_.14.aspx.
14. Dickens JF, Slaven SE, Cameron KL, et al. Prospective Evaluation of Glenoid Bone Loss After First-time and Recurrent Anterior Glenohumeral Instability Events. Am J Sports Med 2019;47(5):1082–9.
15. Milano G, Grasso A, Russo A, et al. Analysis of risk factors for glenoid bone defect in anterior shoulder instability. Am J Sports Med 2011;39(9):1870–6.
16. Griffith JF, Antonio GE, Yung PSH, et al. Prevalence, pattern, and spectrum of gle-noid bone loss in anterior shoulder dislocation: CT analysis of 218 patients. AJR Am J Roentgenol 2008;190(5):1247–54.
17. Shaha JS, Cook JB, Song DJ, et al. Redefining "Critical" Bone Loss in Shoulder Instability: Functional Outcomes Worsen With "Subcritical" Bone Loss. Am J Sports Med 2015;43(7):1719–25. Available at: https://journals.sagepub.com/doi/full/10.1177/0363546515578250.
18. Hettrich CM, Magnuson JA, Baumgarten KM, et al. Predictors of Bone Loss in Anterior Glenohumeral Instability. Am J Sports Med 2023;51(5):1286–94.
19. Pavlov H, Warren RF, Weiss CB, et al. The roentgenographic evaluation of anterior shoulder instability. Clin Orthop 1985;194:153–8.
20. Edwards TB, Boulahia A, Walch G. Radiographic analysis of bone defects in chronic anterior shoulder instability. Arthrosc J Arthrosc Relat Surg 2003;19(7):732–9.
21. Makhni EC, Tramer JS, Anderson MJJ, et al. Evaluating Bone Loss in Anterior Shoulder Instability. J Am Acad Orthop Surg 2022;30(12):563–72.
22. Huysmans PE, Haen PS, Kidd M, et al. The shape of the inferior part of the gle-noid: A cadaveric study. J Shoulder Elbow Surg 2006;15(6):759–63. Available at: https://www.jshoulderelbow.org/article/S1058-2746(05)00261-2/fulltext.
23. Baudi P, Campochiaro G, Rebuzzi M, et al. Assessment of bone defects in ante-rior shoulder instability. Joints 2013;1(1):40–8.

24. Barchilon VS, Kotz E, Barchilon Ben-Av M, et al. A simple method for quantitative evaluation of the missing area of the anterior glenoid in anterior instability of the glenohumeral joint. Skeletal Radiol 2008;37(8):731–6.

25. Dumont GD, Russell RD, Browne MG, et al. Area-based determination of bone loss using the glenoid arc angle. Arthrosc J Arthrosc Relat Surg 2012;28(7): 1030–5.

26. Parada SA, Eichinger JK, Dumont GD, et al. Accuracy and Reliability of a Simple Calculation for Measuring Glenoid Bone Loss on 3-Dimensional Computed Tomography Scans. Arthrosc J Arthrosc Relat Surg 2018;34(1):84–92. Available at: https://linkinghub.elsevier.com/retrieve/pii/S0749806317308046.

27. Rossi LA, Frank RM, Wilke D, et al. Evaluation and Management of Glenohumeral Instability With Associated Bone Loss: An Expert Consensus Statement Using the Modified Delphi Technique. Arthrosc J Arthrosc Relat Surg 2021;37(6):1719–28. Available at: https://linkinghub.elsevier.com/retrieve/pii/S0749806321000116.

28. Huijsmans PE, Haen PS, Kidd M, et al. Quantification of a glenoid defect with three-dimensional computed tomography and magnetic resonance imaging: A cadaveric study. J Shoulder Elbow Surg 2007;16(6):803–9. Available at: https://www.jshoulderelbow.org/article/S1058-2746(07)00325-4/fulltext.

29. Lee RKL, Griffith JF, Tong MMP, et al. Glenoid bone loss: assessment with MR imaging. Radiology 2013;267(2):496–502.

30. Burkhart SS, De Beer JF. Traumatic glenohumeral bone defects and their relationship to failure of arthroscopic Bankart repairs: significance of the inverted-pear glenoid and the humeral engaging Hill-Sachs lesion. Arthrosc J Arthrosc Relat Surg 2000;16(7):677–94.

31. Boileau P, Villalba M, Héry JY, et al. Risk Factors for Recurrence of Shoulder Instability After Arthroscopic Bankart Repair. JBJS 2006;88(8):1755. Available at: https://journals.lww.com/jbjsjournal/abstract/2006/08000/risk_factors_for_recurrence_of_shoulder.10.aspx.

32. Beran MC, Donaldson CT, Bishop JY. Treatment of chronic glenoid defects in the setting of recurrent anterior shoulder instability: a systematic review. J Shoulder Elbow Surg 2010;19(5):769–80.

33. Chen AL, Hunt SA, Hawkins RJ, et al. Management of bone loss associated with recurrent anterior glenohumeral instability. Am J Sports Med 2005;33(6):912–25.

34. Adam M, Attia AK, Alhammoud A, et al. Arthroscopic Bankart repair for the acute anterior shoulder dislocation: systematic review and meta-analysis. Int Orthop 2018;42(10):2413–22.

35. Itoi E, Lee SB, Berglund LJ, et al. The effect of a glenoid defect on anteroinferior stability of the shoulder after Bankart repair: a cadaveric study. J Bone Joint Surg Am 2000;82(1):35–46.

36. Yamamoto N, Muraki T, Sperling JW, et al. Stabilizing Mechanism in Bone-Grafting of a Large Glenoid Defect. JBJS 2010;92(11):2059. Available at: https://journals.lww.com/jbjsjournal/abstract/2010/09010/stabilizing_mechanism_in_bone_grafting_of_a_large.5.aspx.

37. Sugaya H, Moriishi J, Dohi M, et al. Glenoid rim morphology in recurrent anterior glenohumeral instability. J Bone Joint Surg Am 2003;85(5):878–84.

38. Saito H, Itoi E, Sugaya H, et al. Location of the Glenoid Defect in Shoulders with Recurrent Anterior Dislocation. Am J Sports Med 2005;33(6):889–93. Available at: https://journals.sagepub.com/doi/abs/10.1177/0363546504271521.

39. Ernat JJ, Golijanin P, Peebles AM, et al. Anterior and posterior glenoid bone loss in patients receiving surgery for glenohumeral instability is not the same: a

comparative 3-dimensional imaging analysis. JSES Int 2022;6(4):581–6. Available at: https://www.ncbi.nlm.nih.gov/pmc/articles/PMC9264014/.

40. Moroder P, Ernstbrunner L, Pomwenger W, et al. Anterior Shoulder Instability Is Associated With an Underlying Deficiency of the Bony Glenoid Concavity. Arthrosc J Arthrosc Relat Surg 2015;31(7):1223–31.

41. Moroder P, Damm P, Wierer G, et al. Challenging the Current Concept of Critical Glenoid Bone Loss in Shoulder Instability: Does the Size Measurement Really Tell It All? Am J Sports Med 2019;47(3):688–94. Available at:.

42. Bushnell BD, Creighton RA, Herring MM. Bony instability of the shoulder. Arthrosc J Arthrosc Relat Surg 2008;24(9):1061–73.

43. Bollier MJ, Arciero R. Management of glenoid and humeral bone loss. Sports Med Arthrosc Rev 2010;18(3):140–8.

44. Burkhart SS, De Beer JF, Barth JRH, et al. Results of modified Latarjet reconstruction in patients with anteroinferior instability and significant bone loss. Arthrosc J Arthrosc Relat Surg 2007;23(10):1033–41.

45. Peebles LA, Golijanin P, Peebles AM, et al. Glenoid Bone Loss Directly Affects Hill-Sachs Morphology: An Advanced 3-Dimensional Analysis. Am J Sports Med 2022;50(9):2469–75. Available at:.

46. Provencher MT, Midtgaard KS, Owens BD, et al. Diagnosis and Management of Traumatic Anterior Shoulder Instability. J Am Acad Orthop Surg 2021;29(2): e51–61.

47. HALL RH, ISAAC F, BOOTH CR. Dislocations of the shoulder with special reference to accompanying small fractures. J Bone Joint Surg Am. 1959;41-A(3): 489–94.

48. Maio M, Sarmento M, Moura N, et al. How to measure a Hill-Sachs lesion: a systematic review. EFORT Open Rev 2019;4(4):151–7.

49. Rowe CR, Zarins B, Ciullo JV. Recurrent anterior dislocation of the shoulder after surgical repair. Apparent causes of failure and treatment. J Bone Joint Surg Am 1984;66(2):159–68.

50. Flatow EL, Miniaci A, Evans PJ, et al. Instability of the shoulder: complex problems and failed repairs: Part II. Failed repairs. Instr Course Lect 1998;47:113–25.

51. Cho SH, Cho NS, Rhee YG. Preoperative analysis of the Hill-Sachs lesion in anterior shoulder instability: how to predict engagement of the lesion. Am J Sports Med 2011;39(11):2389–95.

52. Montgomery WHJ, Wahl M, Hettrich C, et al. Anteroinferior bone-grafting can restore stability in osseous glenoid defects. J Bone Joint Surg Am 2005;87(9): 1972–7.

53. Elkinson I, Giles JW, Faber KJ, et al. The effect of the remplissage procedure on shoulder stability and range of motion: an in vitro biomechanical assessment. J Bone Joint Surg Am 2012;94(11):1003–12.

54. Bhatia S, McGill K, Ghodara N, et al. *Radiographic and arthroscopic evaluation of glenoid and humeral head bone loss*. In: Provencher M, Romeo A, editors. Shoulder instability: a comprehensive approach. Philadelphia, PA: Elsevier Saunders; 2012. p. 178–83.

55. Trivedi S, Pomerantz ML, Gross D, et al. Shoulder instability in the setting of bipolar (glenoid and humeral head) bone loss: the glenoid track concept. Clin Orthop 2014;472(8):2352–62.

56. Widjaja AB, Tran A, Bailey M, et al. Correlation between Bankart and Hill-Sachs lesions in anterior shoulder dislocation. ANZ J Surg 2006;76(6):436–8.

57. Nakagawa S, Ozaki R, Take Y, et al. Relationship Between Glenoid Defects and Hill-Sachs Lesions in Shoulders With Traumatic Anterior Instability. Am J Sports Med 2015;43(11):2763–73.

58. Kim DS, Yoon YS, Yi CH. Prevalence comparison of accompanying lesions between primary and recurrent anterior dislocation in the shoulder. Am J Sports Med 2010;38(10):2071–6.

59. Di Giacomo G, Itoi E, Burkhart SS. Evolving concept of bipolar bone loss and the Hill-Sachs lesion: from "engaging/non-engaging" lesion to "on-track/off-track" lesion. Arthrosc J Arthrosc Relat Surg 2014;30(1):90–8.

60. Hatta T, Yamamoto N, Shinagawa K, et al. Surgical decision making based on the on-track/off-track concept for anterior shoulder instability: a case-control study. JSES Open Access 2019;3(1):25–8.

61. Shaha JS, Cook JB, Rowles DJ, et al. Clinical Validation of the Glenoid Track Concept in Anterior Glenohumeral Instability. J Bone Joint Surg Am 2016; 98(22):1918–23.

62. Omori Y, Yamamoto N, Koishi H, et al. Measurement of the Glenoid Track In Vivo as Investigated by 3-Dimensional Motion Analysis Using Open MRI. Am J Sports Med 2014;42:1290–5.

63. Arciero RA, Parrino A, Bernhardson AS, et al. The Effect of a Combined Glenoid and Hill-Sachs Defect on Glenohumeral Stability: A Biomechanical Cadaveric Study Using 3-Dimensional Modeling of 142 Patients. Am J Sports Med 2015; 43(6):1422–9. Available at:.

64. Gowd AK, Liu JN, Cabarcas BC, et al. Management of Recurrent Anterior Shoulder Instability With Bipolar Bone Loss: A Systematic Review to Assess Critical Bone Loss Amounts. Am J Sports Med 2019;47(10):2484–93.

65. Barrow AE, Charles SJC, Issa M, et al. Distance to Dislocation and Recurrent Shoulder Dislocation After Arthroscopic Bankart Repair: Rethinking the Glenoid Track Concept. Am J Sports Med 2022;50(14):3875–80.

66. Li RT, Kane G, Drummond M, et al. On-Track Lesions with a Small Distance to Dislocation Are Associated with Failure After Arthroscopic Anterior Shoulder Stabilization. J Bone Joint Surg Am 2021;103(11):961–7.

67. Verweij LPE, van Iersel TP, van Deurzen DFP, et al. "Nearly off-track lesions" or a short distance from the medial edge of the Hill-Sachs lesion to the medial edge of the glenoid track does not seem to be accurate in predicting recurrence after an arthroscopic Bankart repair in a military population: a case-control study. J Shoulder Elbow Surg 2023;32(4):e145–52.

68. Jacxsens M, Elhabian SY, Brady SE, et al. Coracoacromial morphology: a contributor to recurrent traumatic anterior glenohumeral instability? J Shoulder Elbow Surg 2019;28(7):1316–25.e1.

69. Owens BD, Campbell SE, Cameron KL. Risk factors for anterior glenohumeral instability. Am J Sports Med 2014;42(11):2591–6.

70. Peltz CD, Zauel R, Ramo N, et al. Differences in glenohumeral joint morphology between patients with anterior shoulder instability and healthy, uninjured volunteers. J Shoulder Elbow Surg 2015;24(7):1014–20.

71. Kıvrak A, Ulusoy İ. Effect of Glenohumeral Joint Bone Morphology on Anterior Shoulder Instability: A Case-Control Study. J Clin Med 2023;12(15).

72. Hohmann E, Tetsworth K. Glenoid version and inclination are risk factors for anterior shoulder dislocation. J Shoulder Elbow Surg 2015;24(8):1268–73.

73. Eichinger JK, Massimini DF, Kim J, et al. Biomechanical Evaluation of Glenoid Version and Dislocation Direction on the Influence of Anterior Shoulder Instability and Development of Hill-Sachs Lesions. Am J Sports Med 2016;44(11):2792–9.

74. Vaswani R, Como C, Fourman M, et al. Glenoid Radius of Curvature and Humeral Head Volume Are Associated With Postoperative Dislocation After Arthroscopic Bankart Repair. Arthrosc Sports Med Rehabil 2021;3(2):e565–71.
75. Lopez CD, Ding J, Bixby EC, et al. Association between shoulder coracoacromial arch morphology and anterior instability of the shoulder. JSES Int 2020;4(4): 772–9.
76. Jacxsens M, Elhabian SY, Brady SE, et al. Thinking outside the glenohumeral box: Hierarchical shape variation of the periarticular anatomy of the scapula using statistical shape modeling. J Orthop Res 2020;38(10):2272–9.
77. Varacallo M, Seaman TJ, Mair SD. StatPearls. In: Biceps Tendon Dislocation and Instability. Treasure Island, FL: StatPearls Publishing; 2023.
78. Warner JJ, McMahon PJ. The role of the long head of the biceps brachii in superior stability of the glenohumeral joint. J Bone Joint Surg Am 1995;77(3):366–72.
79. Hawkes DH, Alizadehkhaiyat O, Fisher AC, et al. Normal shoulder muscular activation and co-ordination during a shoulder elevation task based on activities of daily living: an electromyographic study. J Orthop Res 2012;30(1):53–60.
80. Pagnani MJ, Deng XH, Warren RF, et al. Role of the long head of the biceps brachii in glenohumeral stability: a biomechanical study in cadavera. J Shoulder Elbow Surg 1996;5(4):255–62.
81. Rauck RC, Jahandar A, Kontaxis A, et al. The role of the long head of the biceps tendon in posterior shoulder stabilization during forward flexion. J Shoulder Elbow Surg 2022;31(6):1254–60.
82. Diplock B, Hing W, Marks D. The long head of biceps at the shoulder: a scoping review. BMC Muscoskel Disord 2023;24(1):232. Available at:.
83. Landin D, Myers J, Thompson M, et al. The role of the biceps brachii in shoulder elevation. J Electromyogr Kinesiol 2008;18(2):270–5.
84. Giphart JE, Elser F, Dewing CB, et al. The long head of the biceps tendon has minimal effect on in vivo glenohumeral kinematics: a biplane fluoroscopy study. Am J Sports Med 2012;40(1):202–12.
85. Feuerriegel GC, Lenhart NS, Leonhardt Y, et al. Assessment of Acute Lesions of the Biceps Pulley in Patients with Traumatic Shoulder Dislocation Using MR Imaging. Diagn Basel Switz 2022;12(10):2345.
86. Rugg CM, Hettrich CM, Ortiz S, et al. Surgical stabilization for first-time shoulder dislocators: a multicenter analysis. J Shoulder Elbow Surg 2018;27(4):674–85.
87. Matsen FA, Fu FH, Hawkins R. The Shoulder: A Balance of Mobility and Stability. 1993. Available at: https://www.semanticscholar.org/paper/The-Shoulder%3A-A-Balance-of-Mobility-and-Stability-Matsen-Fu/0598999449ee1fbd360bb131545c 862fcb096f6b.
88. Rodriguez A, Baumann J, Bezold W, et al. Functional biomechanical comparison of Latarjet vs. distal tibial osteochondral allograft for anterior glenoid defect reconstruction. J Shoulder Elbow Surg 2023;32(2):374–82.
89. Patel RM, Walia P, Gottschalk L, et al. The Effects of Latarjet Reconstruction on Glenohumeral Kinematics in the Presence of Combined Bony Defects: A Cadaveric Model. Am J Sports Med 2016;44(7):1818–24.

Evaluating the Athlete with Instability from on the Field to in the Clinic

Jeffrey D. Hassebrock, MD[a], Eric C. McCarty, MD[b],*

KEYWORDS

• Shoulder instability • Dislocation • Athlete • Labrum

KEY POINTS

• Shoulder instability can present with a frank dislocation or a more subtle insidious inset of pain.
• Clinical suspicion, early evaluation, and communication with the athlete are key factors in treating instability appropriately.
• Serial examinations are often helpful for clarifying clinically difficult situations.

INTRODUCTION

Shoulder instability is a relatively common problem encountered in the young athletic population. Previous National Collegiate Athletic Association (NCAA) surveillance literature estimates isolated anterior shoulder instability has an incidence rate of roughly 31.3 injuries per 100,000 athlete exposures and a surgical intervention in 30% of these cases.[1] This leads to significant time missed from sport, performance challenges, augmented training, and can even affect the overall well-being of the athlete.[2,3] This characterization of the burden of shoulder instability in the athlete fails to capture the true burden of pathology as the majority of studies fail to capture multidirectional instability, posterior instability, or more subtle spectrums of instability such as pain with microtrauma and repetitive overuse injuries.[4,5] This suggests a significant burden on the high-level athlete concerning shoulder instability and necessitates physician awareness, attention, and expertise.

Biomechanically, the shoulder is designed with fairly minimal bony constraint that necessitates significant contribution from soft tissues as both dynamic and static stabilizers.[6–9] The high demands that overhead and contact athletes in particular place across this joint, combined with its minimal bony constraint, predispose this joint to instability injuries.[10] Understanding the unique challenges posed by shoulder

[a] Department of Orthopedic Surgery, Mayo Clinic, Phoenix, AZ, USA; [b] Department of Orthopedic Surgery, University of Colorado School of Medicine, Aurora, CO, USA
* Corresponding author. CU sports Medicine, 2150 Stadium Drive, Boulder, CO 80309.
E-mail address: eric.mccarty@cuanschutz.edu

Clin Sports Med 43 (2024) 567–574
https://doi.org/10.1016/j.csm.2024.03.017
0278-5919/24/© 2024 Elsevier Inc. All rights reserved.

instability in the athlete requires a thorough understanding of the underlying mechanism of injury and the functional anatomy of the patient.[11,12]

RECOGNIZING INSTABILITY

Shoulder instability is multifaceted and recognizing that an injury has occurred may be straightforward or may require a high level of index clinical suspicion. Understanding that multiple mechanisms may contribute to glenohumeral instability is key. Traumatic dislocations typically present with a fixed deformity in a position of relative risk. Primary traumatic anterior instability presents with the abducted and externally rotated position of risk, and typically, the athlete will have fixed external rotation of their injured extremity.[13] Traumatic posterior dislocation requires stress in an adducted and internally rotated position and will present with the opposite, the athlete holding their arm in an internally rotated position.[14]

Often the presentation can be more subtle with a subluxation event or spontaneous relocation event where the glenohumeral shifted out of position but relocated prior to initial evaluation. Athletes often describe a brief sensation of shoulder slipping or "popping" out of place.[15] Finally, repetitive overhead athletes may experience pain as the sole indicator of abnormal glenohumeral joint motion secondary to repetitive microtrauma and high demands leading to subtle subluxation during their sport-specific exercises.[7,16]

It is important to maintain a broad differential during initial examination including fracture, soft tissue other than labral injury, and evaluate for other life-threatening concomitant injuries. Removing the athlete from the field of play to a controlled location (sideline evaluation tent or medical area) is a crucial first step in managing initial shoulder instability evaluation.

ON FIELD EVALUATION AND INITIAL MANAGEMENT

The immediate sideline evaluation of an injured athlete aims to rule out critical medical emergencies and progresses to pain alleviation and further injury prevention. Practitioners should be quick to recognize visible deformity, pain/guarding, apprehension, and recurrent instability. In the setting of fixed deformity, a reduction maneuver should be attempted to relocate the joint and prevent ongoing cartilaginous injury and soft tissue trauma (**Fig. 1**).[17] This reduction should be done soon after the dislocation occurs. If it is during a game, taking the player to a more private area such as a sideline tent or to the locker room is preferred. If it is during the practice, then reducing it there on the playing surface is appropriate. This can be attempted by the health care professional in attendance (physician, physician assistant, athletic trainer, and so forth). Several reduction maneuvers exist, but the general principles require scapular stabilization, muscle relaxation through fatigue, and gentle traction, with subsequent atraumatic relocation of the deformity.[18] This is effective for both anterior and posterior dislocations. Irreducibility should prompt urgent imaging and repeated evaluation. It is also critically important to assess neurovascular integrity both before and after reduction with specific attention paid to axillary nerve function. The goal of reduction is to achieve a stable concentric reduction with full passive range of motion.

Athletes may also present with spontaneous relocation or a subluxation event. This typically manifests as significant pain and guarding. The inability to perform full range of motion with good strength should raise clinical suspicion and prompt further evaluation.[19] Additionally, the inability of an athlete to maintain strength throughout a functional range of motion should preclude return to sport from a sideline evaluation standpoint. Serial examinations may be necessary to help determine the degree of

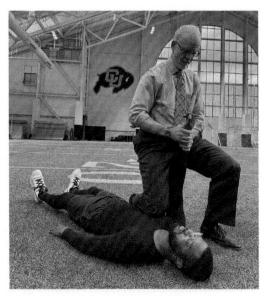

Fig. 1. On field reduction maneuver in the supine athlete.

injury as well as assess for improvement and return to play.[20] In the setting of frank instability, the initial management after reduction should include immobilization and pain management.[20,21] Imaging such as radiographs are then obtained to assess the joint and rule out a fracture. Commonly, advanced imaging is done to assess more completely the extent of the injury to the labrum and cartilage as well as any associated injuries.

TRANSITIONING TO CLINICAL ASSESSMENT

Athletes may present to the clinic either in continuity from a sideline event or as a first time in office evaluation after unknown outside initial sideline management. In either scenario initial clinical office evaluation should begin with a thorough history.[22] It is important to understand the athlete's sport, their time in season, expected demands, prior history of injuries or instability, and expectations as a baseline for establishing a treatment. Special consideration should be paid to the number of subluxations or dislocations experienced by the patient as outcomes/recurrence/management is intimately associated with the number of dislocations an athlete has experienced.[23] It is also important to discuss the position and force placed upon the upper extremity when the injury occurred to aid in the understanding of directional instability. In the setting of chronic repetitive overhead athletes presenting only with pain, the specific portions of their sport that reproduce the discomfort should be discussed to help identify the source of the subtle instability.

After a thorough history, attention should be paid to physical examination. Range of motion both active and passive should be documented in a controlled manner to not provoke another dislocation. The contralateral upper extremity should be evaluated as well as the entire kinetic chain in athletes with repetitive overhead throwing injuries. Strength testing should be performed and palpation of the external surface anatomy is helpful to determine areas of potential bony injury. A Beighton's score to document ligamentous laxity should be obtained. Clinical history and a description of the injury should help drive special testing. In the setting of suspected anterior instability, a load and shift test, apprehension, and relocation tests should be performed. In the setting of posterior instability, a jerk test, Kim's test, and a posterior load and shift or push–pull test should be performed.[24] Superior instability should be suspected with a positive O'Brien's and dynamic labral shear tests and a pure inferior instability is suggested by a positive Gagey test. Again, asking the athlete to demonstrate provocative positions of pain and subjective instability can be extremely helpful in the more subtle presentations.

In all cases, it is important to discuss concerns and expectations with the patient from the onset as athletes may perceive these injuries differently, and this can affect not only rehabilitation but also mental well-being without proper contextualization and open lines of communication between the physician and the athlete.[20]

IMAGING

After a thorough history and physical examination, imaging should be obtained. Standard radiographic assessment should be performed for all shoulder instability athletes.[25] This includes a glenohumeral anteroposterior view (Grashey) as well as a scapular Y view and an axillary lateral (**Fig. 2**). The glenohumeral joint should be critically assessed for concentric reduction on all views. Additionally, each view should be critically assessed for change in the humeral head contour suggesting prior impaction injury from dislocation (Hill Sachs) or loss of glenoid bone stock from either attritional changes or acute fracture (boney Bankart).[26]

Advanced imaging modalities are available and widely used in the setting of shoulder instability to both better elucidate the pathology and to help with dictating treatment. In the setting of radiographs demonstrating bone loss, a computed tomography (CT) scan is the next advanced imaging modality of choice. This allows for precise measurement of bone loss on both the humeral side and the glenoid

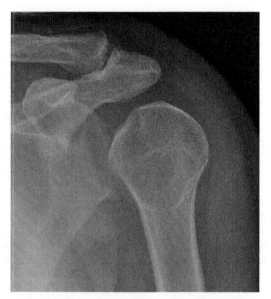

Fig. 2. Anteroposterior (AP) radiograph of a left shoulder demonstrating a "lightbulb" sign or internal rotation from a posterior dislocation.

side.[27] In addition to age, contact, and level of sport, bone loss has been shown to be an important factor in the natural history of traumatic glenohumeral dislocations as well as outcomes after operative intervention.[28,29] This makes accurate representation of bone stock crucial for counseling these athletes on their risk–benefit profiles with different treatment strategies.[30]

In addition to CT advanced imaging, MRI is a commonly utilized form of advanced imaging (**Fig. 3**). This allows for an accurate assessment of soft tissue injury. In the setting of minimal boneless or chronic microtrauma leading to suspected labral pathology, an MRI is an invaluable tool for assessing labral pathology, capsular abnormalities, and the surrounding musculature of the glenohumeral joint.[31] Some literature has advocated for the addition of intra-articular contrast medium when assessing for labral and partial thickness rotator cuff pathology, and prior studies have demonstrated a significant increase in MRI sensitivity with these injuries utilizing contrast when compared to isolated lower magnetic field MRIs.[32,33] However, with increasing magnetic field power, the use of contrast in routine shoulder MRIs for instability is debated. Ultrasonography has also been utilized as an adjunct imaging modality. While useful for visualizing the rotator cuff and dynamic evaluations, the surgical utility of ultrasound for the evaluation of labral pathology is still unclear.[34]

In conclusion, radiographs, CT, MRI, and ultrasound each offer unique advantages to the assessment of an athlete with shoulder instability. A comprehensive understanding of each modality is essential to determine which, if any, additional imaging is going to be beneficial from a diagnostic and prognostic standpoint.

BIOMECHANICAL CONSIDERATIONS

Often the mechanism, or traumatic event, sufficiently explains the source of instability experienced by an athlete. This is more common in contact or high-energy athletes who experience a traumatic dislocation requiring a reduction. However, as previously discussed, the diagnosis can be more difficult when microinstability in the repetitive overhead athlete is the source of the painful chief complaint.[16] The complex nature of the kinetic chain and the adaptive changes athletes undergo to throw overhead with velocity requires the additional consideration.[35,36] Consideration of compounding

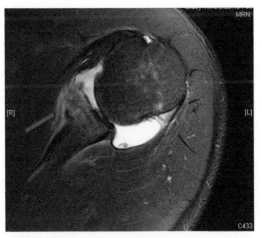

Fig. 3. Axial T2 MRI slice of a left shoulder demonstrating an anterior bone/capsular disruption (*red arrow*) from anterior dislocation.

functional impairments throughout the kinetic chain and the role that fatigue plays in loss of dynamic stabilization are crucial in understanding the throwing shoulder's instability.[37] Treating physicians should be acutely aware of the role the rehabilitation plays in managing these patients as well as the limitations that surgical intervention has in return of these complex patients to play.[38,39]

DISCUSSION

While the treatment options vary for glenohumeral shoulder instability widely depending upon age, laxity, bone loss, chronicity, number of dislocations, sport, level of competition and other factors, the initial management of these patients should be systematic and methodical.[40,41] Prompt evaluation begins on the sideline with a high index of suspicion secondary to high incidence rates among young competitive athletes. Sideline assessment should focus on eliminating life-threatening or limb-threatening conditions from the differential and proceeding with prompt reduction of residual deformities. Careful monitoring and documentation of neurovascular status should be performed with any attempt at reduction and failure should prompt urgent imaging and elevation of level of care. After reduction treatment should focus on a brief period of immobilization for comfort and pain control followed by office evaluation with radiographs and advanced imaging as appropriate. In the setting of subluxation or questionable microinstability, sideline assessment should include a careful assessment of passive and active range of motion as well as strength. Deficits in either strength or motion indicate an inability to return safely and are an indication for further evaluation.

SUMMARY

Shoulder instability is a common upper extremity injury among young athletic populations. Prompt recognition and evaluation is crucial for triaging appropriate intervention and eventual return to sport. Clinicians should maintain a high level of suspicion, especially among young contact or overhead athletic populations.

CLINICS CARE POINTS

- Reduce residual deformities appropriately, monitor neurovascular status throughout.
- Maintain a high clinical suspicion for pain as leading complaint for subluxations or microinstability.
- Establish and maintain open communication with the athlete concerning diagnosis and management options for shared decision-making.

DISCLOSURE

The authors have nothing to disclose.

REFERENCES

1. Trojan JD, Meyer LE, Edgar CM, et al. Epidemiology of shoulder instability injuries in collision collegiate sports from 2009 to 2014. Arthrosc J Arthrosc Relat Surg 2020;36(1):36–43.

2. Cameron KL, Mauntel TC, Owens BD. The epidemiology of glenohumeral joint instability: incidence, burden, and long-term consequences. Sports Med Arthrosc Rev 2017;25(3):144–9.

3. Galvin JW, Ernat JJ, Waterman BR, et al. The epidemiology and natural history of anterior shoulder instability. Curr Rev Musculoskelet Med 2017;10(4):411–24.

4. Anderson MJJ, Mack CD, Herzog MM, et al. Epidemiology of shoulder instability in the National Football League. Orthopaedic Journal of Sports Medicine 2021; 9(5). 23259671211007744.

5. Zacchilli MA, Owens BD. Epidemiology of shoulder dislocations presenting to emergency Departments in the United States. JBJS 2010;92(3):542.

6. DeFroda SF, Donnelly JC, Mulcahey MK, et al. Shoulder instability in women compared with men: epidemiology, pathophysiology, and special considerations. JBJS Reviews 2019;7(9):e10.

7. DeFroda SF, Goyal D, Patel N, et al. Shoulder instability in the overhead athlete. Curr Sports Med Rep 2018;17(9):308.

8. Lugo R, Kung P, Ma CB. Shoulder biomechanics. Eur J Radiol 2008;68(1):16–24.

9. Wang VM, Flatow EL. Pathomechanics of acquired shoulder instability: A basic science perspective. J Shoulder Elbow Surg 2005;14(1Supplement):S2–11.

10. Owens BD, Dawson L, Burks R, et al. Incidence of shoulder dislocation in the united states military: demographic considerations from a high-risk population. JBJS 2009;91(4):791.

11. Terry GC, Chopp TM. Functional anatomy of the shoulder. J Athl Train 2000;35(3): 248–55.

12. Wilk KE, Macrina LC, Fleisig GS, et al. Deficits in glenohumeral passive range of motion increase risk of shoulder injury in professional baseball pitchers: a prospective study. Am J Sports Med 2015;43(10):2379–85.

13. Cutts S, Prempeh M, Drew S. Anterior shoulder dislocation. Annals 2009; 91(1):2–7.

14. Rouleau DM, Hebert-Davies J, Robinson CM. Acute traumatic posterior shoulder dislocation. J Am Acad Orthopaedic Surg. 2014;22(3):145.

15. Bottoni CR, Franks BR, Moore JH, et al. Operative stabilization of posterior shoulder instability. Am J Sports Med 2005;33(7):996–1002.

16. Chambers L, Altchek DW. Microinstability and internal impingement in overhead athletes. Clin Sports Med 2013;32(4):697–707.

17. McCarty EC, Ritchie P, Gill HS, et al. Shoulder instability: return to play. Clin Sports Med 2004;23(3):335–51.

18. Baykal B, Sener S, Turkan H. Scapular manipulation technique for reduction of traumatic anterior shoulder dislocations: experiences of an academic emergency department. Emerg Med J 2005;22(5):336–8.

19. Skelley NW, McCormick JJ, Smith MV. In-game management of common joint dislocations. Sports Health 2014;6(3):246–55.

20. Wolf BR, Tranovich MA, Marcussen B, et al. Team approach: treatment of shoulder instability in athletes. JBJS Reviews 2021;9(11). e21.00087.

21. Bahr R, Craig EV, Engebretsen L. The clinical presentation of shoulder instability including on field management. Clin Sports Med 1995;14(4):761–76.

22. Albertson BS, Trasolini NA, Rue JPH, et al. In-season management of shoulder instability: how to evaluate, treat, and safely return to sport. Curr Rev Musculoskelet Med 2023;16(7):295–305.

23. Owens BD, Dickens JF, Kilcoyne KG, et al. Management of mid-season traumatic anterior shoulder instability in athletes. J Ame Acad Orthop Surg 2012;20(8):518.

24. Haley CCA. History and physical examination for shoulder instability. Sports Med Arthrosc Rev 2017;25(3):150–5.
25. Nguyen D. Anatomy, examination, and imaging of the shoulder. Operat Tech Orthop 2008;18(1):2–8.
26. De Filippo M, Schirò S, Sarohia D, et al. Imaging of shoulder instability. Skeletal Radiol 2020;49(10):1505–23.
27. Rerko MA, Pan X, Donaldson C, et al. Comparison of various imaging techniques to quantify glenoid bone loss in shoulder instability. J Shoulder Elbow Surg 2013; 22(4):528–34.
28. Burkhart SS, De Beer JF. Traumatic glenohumeral bone defects and their relationship to failure of arthroscopic Bankart repairs: Significance of the inverted-pear glenoid and the humeral engaging Hill-Sachs lesion. Arthrosc J Arthrosc Relat Surg 2000;16(7):677–94.
29. Shaha JS, Cook JB, Song DJ, et al. Redefining "critical" bone loss in shoulder instability: functional outcomes worsen with "subcritical" bone loss. Am J Sports Med 2015;43(7):1719–25.
30. Bergin D. Imaging shoulder instability in the athlete. Magnetic Resonance Imaging Clinics 2009;17(4):595–615.
31. Seeger LL, Gold RH, Bassett LW. Shoulder instability: evaluation with MR imaging. Radiology 1988;168(3):695–7.
32. Magee T. 3-T MRI of the shoulder: Is MR arthrography necessary? Am J Roentgenol 2009;192(1):86–92.
33. Major N, Browne J, Domzalski T, et al. Evaluation of the glenoid labrum with 3-T MRI: Is intraarticular contrast necessary? Am J Roentgenol 2011;196:1139–44.
34. Daenen B, Houben G, Bauduin E, et al. Ultrasound of the shoulder. J Belg Radiol 2007;90(5):325–37.
35. Fleisig GS, Andrews JR, Dillman CJ, et al. Kinetics of baseball pitching with implications about injury mechanisms. Am J Sports Med 1995;23(2):233–9.
36. Limpisvasti O, ElAttrache NS, Jobe FW. Understanding shoulder and elbow injuries in baseball. JAAOS - Journal of the American Academy of Orthopaedic Surgeons 2007;15(3):139.
37. Kvitne RS, Jobe FW, Jobe CM. Shoulder instability in the overhand or throwing athlete. Clin Sports Med 1995;14(4):917–35.
38. Altchek DW, Dines DM. Shoulder injuries in the throwing athlete. JAAOS - Journal of the American Academy of Orthopaedic Surgeons. 1995;3(3):159.
39. Jaggi A, Lambert S. Rehabilitation for shoulder instability. Br J Sports Med 2010; 44(5):333–40.
40. Hohmann E. Editorial commentary: delphi expert consensus clarifies evidence-based medicine for shoulder instability and bone loss. Arthrosc J Arthrosc Relat Surg 2021;37(6):1729–30.
41. Rossi LA, Frank RM, Wilke D, et al. Evaluation and management of glenohumeral instability with associated bone loss: an expert consensus statement using the modified delphi technique. Arthrosc J Arthrosc Relat Surg 2021;37(6):1719–28.

Current Imaging of Anterior and Posterior Instability in the Athlete

Charles Qin, MD, Grant Jones, MD*

KEYWORDS

• Imaging • Shoulder instability • Athlete

KEY POINTS

- Careful assessment of imaging plays an important role in deciding the optimal treatment approach for shoulder instability.
- Orthogonal radiographs are critical to not miss the presence of dislocation, particularly posterior.
- Certain associated soft tissue pathologies such as humeral avulsion of the inferior gleno-humeral ligament lesions must not be missed in the assessment of shoulder instability, and thus a contrast study should be considered if there is uncertainty of the diagnosis.
- Computed tomographic scans and the development of 3D reconstructions have allowed for a more nuanced approach to quantifying humeral and glenoid-sided bone loss.

INTRODUCTION

The last two decades have seen tremendous advancements in technology available for shoulder stabilization surgery.[1] As the orthopedic surgeon's armamentarium to treat shoulder instability has grown, so has imaging modalities such as computed tomography (CT) and MRI that are workhorses in the evaluation of shoulder instability. Concepts such as glenoid track in the setting of bipolar lesions and critical bone loss have been refined with the advancements in imaging. Accordingly, it is vital that the orthopedic surgeon be facile in utilizing and interpreting the basic and advanced imaging of an unstable shoulder.

Recognition of relevant pathology is critical to planning a surgical treatment that minimizes the risk for recurrent instability. The purpose of this review is to (1) discuss the use of radiography, CT, and MRI in evaluating shoulder instability and (2) demonstrate how various imaging modalities are useful in identifying critical pathologies in the shoulder that are relevant for treatment.

Department of Orthopaedics, Sports Medicine Research Institute, Wexner Medical Center, The Ohio State University, Columbus, OH, USA
* Corresponding author. 2835 Fred Taylor Drive, Columbus, OH 43202.
E-mail address: grant.jones@osumc.edu

Clin Sports Med 43 (2024) 575–584
https://doi.org/10.1016/j.csm.2024.03.018
0278-5919/24/© 2024 Elsevier Inc. All rights reserved.

RADIOGRAPHS

Radiographs remain the first-line imaging modality used in the evaluation of shoulder instability. They can be useful to assess bony alignment as well as the presence of bony lesions or fractures of the glenoid or humerus, as well as confirm a reduced joint following a closed reduction procedure in the acute or traumatic setting. While they are available and relatively inexpensive, they do not provide sufficient detail with regards to glenoid and humeral bone loss, may under-recognize a bony Bankart lesion, and do not provide any detail about the soft tissue structures of the shoulder. Nonetheless, it is standard practice to obtain a 4 view radiographic series including the anteroposterior (AP), scapular Y, Grashey, and axillary views of the shoulder. In patients who are not able to abduct the arm, a Velpeau view may be an acceptable substitute. The researchers believe that an orthogonal view, whether Velpeau or axillary, is critical to have unambiguous evidence of the AP glenohumeral alignment. The Velpeau view is taken with the patient standing but bent 30° backwards whereas the axillary view is taken with the patient seated and the arm abducted enough such that the glenohumeral joint is central to the image detector (**Fig. 1**). Indirect signs of posterior dislocation have been described including the trough sign that demonstrates anterior humeral head impaction against the glenoid or the lightbulb sign (**Fig. 2**).[2] Despite these signs, the treating provider still may have doubt whether a dislocation is present. If that is the case, the provider should obtain cross-sectional imaging to confirm the diagnosis as cases of traumatic posterior dislocation can be missed leading to inferior outcomes.[3]

There are additional views that have been described in the evaluation of glenohumeral instability including the Stryker notch and west point views, which increase the recognition of Hill–Sachs and Bankart lesions, respectively. The Stryker notch view is obtained with the arm extended and the palm of the hand placed behind the patient's head. The west point view is obtained with the patient prone and the arm abducted 90° from the long axis of the body. Finally, Ikemoto and colleagues described the Bernageau profile view in 2010 whereby the distance between the anterior and posterior glenoid rims were measured for the injured and uninjured shoulders to assess bone loss. This view was obtained with the arm forward flexed to 160°, the chest in contact with the radiographic cassette at 70° and the X-ray tube angulated

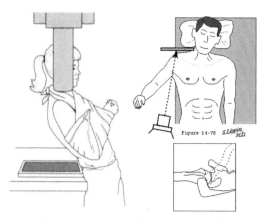

Fig. 1. The Velpeau view with the patient standing but bent 30° backwards (*left*) the axillary view with the patient seated and their arm abducted enough such that the glenohumeral joint is central to the image detector (*right*).

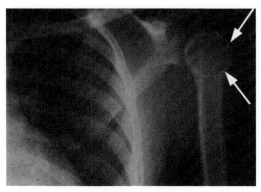

Fig. 2. "Lightbulb" sign suggestive of posterior dislocation.

30° in the craniocaudal direction. This view allows for dedicated assessment of the anterior glenoid rim which is difficult to obtain in standard views (**Fig. 3**). Ikemoto and colleagues[4] reported that this view was an acceptable substitute to CT in up to 80% cases.

COMPUTED TOMOGRAPHIC SCAN

In almost all situations, CT scan is critical to understanding the bony pathology present in shoulder instability. Bony Bankart lesions that are anteroinferior glenoid rim fractures seen in anterior shoulder instability are best detected on CT. CT is also useful

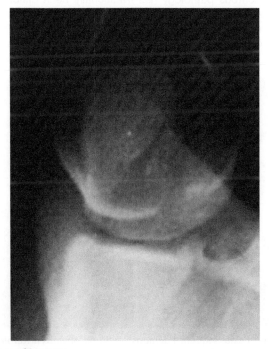

Fig. 3. Bernageau profile view.

to characterize the displacement and size of these lesions, both of which are critical in deciding how to address them. CT is also critical when applying the glenoid track concept in the setting of bipolar bone lesions. Glenoid bone loss and glenoid diameter can be measured through best fit circle technique on a 2D or 3D sagittal image of the glenoid fossa. Furthermore, CT evaluation of the Hill–Sachs lesion has been shown to be as accurate as arthroscopy evaluation. In the case of posterior instability, posterior bone loss of the glenoid and the presence, depth, and width of a reverse Hill–Sachs lesion can be evaluated. Often, posterior instability can be nontraumatic and related to anatomic differences such as glenoid hypoplasia and retroversion which is best assessed on CT.[5] Thin slice CT with multiplanar reformatting has allowed for 3D reconstructions that allow the most meticulous inspection of any bony pathology present in the unstable shoulder.

MRI AND MAGNETIC RESONANCE ARTHROGRAPHY

MRI is critical to assessing the soft tissue structures of the shoulder and the various pathologies associated with shoulder instability. Noncontrast MRI allows detection of labral tears in 70% of cases.[6] In noncontrast MRI, labral pathology is best assessed on proton density and T2-fat suppressed sequences. The abduction and external rotation (ABER) shoulder position has been used in an additional sequence to help increase the sensitivity of detecting anteroinferior labral (**Fig. 4**).[7,8]

T2 sequences can be useful in identifying the hyperintense signal of bone marrow edema that can represent an impaction fracture when assessing for Hill–Sachs and reverse Hill–Sachs lesions. MRI can also be useful in the setting of an irreducible posterior dislocation to identify the interposed tissue blocking closed reduction, which is commonly the rotator cuff, the biceps tendon, or avulsed capsule.[2]

Labral and ligamentous pathology has traditionally been difficult to conclusively discern on images provided by an 1.5 Tesla (T) MR machine. This is in large part due to lack of great definition of the chondral–labral interface. The use of intra-articular contrast can be instrumental in defining any separations at this interface.

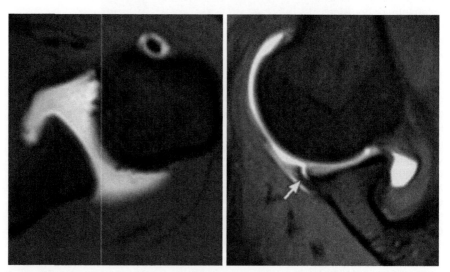

Fig. 4. MR arthrogram axial sequence demonstrating no obvious anteroinferior labral tear on the left panel. A tear can be visualized in the ABER position on the right panel.

However, with improvements in shoulder coil design and fast spin-echo imaging sequences 1.5 T MRI can be adequate. 3T MRI leads to further improvements with recent evidence supporting its use and potentially as an acceptable substitute to magnetic resonance arthrography (MRA).[9]

Ultimately, MRA remains the gold standard for the imaging evaluation of shoulder instability.[10] MRA is an MRI performed after the shoulder joint has been injected with a contrast agent such as diluted gadolinium. The distention of the dye outlines the cartilage, ligaments, and labrum which improves its sensitivity in detecting tears over traditional noncontrast MRI. In the acute situation with effusion present, a noncontrast study may suffice. The authors recommend an MRA in the subacute or chronic setting or if suspicious for a humeral avulsion of the inferior glenohumeral ligament (HAGL). Regardless of whether the orthopedic surgeon chooses to order contrast or noncontrast MRI, it is critical that he or she discuss with the collaborating musculoskeletal imaging radiologist beforehand to ensure the correct imaging sequences are obtained and that they are adequate to identify the pathology in question.

3D MRI is a new emerging technology in the field of shoulder instability. With 3D MRI, image postprocessing creates 3D reformatting of osseous structures with concomitant assessment of soft tissue structures, avoiding the need from radiation associated with a 3D CT. 3D MRI, in one clinical study, has been shown to be as accurate in assessing glenoid bone loss as arthroscopic assessment. Sequence acquisition times are admittedly slower for 3D MRI and may represent a barrier for inclusion into current clinical practice.[11]

GLENOID BONE LOSS

Initial radiographs can clue the orthopedic surgeon in on any significant fractures or bone loss in the setting of anterior or posterior shoulder instability. However, further evaluation with CT and potential MRI is needed to characterize the extent and size of bone loss that is essential to surgical planning. In the case of anterior shoulder instability, assessing the CT for critical bone loss is critical when deciding between a soft tissue or bony stabilization procedure. Critical bone loss, the maximum amount of anteroinferior bone loss after which a soft tissue labral repair and capsulorraphy portends worse outcomes compared to Laterjet or other bone block procedures, has been reported to be as low as 13.5%.[12] While this number is an ongoing source of debate, the methodology to measure glenoid bone loss relative to the native glenoid width must be straightforward and reproducible. There are 2 commonly described techniques. The "circle method" assumes that normal inferior glenoid contour is a true circle and a best fit circle drawn with the existing glenoid contour can be used to determine the native glenoid width and the defect width (**Fig. 5**). Bone loss is then defined as the ratio of the defect width to the native glenoid width. Variations, including the "Sugaya method," have been described with the use of an en face 3D CT sagittal view of the glenoid and shown to be an accurate alternative.[13] The other technique has been described by Giles and colleagues who attempted to apply an MRI-based formula that calculates native glenoid width in relation to glenoid height which is typically unchanged in cases of shoulder instability to CT data. Ultimately, they concluded that the most accurate method to quantify bone loss was to apply a CT-based formula to CT data.[14]

These two methodologies can be used in the setting of posterior bone loss as well. The key difference is that there is even less consensus on critical bone loss in the setting of posterior instability. Preliminary laboratory data suggest that a shoulder with greater than 20% bone loss remains unstable after isolated soft tissue repair.[15]

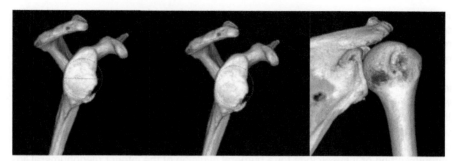

Fig. 5. Best fit circle method to estimate glenoid bone loss in the setting anterior instability. The left panel demonstrates a perfect circle estimation of the true glenoid diameter. The middle panel demonstrates the amount of bone loss according to the perfect circle method. The right panel demonstrates the Hill–Sachs interval, which is the width of the Hill–Sachs lesion in addition to the osseous bridge between the lateral most aspect of the Hill–Sachs and the medial most insertion point of the rotator cuff.

In addition, as opposed to traumatic bone loss which is characteristic in anterior dislocation, glenoid dysplasia and retroversion may be the primary driving factors in posterior instability. In cases of anterior instability with bone loss, the authors recommend 3D CT evaluation of glenoid bone loss when available with the circle method. We have encountered scenarios in which the 2D CT images are not formatted perfectly to the plane of the glenoid face, and therefore has underestimated the true extent of missing bone. A 3D CT with humeral subtraction affords the surgeon the ability to assess the bone loss in all planes and to be able to plan both dimensions and morphology of bone block needed in cases exceeding critical bone loss. In the setting of posterior instability, the authors recommend obtaining an MRI to assess glenoid morphology and if there is any concern about posterior bone loss or dysplasia, to obtain a CT scan to characterize further.

HUMERAL BONE LOSS

An impaction fracture of the posterolateral humeral head in anterior dislocation (ie, Hill–Sachs deformity) and anterior humeral head in posterior dislocation (ie, reverse Hill–Sachs deformity) is crucial to recognize. While they can be subtle on radiographs, these bony lesions may be more readily identified on MRI or CT. Increased number of dislocations and long-term instability can lead to larger deformities. First described in 2007, the glenoid track concept describes the possibility of bipolar lesions engaging as the glenoid contact shifts from inferomedial to superolateral with elevation of the arm.[16] The glenoid track "calculator" has since been developed by inputting the Hill–Sachs interval, native glenoid diameter, and bone loss into a formula to characterize bipolar lesions as "on-track" or "off-track". For posterior dislocations, the authors are not aware of any standardized method of characterizing reverse Hill–Sachs lesions on imaging. Moroder and colleagues[17] has described the "gamma angle" in a series of 102 reverse Hill–Sachs which accounted for the depth and location of the Hill–Sachs into one measurement and found that higher gamma angles were associated with chronic locked posterior dislocations.

LABRAL TEARS AND VARIANTS

During anterior dislocation, tears of the anteroinferior labrum can occur either with intact periosteum (ie, Perthes lesion) or with an associated tear of the periosteum (ie,. soft tissue Bankart lesion). This usually results from significant tension of the inferior glenohumeral ligament (IGHL) during dislocation with those forces transferred to the labrum leading to tearing. Posterior dislocations are similarly associated with posterior labral tears. Traditionally, the Kim lesion describes an incomplete avulsion of the posterior labrum. More recently, Kim and colleagues[18] introduced a new classification of posterior labral tears based on MRA findings and reported on its correlation with arthroscopic findings (**Fig. 6**). Increased signal on T2 sequences at the interface between labrum and glenoid cartilage can be suggestive of these tears. However, suboptimal definition of this interface on noncontrast MRI sequences can make identification of these lesions difficult. As mentioned in a prior section, use of contrast can help delineate chondral–labral separation as well as the use of ABER arms positioning which tensions the IGHL. In the setting of posterior instability, MRA can demonstrate loss of posterior labral height as well as incomplete extrusion of contrast at the posterior labral–chondral junction. In some cases, the Bankart lesion can put tension on adjacent cartilage leading to damage. This is termed glenolabral articular disruption (GLAD). GLAD lesions can be recognized on the same sequences used to evaluate labrum. Typically increased signal on T2 sequences or contrast in the case of MRA can extend into the cartilage adjacent to a labral tear. To the author's knowledge, a reciprocal lesion of the posterior cartilage in posterior dislocations has not been named in the literature.

MRI is also helpful in assessing anterior labrum periosteal sleeve avulsion (ALPSA) lesions. As described by its name, the ALPSA lesion occurs when the labrum has displaced medially onto the glenoid neck typically in chronic settings. Often, depending on the chronicity there can be significant changes to the labral morphology and this is critical to assess when anticipating the quality and mobility of tissue for a soft tissue labral repair. The degree of displacement of an ALPSA lesion is best assessed on axial and sagittal images.

HUMERAL AVULSION OF INFERIOR GLENOHUMERAL LIGAMENT

The anterior band of the IGHL is the primary anterior stabilizer and experiences significant tension during anterior dislocation. While the adjacent labrum and scapular

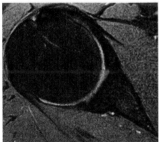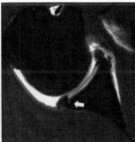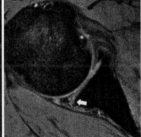

Fig. 6. MRA images of different posterior labral tears. The left panel demonstrates a type 1 tear without obvious detachment of the labrum from the glenoid surface. The middle panel demonstrates a type 2 tear with superficial and partial detachment (*arrowhead*). The right panel demonstrates a type 3 tear with complete detachment and contrast extravasation into the chondrolabral space (*arrowhead*). (*From*: Kim JH, Ahn J, Shin SJ. Occult, Incomplete, and Complete Posterior Labral Tears Without Glenohumeral Instability on Imaging Underestimate Labral Detachment. Arthroscopy. Jan 2024;40(1):58–67. https://doi.org/10.1016/j.arthro.2023.06.015.)

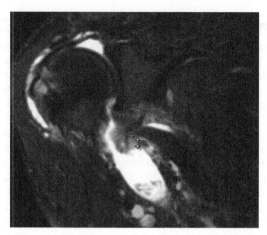

Fig. 7. HAGL lesion.

periosteum more commonly fails, the IGHL can fail at the humeral attachment which is termed a HAGL lesion. MRI is the imaging modality of choice for HAGL lesions. The IGHL is best identified on an arthrogram. In acute settings following dislocation, the joint effusion serves as a "traumatic arthrogram" and serves the same purpose as contrast in delineating the band like structure that is the IGHL. In the acute setting, all sequences on MRI but classically the coronal sequence will demonstrate contrast or joint effusion extending beyond the axillary recess because of the fully torn IGHL **(Fig. 7)**. In the subacute setting, effusion from the acute HAGL lesion will be replaced by scar and granulation tissue making identification more difficult. Posterior HAGL lesions represent a significant capsular injury in posterior instability cases. They are important but difficult to identify on MRI as only 50% of posterior HAGL lesions were identified preoperatively in one study **(Fig. 8)**. They can be partial or complete tears from the humeral attachment, or detached from both the glenoid and humeral side.[19] They have been associated with increased chondrolabral retroversion, as this may increase the translational forces that the posterior capsule is subjected to during instability events.

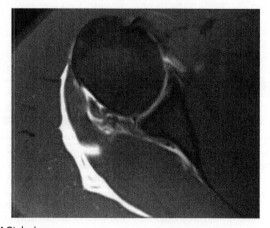

Fig. 8. Reverse HAGL lesion.

SUMMARY

We have reviewed the main concepts for current imaging of anterior and posterior instability, including the most common imaging findings as well as imaging modalities. An understanding of these concepts is critical for managing this complex issue.

CLINICS CARE POINTS

- A thorough understanding and interpretation of imaging is critical in the treatment of shoulder instability.
- The use of contrast and 3D reconstructions in imaging modalities may help enhance our assessment of shoulder instability.

DISCLOSURE

The authors report no relevant disclosures.

REFERENCES

1. Wolf BR, Tranovich MA, Marcussen B, et al. Team Approach: Treatment of Shoulder Instability in Athletes, JBJS Rev, 9 (11), 2021, 213-224.
2. Rouleau DM, Hebert-Davies J, Robinson CM. Acute traumatic posterior shoulder dislocation. J Am Acad Orthop Surg 2014;22(3):145–52.
3. Moussa ME, Boykin RE, Earp BE. Missed locked posterior shoulder dislocation with a reverse Hill-Sachs lesion and subscapularis rupture. Am J Orthoped 2013;42(12):E121–4.
4. Ikemoto RY, Nascimento LG, Bueno RS, et al. ANTERIOR GLENOID RIM EROSION MEASURED BY X-RAY EXAM: A SIMPLE WAY TO PERFORM THE BERNAGEAU PROFILE VIEW. Rev Bras Ortop 2010;45(6):538–42.
5. Provencher MT, LeClere LE, King S, et al. Posterior instability of the shoulder: diagnosis and management. Am J Sports Med 2011;39(4):874–86.
6. Kompel AJ, Li X, Guermazi A, et al. Radiographic Evaluation of Patients with Anterior Shoulder Instability. Curr Rev Musculoskelet Med 2017;10(4):425–33.
7. Schreinemachers SA, van der Hulst VP, Jaap Willems W, et al. Is a single direct MR arthrography series in ABER position as accurate in detecting anteroinferior labroligamentous lesions as conventional MR arthography? Skeletal Radiol 2009; 38(7):675–83.
8. Tian CY, Cui GQ, Zheng ZZ, et al. The added value of ABER position for the detection and classification of anteroinferior labroligamentous lesions in MR arthrography of the shoulder. Eur J Radiol 2013;82(4):651–7.
9. Magee TH, Williams D. Sensitivity and specificity in detection of labral tears with 3.0-T MRI of the shoulder. AJR Am J Roentgenol 2006;187(6):1448–52.
10. Subhas N, Benedick A, Obuchowski NA, et al. Comparison of a Fast 5-Minute Shoulder MRI Protocol With a Standard Shoulder MRI Protocol: A Multiinstitutional Multireader Study. AJR Am J Roentgenol 2017;208(4):W146–54.
11. Gyftopoulos S, Beltran LS, Yemin A, et al. Use of 3D MR reconstructions in the evaluation of glenoid bone loss: a clinical study. Skeletal Radiol 2014;43(2):213–8.
12. Shaha JS, Cook JB, Song DJ, et al. Redefining "Critical" Bone Loss in Shoulder Instability: Functional Outcomes Worsen With "Subcritical" Bone Loss. Am J Sports Med 2015;43(7):1719–25.

13. Sugaya H. Techniques to evaluate glenoid bone loss. Curr Rev Musculoskelet Med 2014;7(1):1–5.
14. Giles JW, Owens BD, Athwal GS. Estimating Glenoid Width for Instability-Related Bone Loss: A CT Evaluation of an MRI Formula. Am J Sports Med 2015;43(7): 1726–30.
15. Nacca C, Gil JA, Badida R, et al. Critical Glenoid Bone Loss in Posterior Shoulder Instability. Am J Sports Med 2018;46(5):1058–63.
16. Yamamoto N, Itoi E, Abe H, et al. Contact between the glenoid and the humeral head in abduction, external rotation, and horizontal extension: a new concept of glenoid track. J Shoulder Elbow Surg 2007;16(5):649–56.
17. Moroder P, Tauber M, Scheibel M, et al. Defect Characteristics of Reverse Hill-Sachs Lesions. Am J Sports Med 2016;44(3):708–14.
18. Kim JH, Ahn J, Shin SJ. Occult, Incomplete, and Complete Posterior Labral Tears Without Glenohumeral Instability on Imaging Underestimate Labral Detachment. Arthroscopy 2024;40(1):58–67.
19. Rebolledo BJ, Nwachukwu BU, Konin GP, et al. Posterior Humeral Avulsion of the Glenohumeral Ligament and Associated Injuries: Assessment Using Magnetic Resonance Imaging. Am J Sports Med 2015;43(12):2913–7.

Anterior Instability

Anterior Instability

Decision Making of the In-season Athlete with Anterior Shoulder Instability

Garrett V. Christensen, MD[a],*, Olivia C. O'Reilly, MD[a],
Brian R. Wolf, MD, MS[a]

KEYWORDS

- In-season injury • Bankart tear • Arthroscopic shoulder surgery • Hill–Sachs lesion
- Bony Bankart lesion • Return to sport • Remplissage • Latarjet procedure

KEY POINTS

- In-season management of anterior shoulder instability is complex and can be managed initially nonoperatively or operatively depending on an athlete's goals, timing within the season, eligibility, and severity of injury.
- Nonoperative management of in-season anterior shoulder instability leads to high rates of return to sport; however, there are high rates of recurrent instability, particularly in contact sport athletes.
- Operative management of anterior shoulder instability with one of several stabilization procedures significantly decreases risk of recurrence; however, this is often a season-ending option.
- Procedure choice is based on several patient factors, including but not limited to athlete age, sport of choice, prior surgery, and amount of glenoid and humeral head bone loss.

INTRODUCTION

The shoulder is a ball-and-socket joint that relies on an interdependence of static and dynamic stabilizers to maintain function. Injury to any of these structures can lead to instability, both subluxation and frank dislocation. Anterior shoulder instability can occur with non-sport trauma but is also common in contact and overhead athletes. Shoulder instability can lead to pain, cartilage and bone loss, neurovascular injury, and, importantly in athletes, loss of playing time.

Given its relatively shallow socket and wide range of motion, the shoulder is the most commonly unstable joint in the body, particularly in the young contact athlete (**Fig. 1**).[1] Management of anterior shoulder instability is further complicated when the athlete sustains the injury during the season. In those with a first-time dislocation

a Department of Orthopedics and Rehabilitation, University of Iowa Hospitals and Clinics, Iowa city, IA, USA
* Corresponding author. 200 Hawkins Drive, Iowa city, IA 52242.
E-mail address: garrett-christensen@uiowa.edu

Clin Sports Med 43 (2024) 585–599
https://doi.org/10.1016/j.csm.2024.03.019
0278-5919/24/Published by Elsevier Inc.

sportsmed.theclinics.com

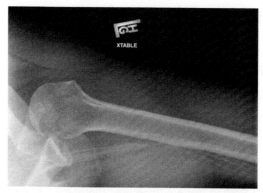

Fig. 1. Axillary lateral view of a left shoulder with an anterior shoulder dislocation. There is also evidence of a Hill–Sachs lesion of the posterolateral humeral head.

or subluxation, there are multiple treatment options. There is literature to support immediate surgical stabilization to prevent further instability and subsequent damage to the glenohumeral joint, ligaments, and capsule. Conversely, many team physicians work with athletes and training staff to pursue nonoperative treatment, with expedited rehabilitation until the injured extremity has similar strength and range of motion compared to the uninjured extremity.[2]

Recurrent instability is common in nonoperative management strategies. Previous literature demonstrates with each instability event, the athlete can further damage the joint and potentially worsen bone loss from the glenoid and/or humeral head.[3,4] For these reasons, it is crucial that the athlete, family, and provider understand and discuss the risks and benefits of each treatment pathway and come to an informed decision on which to pursue. These choices depend on timing of injury during the season, type of instability event (dislocation vs subluxation), presence of osseous injury, and the sport being played, including position-specific activity.[5] Other factors include the athlete's short-term and long-term goals, risk-tolerance, and eligibility.

ON-FIELD MANAGEMENT

The on-field management of a suspected anterior shoulder dislocation begins with an understanding of injury mechanism followed by a thorough physical examination. A provider will often find an athlete with an externally rotated extremity and acute shoulder pain. In some instances, a subluxation or dislocation will reduce prior to evaluation, in which the physical examination may be largely normal aside from shoulder pain and apprehension. In a frankly dislocated shoulder, there may be visual asymmetry compared to the contralateral side or anterior prominence about the involved shoulder. Other clues might include a sulcus superiorly or posteriorly with a palpable cavity or subjective feeling of instability by the athlete.

The provider should perform and document a complete neurovascular examination of the affected extremity and compare this to the well-arm, as neurovascular injuries, particularly axillary nerve injuries, can occur. Palpable crepitus or step-offs of the proximal humerus, clavicle, or scapula can clue one into a possible fracture. Other areas of pain should also be investigated, as shoulder instability may occur in tandem with sternoclavicular joint or elbow injuries. The provider should discuss with the athlete about any history of shoulder injuries, instability, or hyperlaxity.

If the provider is confident that the athlete sustained an anterior shoulder dislocation with low suspicion of associated fracture or other injury, it is reasonable and recommended to attempt a reduction prior to any further workup or imaging. After a thorough examination, a timely reduction is helpful as a delay can lead to muscle spasm and increased difficulty of reduction. Reduction maneuvers are generally performed in the locker room or training room but can also be attempted on the field or sideline by a qualified provider.

Many reduction maneuvers have been described and it is recommended that providers know how to perform at least a couple different techniques. The authors' preferred techniques are the Stimson, Milch, and Cunningham techniques. The Stimson technique utilizes weights to pull traction on the shoulder in a prone patient with their arm off the table. The Milch technique utilizes gentle shoulder external rotation, abduction, and anterior to posterior pressure on the humeral head. Lastly, the Cunningham technique is described as very gently pulling traction on an adducted shoulder while massaging the trapezius, deltoid, and biceps to allow for muscle relaxation.

Generally, the athlete should not return to play for the duration of the game or practice if they suffered a true dislocation requiring relocation; however, there are circumstances in athletes with recurrent instability, usually subluxation events, in which return is considered within that game or practice if the athlete has maintained motion and strength. Immobilization acutely with a sling may provide comfort for the athlete but is not recommended for longer than 1 week.[6]

POSTINJURY CARE

Treatment of first-time shoulder instability requires thought and consideration as well as discussion with the athlete, family members, physician, athletic trainers, and coaches. In some instances, an agent may be involved. Operative and nonoperative options should be discussed and the risks and benefits of both options clarified. Operative versus nonoperative management of acute anterior shoulder instability has been studied at length. There are risks and benefits to both treatment pathways and the patient must make the best decision for them and their goals.

IMAGING

Postinjury shoulder imaging should start with a true anteroposterior, axillary lateral, and west point view radiographs. This series will allow the provider to evaluate for glenoid defects or fractures of the clavicle, scapula, or humerus. A provider can ensure adequate reduction as well as preliminarily gauge glenoid or humeral bony lesions (**Fig. 2**). Stryker notch radiographs are also available to further characterize Hill–Sachs lesions, but these are not often part of a routine series.

While there is no consensus on timing of advanced imaging, MRI is helpful in identifying pathology of the labrum, capsule injury such as humeral avulsion of glenohumeral ligament lesions, and glenoid and humeral osteochondral lesions. In our experience, obtaining an MRI acutely has been useful given the traumatic hemarthrosis which can act as a natural contrast agent. In the subacute setting, a MR arthrogram with intraarticular contrast is utilized, as non-arthrogram MRI studies have been shown to be less sensitive at detecting labral pathology.[7] Unfortunately, MRI has been shown to be inconsistent in measuring glenoid and humeral bone loss and should be used with caution when evaluating bony defects.[8] MRI findings that, in the authors opinion, would push treatment recommendation to early surgery include significant full or partial-thickness rotator cuff tears, acute bony Bankart lesions, or

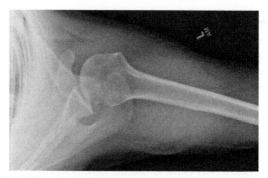

Fig. 2. Postreduction axillary lateral radiograph of a left shoulder with evidence of a Hill–Sachs lesion.

large Hill–Sachs lesions measuring greater than 25% of the circumference of the articular surface.

Finally, in those with radiographic evidence of glenoid bone loss or significant Hill–Sachs lesions, a computed tomography (CT) scan is useful to characterize associated bone loss and help guide decision making (**Fig. 3**). Some authors advocate for obtaining CT scans on all traumatic shoulder dislocations, as plain radiographs may underestimate the degree of bone loss.[9] There are several described methods to measure glenoid bone loss on CT, including area-based as well as linear-based methods.[10] In area-based measurement, an en face view of the glenoid is obtained, and a best-fit circle is drawn to obtain the area of the native glenoid articular surface. Next, an area measurement is made of the anterior glenoid bony defect and a measurement of defect area/total glenoid area is performed. A linear-based measurement uses the same en face view of the glenoid and starts with a best fit circle, as discussed earlier. A horizontal line is drawn from the anterior-most aspect of the best fit circle to the anterior aspect of the glenoid bone. Bone loss is then calculated as width of bony defect/total anterior to posterior glenoid width. The advantage of the linear-based method is that these measurements can be done in nearly all radiograph-viewing software, while area-based measurements often require more advanced technology.

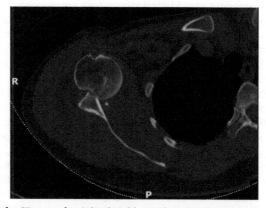

Fig. 3. Axial slice of a CT scan of a right shoulder with an irreducible anterior shoulder dislocation. There is significant anterior glenoid bone loss and a large, engaging Hill–Sachs lesion.

It is the author's opinion that acute bony Bankart lesions, glenoid bony defects of any chronicity measuring greater than 25% of the glenoid width, and Hill–Sachs lesions measuring greater than 25% of the humeral articular width are better served with an early stabilization procedure. While nonoperative management and return to sport is an acceptable option for these athletes, the likelihood of recurrent instability and failure of nonoperative treatment is high.

GLENOID TRACK

In 2007, Yamamoto and colleagues made the first description of glenoid track.[11] This was an attempt to quantify the size of Hill–Sachs lesions that need surgical intervention. They found that in high-risk positions (ie, shoulder external rotation, abduction, and extension) there is a defined area of humeral head cartilage that contacts the glenoid. This was termed as the glenoid track. If a Hill–Sachs lesion was large enough that in external rotation, abduction, and extension, it extended medially in front of the anterior rim of the glenoid, it was at risk of dislocation, and this was termed an "engaging Hill–Sachs lesion." Those Hill–Sachs lesions that are small enough to remain within the glenoid track in high-risk positions were termed "non-engaging Hill–Sachs lesions" and conferred a lower risk of instability.

Di Giacomo and colleagues further clarified and recommended the more accurate terminology of "on-track" or "off-track" lesions.[12] An on-track lesion describes a smaller Hill–Sachs lesion that remains within the glenoid track and is at lower risk of instability. The authors proposed a treatment algorithm based on the amount of glenoid bone loss and whether the Hill–Sachs lesion is on-track or off-track (**Table 1**).

NONOPERATIVE MANAGEMENT

Athletes who wish to return to play during the index season in which they have shoulder instability generally elect for nonoperative management. Studies consistently support that most athletes can return to sport after a short period of relative rest and rehabilitation. Buss and colleagues reported on their series of 30 athletes who sustained in-season anterior shoulder instability and observed that these athletes missed, on average, 10 days of play. Around 90% of these athletes were able to return to their sport that season, though 10 of those that returned (37%) had a recurrent instability event that season.[13]

Dickens and colleagues reported the results of their prospective study of collegiate athletes with in-season anterior shoulder instability and found that 73% were able to

Table 1			
Proposed treatment algorithm			
Group	**Glenoid Defect Size**	**Hill–Sachs Lesion**	**Proposed Treatment**
I	<10%–15%	On-track lesion	Arthroscopic or open Bankart repair
II	<10%–15%	Off-track lesion	Arthroscopic Bankart repair plus remplissage or open Bankart repair with capsular shift
III	≥25%	On-track lesion	Latarjet
IV	≥25%	Off-track lesion	Latarjet with possible humeral procedure (bone grafting or remplissage) depending on engagement after Latarjet

Adapted from Di Giacomo G, Itoi E, Burkhart SS. Evolving concept of bipolar bone loss and the Hill-Sachs lesion: from "engaging/non-engaging" lesion to "on-track/off-track" lesion. Arthroscopy. 2014;30(1):90-98. https://doi.org/10.1016/j.arthro.2013.10.004

return to sport during the index season.[14] Twenty-one of 33 athletes who returned to play had a recurrent instability event (64%). Despite this, 67% of the athletes who returned to sport were able to complete the season. In this cohort, median time lost to competition after instability was just 5 days. The most common reason for inability to return to sport was failure to attain sufficient shoulder function. These athletes who could not return to sport were all involved in contact sports.[14] Shanley and colleagues followed 129 high school athletes with instability through the next season and found that 85% of those treated nonoperatively were able to play through the next season without missing time related to their shoulder instability.[15]

These studies and several others demonstrate reasonably high rates of return to sport; however, this is not without risk to the athlete. Each occurrence of instability puts the athletes' neurovascular structures and joint at risk. Axillary nerve injuries have been reported in 5% to 35% of first-time dislocations, and though more seldom, they also occur in the setting of recurrent instability.[16,17] It is our clinical experience that axillary nerve injuries are uncommon and transient, however, they do occur, and athletes and families should be aware of this risk.

In addition, studies have illuminated the correlation between number of instability events and worsened glenohumeral bone loss. Rugg and colleagues found that patients with a single dislocation had, on average, 6.9% glenoid bone loss, while those with 2 or more dislocations had glenoid bone loss approaching 20%.[3] Dickens and colleagues reported on a prospectively followed cohort of over 700 athletes and monitored for instability. They found first time dislocators had an average of 6.8% glenoid bone loss.[18] This contrasted with those who had recurrent instability in which the average bone loss was 22.8%. Hettrich and colleagues evaluated nearly 900 patients with anterior shoulder instability and found the factor most associated with glenoid bone loss and Hill–Sachs lesions of the humerus was an increasing number of dislocations.[4]

Overall, the data suggest initial nonoperative management of anterior shoulder instability is a reasonable option for those who wish to finish the season. These data do, though, clarify that recurrent instability is prevalent and those who have recurrent instability events generally develop greater bone loss. This can complicate treatment options for athletes, as increased glenoid bone loss makes subsequent arthroscopic Bankart repair more likely to fail.[19,20] In these cases, the athlete may need more invasive techniques, such as a Latarjet or other bone block grafting procedures (**Box 1**).

Timing of instability within the season, as well as position played, should also be factored in when evaluating a patient and making treatment decisions. A football

---

Box 1
Relative indications for early nonoperative management with return to sport for athletes with in-season anterior shoulder instability

- First-time instability
- Subluxation event versus frank dislocation
- Normal postreduction radiographs without evidence of bony Bankart lesion or significant Hill–Sachs lesion
- Normal neurovascular examination
- Progress with rehabilitation and a pain-free shoulder with range of motion that is symmetric to the contralateral upper extremity
- Instability early in the season with adequate time for rehabilitation
- Athlete's final year of eligibility
- Ability to perform sport-specific drills/activities

linebacker who has an instability event in the second game of the season will be counseled differently than a softball player with instability in the playoffs. As detailed earlier, several days to weeks of rehabilitation is recommended prior to returning to sport, and an injury near the end of the season may limit an athlete's ability to rehab appropriately. In these cases, we generally recommend early stabilization.

An athlete's sport and position should be factored into decision making, as well. Overhead and throwing athletes, for example, often place their shoulders in positions of risk for instability. These athletes generally need more time for rehabilitation and progression through sport-specific drills can be slower. In some cases, return to sport within the season may not be possible due to pain or feelings of instability. Position differences also play a role in decision making, as a wide receiver in football may find it more difficult to return to the same level of play as a running back.

Bracing

There are several braces on the market (Sully, Aryse, Duke, etc.) each with the goal of limiting positions of risk (ie, shoulder abduction, extension, and external rotation; **Fig. 4**). These braces, though, have not proven to reduce risk of recurrent instability. Chu and colleagues and Ulkar and colleagues both performed biomechanical studies showing bracing to be positive in improving joint position sense in those with prior instability;

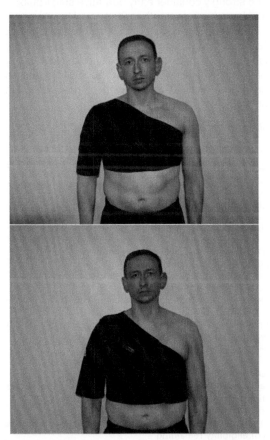

Fig. 4. Example of a Sully brace (top) and an Aryse SFast brace (bottom) for shoulder instability.

however, no studies have shown bracing to decrease risk of recurrent instability.[21–24] Bracing is a useful tool and may help athletes feel more comfortable returning to sport, but the clinical effectiveness in terms of recurrent instability is still unknown. No brace has been shown superior to another.[25,26] Unfortunately, many of the available braces are cumbersome and may not be tolerated by elite athletes. In addition, braces are often not practical in overhead or throwing athletes. Braces, though, have the potential to increase an athlete's confidence and should be discussed on an individualized basis as part of the nonoperative versus operative discussion.

OPERATIVE MANAGEMENT

In some scenarios, an athlete may be near the end of the season, have multiple years of eligibility remaining, or may be risk-averse and decide not to return to sport that season. In addition, injury-specific factors like fractures, irreducible dislocations, large osseous defects, among others may be present. In these cases, early surgery is recommended to decrease risk of recurrent instability. Specific procedure selection is guided by patient factors, such as age, presence of bony defects, sport type, competition level, and future goals.

In our opinion, most athletes can return to play; however, there are factors that would make us more strongly consider early operative stabilization. Acute bony Bankart lesions or glenoid bone loss greater than 25% is unlikely to provide the athlete with a stable shoulder. In addition, significant rotator cuff pathology or associated fracture is likely to do better when treated acutely. Failed trial of rehabilitation with decreased range of motion and persistent pain, or the inability of an athlete to perform their sport-specific tasks would be other factors that might support early surgery (**Box 2**). Lastly, if an athlete suffered repeat dislocation requiring manual reduction, then increasing consideration of surgical intervention is warranted.

Arthroscopic Stabilization procedures

Previous literature has shown operative stabilization to decrease the risk of recurrent instability. Arciero and colleagues published their prospective series of nonoperative

---

Box 2
Absolute and relative indications for early surgical management without return to play

Indications for early surgery
Absolute
- Significant partial-thickness or full-thickness rotator cuff tear
- Glenoid bony defect greater than 25%
- Hill–Sachs lesion greater than 25% humeral head articular surface
- Associated fracture (humeral, clavicle, etc.)
- Irreducible dislocations or nonconcentric reductions due to interposed tissue/incarcerated fragments
- Failed trial of rehabilitation with continued pain, inability to obtain symmetric range of motion and strength compared to contralateral extremity
- Inability to perform sport-specific drills

Relative
- Acute bony Bankart injury
- Recurrent instability events within the same season, especially repeat dislocation requiring manual reduction
- Overhead or throwing athletes unable to perform in their sport
- Injury occurs late in the season without time for adequate rehabilitation
- Multiple years of eligibility remaining
- Contact sport athletes

versus operative treatment of first-time shoulder dislocators.[27] They observed that in the nonoperative group, defined as 4 weeks of immobilization followed by rehabilitation, 80% of athletes had recurrent instability, while in the arthroscopic stabilization group, only 14% had recurrent instability at nearly 3 year follow-up. In a prospective, randomized study evaluating nonoperative versus operative management of first-time dislocations, Bottoni and colleagues found that 75% of nonoperatively treated athletes had recurrent instability compared to 11% of those treated with arthroscopic stabilization.[28] Hurley and colleagues performed a meta-analysis encompassing 10 prospective studies including 569 patients with first-time anterior shoulder dislocations and found that 10% of those treated with arthroscopic Bankart repair recurred while 67% of those treated nonoperatively had another instability event.[29]

Stabilization procedures come in several varieties. The most common is arthroscopic Bankart repair, which accounts for nearly 90% of stabilization procedures performed in the United States today in place of open Bankart repair which was the gold standard previously.[30–37]

Other surgical adjuncts may help decrease recurrence in the setting of arthroscopic stabilization. Di Giacomo and colleagues advocate for remplissage in cases of subcritical glenoid bone loss with Hill–Sachs lesions.[12] Remplissage is a soft tissue surgical technique to anchor the infraspinatus tendon into a Hill–Sachs lesion on the posterosuperior humeral head, effectively filling the void caused by the lesion and making dislocation more difficult. Many authors have evaluated the risks and benefits of remplissage and the data, taken together, do support the use of remplissage in some cases of large, engaging Hill–Sachs lesions, particularly when the anterior glenoid bone loss is subcritical.[38–41]

More recently in the literature there have been descriptions of arthroscopic Latarjet and bone grafting procedures.[42,43] Preliminary data are positive; however, these procedures have a steep learning curve and have not been widely adopted.[44]

Open Stabilization Procedures

Although much less common today, open Bankart repair plus or minus capsular shift is a classic way to deal with anterior shoulder instability. Labral repair with anchors in addition to capsular tightening through either a subscapularis tenotomy or split is a powerful way to treat anterior instability. Neviaser and colleagues reported on 127 patients, including 107 athletes, with mean follow up of 17 years.[45] They reported 1 (0.8%) recurrent dislocation and 1 (0.8%) recurrent subluxation with 98 of 107 athletes returning to sport. Pagnani reported on 103 patients, with 83 athletes, who underwent open capsular and labrum repair.[46] At a minimum of 2 year there was a 2% (2 of 103) rate of recurrent instability with one dislocation and one subluxation. Two of 83 contact athletes had recurrence.

Other open procedures continue to be useful in some circumstances, as patients with significant Hill–Sachs lesions, multiple dislocations, or glenoid bone defects have increased risk of recurrent instability with isolated arthroscopic Bankart repair.[47,48] For these patients, open Latarjet or allograft bone block procedures may decrease risk of recurrence. Many authors have attempted to identify a critical amount of glenoid bone loss to identify which patients benefit most from these bony procedures.

Current data support consideration of the bony procedures in those with 13% to 20% or more glenoid bone loss.[19] Other factors that might support primary Latarjet or bone block procedure include competitive contact sport participation, generalized ligamentous laxity, multiple dislocations, or younger age.[49] These procedures have a higher risk profile than arthroscopic procedures, as neurovascular injury, screw breakage, graft resorption or fracture, and wound dehiscence can occur.[50,51] Despite this, patients who are indicated for Latarjet return to sport at high rates and have improved patient-reported outcome scores and low rates of recurrent instability.[49,52,53]

PSYCHOLOGICAL READINESS FOR RETURN TO PLAY

Not only does an athlete need to prove physical readiness to return to play after shoulder instability, but they also need to be psychologically prepared to return to play. Gerometta and colleagues proposed and validated a psychological readiness assessment for athletes modeled after the Anterior Cruciate Ligament-Return to Sport after Injury scale. It is termed the Shoulder Instability-Return to Sport after Injury scale (SIRSI). The SIRSI asks an athlete a series of questions on a Likert-type scale to evaluate their mental readiness and safety to return to play. The SIRSI has been shown to predict with high accuracy an athlete's ability to return to sport. It is our recommendation that team physicians and trainers work in conjunction with athletes to ensure not only their physical but mental readiness to return to play regardless of whether they undergo operative or nonoperative management for their shoulder instability.[54,55]

DISCUSSION

Treatment of an in-season anterior shoulder dislocation is a dilemma requiring thought and shared decision making. Multiple factors should be considered including timing of the injury during the season, type of instability event (dislocation vs subluxation), any osseous involvement (both fracture and attritional bone loss), and sport-specific characteristics (level of competition, position, etc.)[5] Other factors include the athlete's short-term and long-term goals, risk-tolerance, and eligibility. Initial nonoperative management is a reasonable option for most athletes, and return to sport rates are high, but the athlete must understand that recurrent instability is likely. Each additional instability event increases the likelihood of bony lesions of the glenoid and/or humerus, which may make the shoulder more unstable, and complicates future operative planning.

Nonoperative management includes rest from competition, targeted physical therapy focusing on regaining shoulder range of motion and strength, and possible bracing modalities. Bracing can be helpful, and some athletes prefer to brace; however, no substantial data support the use of bracing for decreasing recurrence rates.

After the season, operative stabilization is recommended. In those without significant glenoid or humeral bony defects, arthroscopic Bankart repair significantly decreases risk of recurrent instability. In those with bony defects, a Latarjet procedure, allograft bone block procedure, or arthroscopic Bankart repair with remplissage should be considered. Each of the surgical options listed earlier lead to low rates of recurrent instability with high rates of return to sport.

SUMMARY

Management of anterior shoulder instability in an in-season athlete is complex and requires shared decision making among all parties involved. Return to sport rates are high, even in contact and overhead athletes; however, recurrence rates are also high, so athletes should be made aware of this risk prior to returning to sport. It is generally safe for athletes to return to their sport when the injured shoulder has similar strength and range of motion compared to the uninjured extremity. In those with recurrent instability, several arthroscopic and open surgical options are available depending on age, glenoid and humeral bony defects, surgeon preference, eligibility, among other factors. Operative stabilization continues to be very successful at decreasing rates of recurrent instability.

CLINICS CARE POINTS

- Carefully selected athletes with in-season anterior shoulder instability can return to sport at high rates; however, they should know that recurrent instability rates are also high.

- In-season athletes who are near the end of the season or have multiple years of eligibility remaining should consider early operative stabilization. These procedures are safe, have high rates of return to sport, and significantly decrease recurrent instability rates.

- Athletes who elect nonoperative treatment are considered safe to perform an expedited physical therapy program and return to sport when they are (1) pain-free and (2) have symmetric range of motion and strength compared to the contralateral side.

DISCLOSURE

B.R. Wolf is a board or committee member for the American Orthopedic Society for Sports Medicine, the American Board of Orthopedic Surgery, and the Mid-America Orthopedic Association. He is on the Editorial or Governing Board for the Orthopedic Journal of Sports Medicine. He receives IP royalties, is a paid consultant, or paid presenter/speaker for CONMED Linvatec. G.V. Christensen and O.C. O'Reilly certify that they have no disclosures.

REFERENCES

1. Abrams R, Akbarnia H. Shoulder dislocations overview. In: StatPearls. Treasure Island (FL): StatPearls Publishing; 2023.
2. Kuhn JE. Treating the initial anterior shoulder dislocation–an evidence-based medicine approach. Sports Med Arthrosc Rev 2006;14(4):192–8.
3. Rugg CM, Hettrich CM, Ortiz S, Wolf BR, MOON Shoulder Instability Group, Zhang AL. Surgical stabilization for first-time shoulder dislocators: a multicenter analysis. J Shoulder Elbow Surg 2018;27(4):674–85.
4. Hettrich CM, Magnuson JA, Baumgarten KM, et al. Predictors of bone loss in anterior glenohumeral instability. Am J Sports Med 2023;51(5):1286–94.
5. Wolf BR, Tranovich MA, Marcussen B, et al. Team approach: treatment of shoulder instability in athletes. JBJS Rev 2021;9(11). https://doi.org/10.2106/JBJS. RVW.21.00087.
6. Paterson WH, Throckmorton TW, Koester M, et al. Position and duration of immobilization after primary anterior shoulder dislocation: a systematic review and meta-analysis of the literature. J Bone Joint Surg Am 2010;92(18):2924–33.
7. Smith TO, Drew BT, Toms AP. A meta-analysis of the diagnostic test accuracy of MRA and MRI for the detection of glenoid labral injury. Arch Orthop Trauma Surg 2012;132(7):905–19.
8. Vopat ML, Peebles LA, McBride T, et al. Accuracy and reliability of imaging modalities for the diagnosis and quantification of hill-sachs lesions: a systematic review. Arthroscopy 2021;37(1):391–401. https://doi.org/10.1016/j.arthro.2020. 08.005.
9. Delage Royle A, Balg F, Bouliane MJ, et al. Indication for computed tomography scan in shoulder instability: sensitivity and specificity of standard radiographs to

predict bone defects after traumatic anterior glenohumeral instability. Orthop J Sports Med 2017;5(10). 2325967117733660.

10. Chalmers PN, Christensen G, O'Neill D, et al. Does bone loss imaging modality, measurement methodology, and interobserver reliability alter treatment in glenohumeral instability? Arthroscopy 2020;36(1):12–9. https://doi.org/10.1016/j.arthro.2019.06.025.

11. Yamamoto N, Itoi E, Abe H, et al. Contact between the glenoid and the humeral head in abduction, external rotation, and horizontal extension: a new concept of glenoid track. J Shoulder Elbow Surg 2007;16(5):649–56. https://doi.org/10.1016/j.jse.2006.12.012.

12. Di Giacomo G, Itoi E, Burkhart SS. Evolving concept of bipolar bone loss and the Hill-Sachs lesion: from "engaging/non-engaging" lesion to "on-track/off-track" lesion. Arthroscopy 2014;30(1):90–8. https://doi.org/10.1016/j.arthro.2013.10.004.

13. Buss DD, Lynch GP, Meyer CP, et al. Nonoperative management for in-season athletes with anterior shoulder instability. Am J Sports Med 2004;32(6):1430–3. https://doi.org/10.1177/0363546503262069 [published correction appears in Am J Sports Med. 2004 Oct-Nov;32(7):1780].

14. Dickens JF, Owens BD, Cameron KL, et al. Return to play and recurrent instability after in-season anterior shoulder instability: a prospective multicenter study. Am J Sports Med 2014;42(12):2842–50. https://doi.org/10.1177/0363546514553181.

15. Shanley E, Thigpen C, Brooks J, et al. Return to sport as an outcome measure for shoulder instability: surprising findings in nonoperative management in a high school athlete population. Am J Sports Med 2019;47(5):1062–7. https://doi.org/10.1177/0363546519829765.

16. Perlmutter GS, Apruzzese W. Axillary nerve injuries in contact sports: recommendations for treatment and rehabilitation. Sports Med 1998 Nov;26(5):351–61.

17. Hardie CM, Jordan R, Forker O, et al. Prevalence and risk factors for nerve injury following shoulder dislocation. Musculoskelet Surg 2023;107(3):345–50. https://doi.org/10.1007/s12306-022-00769-4.

18. Dickens JF, Slaven SE, Cameron KL, et al. Prospective evaluation of glenoid bone loss after first-time and recurrent anterior glenohumeral instability events. Am J Sports Med 2019;47(5):1082–9. https://doi.org/10.1177/0363546519831286.

19. Boileau P, Villalba M, Héry JY, et al. Risk factors for recurrence of shoulder instability after arthroscopic Bankart repair. J Bone Joint Surg Am 2006;88(8):1755–63. https://doi.org/10.2106/JBJS.E.00817.

20. Balg F, Boileau P. The instability severity index score. A simple pre-operative score to select patients for arthroscopic or open shoulder stabilisation. J Bone Joint Surg Br 2007;89(11):1470–7. https://doi.org/10.1302/0301-620X.89B11.18962.

21. Chu JC, Kane EJ, Arnold BL, et al. The effect of a neoprene shoulder stabilizer on active joint-reposition sense in subjects with stable and unstable shoulders. J Athl Train 2002;37(2):141–5.

22. Ulkar B, Kunduracioglu B, Cetin C, et al. Effect of positioning and bracing on passive position sense of shoulder joint. Br J Sports Med 2004;38(5):549–52. https://doi.org/10.1136/bjsm.2002.004275.

23. Kwapisz A, Shanley E, Momaya AM, et al. Does functional bracing of the unstable shoulder improve return to play in scholastic athletes? returning the unstable shoulder to play. Sport Health 2021;13(1):45–8. https://doi.org/10.1177/1941738120942239.

24. Conti M, Garofalo R, Castagna A, et al. Dynamic brace is a good option to treat first anterior shoulder dislocation in season. Musculoskelet Surg 2017;101(Suppl 2):169–73. https://doi.org/10.1007/s12306-017-0497-5.

25. Owens BD, Dickens JF, Kilcoyne KG, et al. Management of mid-season traumatic anterior shoulder instability in athletes. J Am Acad Orthop Surg 2012;20(8): 518–26. https://doi.org/10.5435/JAAOS-20-08-518.

26. Baker HP, Krishnan P, Meghani O, et al. Protective sport bracing for athletes with mid-season shoulder instability. Sport Health 2023;15(1):105–10. https://doi.org/10.1177/19417381211069069.

27. Arciero RA, Wheeler JH, Ryan JB, et al. Arthroscopic Bankart repair versus nonoperative treatment for acute, initial anterior shoulder dislocations. Am J Sports Med 1994;22(5):589–94. https://doi.org/10.1177/036354659402200504.

28. Bottoni CR, Wilckens JH, DeBerardino TM, et al. A prospective, randomized evaluation of arthroscopic stabilization versus nonoperative treatment in patients with acute, traumatic, first-time shoulder dislocations. Am J Sports Med 2002;30(4): 576–80. https://doi.org/10.1177/03635465020300041801.

29. Hurley ET, Manjunath AK, Bloom DA, et al. Arthroscopic bankart repair versus conservative management for first-time traumatic anterior shoulder instability: a systematic review and meta-analysis. Arthroscopy 2020;36(9):2526–32. https://doi.org/10.1016/j.arthro.2020.04.046.

30. Ahmed AS, Gabig AM, Dawes A, et al. Trends and projections in surgical stabilization of glenohumeral instability in the United States from 2009 to 2030: rise of the Latarjet procedure and fall of open Bankart repair. J Shoulder Elbow Surg 2023;32(8):e387–95. https://doi.org/10.1016/j.jse.2023.03.011.

31. Riff AJ, Frank RM, Sumner S, et al. Trends in shoulder stabilization techniques used in the United States Based on a Large Private-Payer Database. Orthop J Sports Med 2017;5(12). 2325967117745511.

32. Mohtadi NG, Bitar IJ, Sasyniuk TM, et al. Arthroscopic versus open repair for traumatic anterior shoulder instability: a meta-analysis. Arthroscopy 2005;21(6): 652–8. https://doi.org/10.1016/j.arthro.2005.02.021.

33. Freedman KB, Smith AP, Romeo AA, et al. Open Bankart repair versus arthroscopic repair with transglenoid sutures or bioabsorbable tacks for Recurrent Anterior instability of the shoulder: a meta-analysis. Am J Sports Med 2004; 32(6):1520–7. https://doi.org/10.1177/0363546504265188.

34. Harris JD, Gupta AK, Mall NA, et al. Long-term outcomes after Bankart shoulder stabilization. Arthroscopy 2013;29(5):920–33. https://doi.org/10.1016/j.arthro.2012.11.010.

35. Chalmers PN, Mascarenhas R, Leroux T, et al. Do arthroscopic and open stabilization techniques restore equivalent stability to the shoulder in the setting of anterior glenohumeral instability? a systematic review of overlapping meta-analyses. Arthroscopy 2015;31(2):355–63. https://doi.org/10.1016/j.arthro.2014.07.008.

36. Petrera M, Patella V, Patella S, et al. A meta-analysis of open versus arthroscopic Bankart repair using suture anchors. Knee Surg Sports Traumatol Arthrosc 2010; 18(12):1742–7. https://doi.org/10.1007/s00167-010-1093-5.

37. Bottoni CR, Johnson JD, Zhou L, et al. Arthroscopic versus open anterior shoulder stabilization: a prospective randomized clinical trial with 15-year follow-up with an assessment of the glenoid being "On-Track" and "Off-Track" as a predictor of failure. Am J Sports Med 2021;49(8):1999–2005. https://doi.org/10.1177/03635465211018212 [published correction appears in Am J Sports Med. 2022 Feb;50(2):NP14-NP15].

38. MacDonald P, McRae S, Old J, et al. Arthroscopic Bankart repair with and without arthroscopic infraspinatus remplissage in anterior shoulder instability with a Hill-Sachs defect: a randomized controlled trial. J Shoulder Elbow Surg 2021;30(6): 1288–98. https://doi.org/10.1016/j.jse.2020.11.013.

39. Camus D, Domos P, Berard E, et al. Isolated arthroscopic Bankart repair vs. Bankart repair with "remplissage" for anterior shoulder instability with engaging Hill-Sachs lesion: A meta-analysis. Orthop Traumatol Surg Res 2018;104(6): 803–9. https://doi.org/10.1016/j.otsr.2018.05.011.

40. Frantz TL, Everhart JS, Cvetanovich GL, et al. What are the effects of remplissage on 6-month strength and range of motion after arthroscopic bankart repair? a multicenter cohort study. Orthop J Sports Med 2020;8(2). 2325967120903283.

41. Boileau P, O'Shea K, Vargas P, et al. Anatomical and functional results after arthroscopic Hill-Sachs remplissage. J Bone Joint Surg Am 2012;94(7):618–26. https://doi.org/10.2106/JBJS.K.00101.

42. Lafosse L, Lejeune E, Bouchard A, et al. The arthroscopic Latarjet procedure for the treatment of anterior shoulder instability. Arthroscopy 2007;23(11):1242.e1-5. https://doi.org/10.1016/j.arthro.2007.06.008.

43. Lukenchuk J, Thangarajah T, More K, et al. Arthroscopic anterior glenoid reconstruction using a distal tibial allograft positioned with an intra-articular guide and secured with double-button fixation. Arthrosc Tech 2022;11(6):e1053–7.

44. Lafosse L, Boyle S. Arthroscopic Latarjet procedure. J Shoulder Elbow Surg 2010;19(2 Suppl):2–12. https://doi.org/10.1016/j.jse.2009.12.010.

45. Neviaser RJ, Benke MT, Neviaser AS. Mid-term to long-term outcome of the open Bankart repair for recurrent traumatic anterior dislocation of the shoulder. J Shoulder Elbow Surg 2017;26(11):1943–7. https://doi.org/10.1016/j.jse.2017. 04.013.

46. Pagnani MJ. Open capsular repair without bone block for recurrent anterior shoulder instability in patients with and without bony defects of the glenoid and/or humeral head. Am J Sports Med 2008;36(9):1805–12. https://doi.org/10. 1177/0363546508316284.

47. Rowe CR, Zarins B, Ciullo JV. Recurrent anterior dislocation of the shoulder after surgical repair. Apparent causes of failure and treatment. J Bone Joint Surg Am 1984;66(2):159–68.

48. Burkhart SS, De Beer JF. Traumatic glenohumeral bone defects and their relationship to failure of arthroscopic Bankart repairs: significance of the inverted-pear glenoid and the humeral engaging Hill-Sachs lesion. Arthroscopy 2000;16(7): 677–94. https://doi.org/10.1053/jars.2000.17715.

49. Bessière C, Trojani C, Carles M, et al. The open latarjet procedure is more reliable in terms of shoulder stability than arthroscopic bankart repair. Clin Orthop Relat Res 2014;472(8):2345–51. https://doi.org/10.1007/s11999-014-3550-9.

50. Sobhani A, Taheri SN, Amiri S. Short-term complications of open latarjet procedure for recurrent anterior shoulder dislocation. Med J Islam Repub Iran 2023; 37(60).

51. Gupta A, Delaney R, Petkin K, et al. Complications of the Latarjet procedure. Curr Rev Musculoskelet Med 2015;8(1):59–66. https://doi.org/10.1007/s12178-015-9258-y.

52. Ernat JJ, Rakowski DR, Hanson JA, et al. High rate of return to sport and excellent patient-reported outcomes after an open Latarjet procedure. J Shoulder Elbow Surg 2022;31(8):1704–12. https://doi.org/10.1016/j.jse.2022.01.139.

53. Bishop JY, Hidden KA, Jones GL, et al, MOON Shoulder Group. Factors Influencing Surgeon's Choice of Procedure for Anterior Shoulder Instability: A

Multicenter Prospective Cohort Study. Arthroscopy 2019;35(7):2014–25. https://doi.org/10.1016/j.arthro.2019.02.035.

54. Gerometta A, Klouche S, Herman S, et al. The Shoulder Instability-Return to Sport after Injury (SIRSI): a valid and reproducible scale to quantify psychological readiness to return to sport after traumatic shoulder instability. Knee Surg Sports Traumatol Arthrosc 2018;26(1):203–11. https://doi.org/10.1007/s00167-017-4645-0.

55. Rossi LA, Pasqualini I, Brandariz R, et al. Relationship of the SIRSI Score to Return to Sports After Surgical Stabilization of Glenohumeral Instability. Am J Sports Med 2022;50(12):3318–25. https://doi.org/10.1177/03635465221118369.

Arthroscopic Management of the Contact Athlete with Anterior Instability

Joseph C. Brinkman, MD[a],*, Elizabeth Damitio[b],
John M. Tokish, MD[c]

KEYWORDS

- Shoulder instability • Bankart lesion • Remplissage • Shoulder dislocation
- Distal clavicle autograft • Distal tibia allograft

KEY POINTS

- Anterior glenohumeral instability is one of the most common injuries suffered from sport.
- Most up-to-date literature on outcomes of arthroscopic management in athletes are discussed.
- Despite padding and conditioning, the shoulder joint remains particularly vulnerable to injury, especially in the setting of contact.
- Arthroscopic procedures such as the Bankart repair and remplissage continue to demonstrate favorable results in appropriately selected patients.
- In the setting of bone loss, bony augmentation procedures including the Latarjet and distal tibial allograft are required to restore stability and function.

INTRODUCTION

Anterior glenohumeral instability is one of the most common injuries suffered from sport. Despite padding and conditioning, the shoulder joint remains particularly vulnerable to injury, especially in the setting of contact. The overall rate of anterior instability is reported to be 0.12 injuries per 1000 athlete exposures, although this is increased up to 0.40 to 0.51 in the contact athlete.[1,2] Young athletes with high physical demands are at an increased risk of instability, with rates occurring as high as 3% per year in this susceptible population.[3] Although instability results from trauma in the majority of athletic cases, repetitive overhead activities along with capsular laxity can also predispose to atraumatic dislocation.[4,5] The spectrum of anterior instability ranges between microinstability, subluxation, and complete dislocation (**Fig. 1**A and B). As the

[a] Department of Orthopedic Surgery, Mayo Clinic, Phoenix, AZ, USA; [b] Institute of Protein Design, University of Washington, Seattle, Washington, USA; [c] Department of Orthopedic Surgery Sports Medicine, Mayo Clinic, Phoenix, AZ, USA
* Corresponding author. Mayo Clinic Department of Orthopedic Surgery Sports Medicine, 5881 East Mayo Boulevard, Phoenix, AZ 85054.
E-mail address: brinkman.joseph@mayo.edu

Clin Sports Med 43 (2024) 601–615
https://doi.org/10.1016/j.csm.2024.03.020

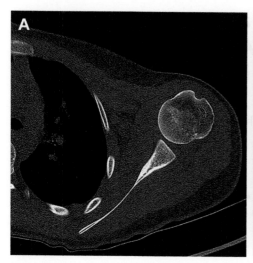 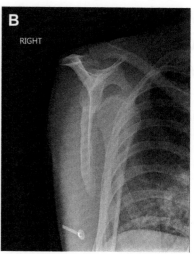

Fig. 1. (*A*) Computed tomography (CT) axial image of resting subluxation of a left shoulder. (*B*) Scapular Y view of a right shoulder demonstrating definitive dislocation of glenohumeral joint.

condition causes pain, disability, and lower quality of life, managing this pathology is imperative in the contact athlete. Owing to the high rates of recurrent instability and progressive injury associated with nonoperative treatment, many athletes elect to undergo surgical intervention.[6,7] Successful treatment requires consideration of restoring stability while minimizing loss of glenohumeral motion. Common treatment strategies involve addressing the pathology that results from anterior shoulder dislocation including labral detachment as well as bony defects to the humeral head and glenoid.

HISTORY OF THE BANKART REPAIR

Bankart[8] first described the lesion of the anteroinferior glenoid in 1923. In his seminal report, he supported surgical fixation of anteroinferior labral detachment as he suggested it was the main feature of anterior shoulder instability. He also described his original technique for Bankart lesion repair. In this open technique, a coracoid osteotomy and subscapularis tenotomy were utilized to gain access to the anterior glenoid. Following, a wide osteotomy was utilized to prepare the glenoid to allow for healing of the labrum that was attached using interrupted silkworm sutures. After repair of the tenotomy and osteotomy, patients were placed in adduction for 4 weeks. This technique was reported to result in favorable although limited outcomes in a series of 4 patients, 2 of whom were soccer players.

MODERN BANKART REPAIR TECHNIQUE

Since originally described, the Bankart repair technique has benefitted from several innovations that have allowed for the procedure to become safer with stronger fixation. Most notably, the modern Bankart repair can be performed arthroscopically, which allows for direct intraoperative visualization of essential shoulder pathology and obviates the need for a coracoid osteotomy, subscapularis tenotomy, or capsulotomy. Innovation has also allowed for fixation to be achieved with suture anchors, precluding the need for bone tunnels and thus allowing for more bone preservation.

ACCESS AND GLENOID PREPARATION

In 2019, Lacheta and colleagues[9] outlined the specifics of a modern arthroscopic Bankart repair using all-suture anchors. The lateral position allows for increased lateral traction and visualization of the lesion from the anterosuperior portal (**Fig. 2**A and B). Traction can be achieved with an axillary roll in place with a 3-point distraction system or jack device as per surgeon preference. Standard posterior, anterosuperior, and anteroinferior portals are utilized, with cannulas positioned in each of the anterior portals. A diagnostic arthroscopy is first performed to evaluate for any coexisting pathology. While viewing through the posterior portal, the capsulolabral tissue can be mobilized with an elevator or electrocautery. Visualization can be further improved by viewing from the anterosuperior portal, allowing for direct evaluation of the anteroinferior glenoid rim. Debridement is then carried down to liberate the labrum down the glenoid neck until a bleeding bed is created. Complete liberation can be confirmed by anteriorly lifting the labrum to directly view between the labrum and glenoid neck to verify the absence of soft tissue adhesions.

LABRAL REPAIR

The capsulolabral tissue is typically fixed using a minimum of 3 suture anchors. The inferior-most anchor is placed first and is typically achieved through the anteroinferior portal. A drill guide is utilized to set the location for the anchors, with labral re-approximation optimized by placing the anchors 1 to 2 mm onto the glenoid face. After drilling, the anchor is inserted into the bone tunnel and started by hand to ensure proper seating before finalizing anchor position. There are multiple methods including knotted and knotless techniques for fixation of the labrum. The senior author's current preference is in the use of an all-suture knotless construct. In this technique, the working suture is retrieved through the anterosuperior portal with a retriever before the capsule is penetrated inferior to the anchor. Using a suture shuttle (suture lasso, Arthrex, Naples, FL, USA), the capsule and labrum are pierced at the desired location, inferior to the anchor, and a nitinol wire is shuttled and retrieved through the anterior superior portal. The working stitch is then placed through the loop and retrograde passed through the labrum. This stitch is then passed through the anchor using the shuttle stitch and this forms a closed loop self-locking stitch around the labrum that can be tightened to the desired tension. Excess suture is then cut with an arthroscopic cutter which completes a knotless construct repair (**Fig. 3**).

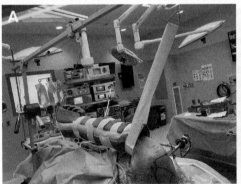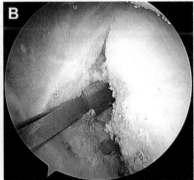

Fig. 2. Arthroscopic view of right shoulder, viewing from anterosuperior portal of a Bankart lesion, pre-repair(A–B).

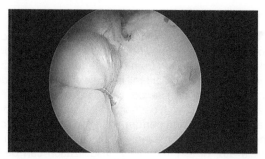

Fig. 3. Arthroscopic view of right shoulder, viewing from anterosuperior portal of a completed Bankart repair.

The aforementioned process is repeated until appropriate repair is achieved. An adequate Bankart repair typically involves 3 to 5 anchors, depending on tear severity and stability required. It is standard to start with the repair inferiorly and work superiorly. Specifically, the inferior anchor is used to tighten the axillary pouch, with subsequent anchors placed at the level of the inferior glenohumeral ligament, middle glenohumeral ligament, and anterosuperior labrum. If a concomitant superior labrum anterior to posterior tear is present, repair can be continued more superiorly. Postoperatively, patients are placed in a sling for 4 weeks while gentle passive range of motion exercises are permitted with limitations in external rotation to approximately 30°. After 4 weeks, the sling is discontinued, and full unrestricted passive range of motion is allowed. Active strengthening is introduced with closed chain exercises followed by open chain exercises at 6 weeks postoperatively. Full return to activities is typically achieved at 4 months postoperatively. Specific to athletes, return to sport after arthroscopic Bankart has been shown to be as high as 98% at a mean of 5.9 months.[10]

BANKART REPAIR OUTCOMES IN ATHLETES

Several studies have evaluated the outcomes of the Bankart repair in athletes. A systematic review by Memon and colleagues[11] in 2018 showed that the procedure resulted in significant pain and functional improvement in the athletes. Pooled analysis showed that 81% of athletes return to sport after arthroscopic Bankart, with 82% of these returning to a competitive level and 66% returning to preinjury level of play. A high rate of return to sport was also noted in a separate systematic review comprising 290 athletes who reported an overall return to sport rate of 91%.[12] In those that do not return to sport, shoulder-related concerns are most commonly noted including persistent instability, fear of reinjury, apprehension, or pain.[13] Long-term studies have shown that favorable clinical results can be expected in athletes as concluded by Bauer and colleagues[14], despite a recurrence rate of nearly 22% at 14 years of follow-up. However, failure has been shown to be higher in the contact athlete. Specifically, contact athletes have been shown to have 3 times the rate of recurrence when compared to noncontact athletes undergoing arthroscopic Bankart repair.[15] Importantly, many series evaluating the outcomes of arthroscopic Bankart repair exclude patients with significant bony defects, as this is a known risk factor for failure.[16]

REMPLISSAGE

One factor that has been associated with Bankart repair failure is the presence of a posterosuperior humeral head defect, otherwise known as a Hill-Sachs lesion.[17]

Burkhart and De Beer[17] first reported the phenomenon in which the Hill-Sachs lesion engages with the glenoid defect, leading to recurrent instability.[18] Due to this, patients with these humeral-sided defects are often considered poor candidates for Bankart repair alone as this would not address the humeral-sided defect. Several treatment options exist to treat this humeral-sided bone loss by filling or offloading the defect, including osteoarticular allografts, bone plugs, dis-impaction, rotational osteotomies, and prosthetic humeral head replacement.[19] However, the most widely used method for addressing humeral head defects is the arthroscopic remplissage procedure. Originally described by Connolly[20] followed by Purchase[21] and modified by Koo,[22] the remplissage procedure involves filling the Hill-Sachs lesion through tenodesis of the posterior capsule and infraspinatus tendon.

REMPLISSAGE TECHNIQUE

In 2016, Tokish and colleagues[23] reported an arthroscopic remplissage technique for moderate-sized Hill-Sachs lesions. With the patient in the lateral decubitus position, the posterior portal is established first prior to creating the anterosuperior and mid-glenoid portals under direct visualization. A diagnostic arthroscopy is first performed, with specific attention paid to the glenoid to confirm that no significant glenoid bone loss is present. Standard arthroscopic technique is utilized to liberate and prepare the glenoid and Bankart lesion for labral repair. For improved visualization of the Hill-Sachs lesion, the arm can be taken into abduction and the arthroscope can be placed into the anterosuperior portal. Dynamic assessment in this position can improve the assessment of the glenoid track and engagement of the Hill-Sachs lesion.[24] During concomitant Bankart repair, some authors may choose to delay the final Bankart repair to best visualize the Hill-Sachs lesion and avoid anterior shear forces from a remplissage on a completed Bankart repair.

Alexander and colleagues[25] have reported a technique in which this double pulley technique is created with knotless, all-suture anchors. The Hill-Sachs lesion is first biologically prepared for infraspinatus healing with a shaver, rasp, or bone cutter (**Fig. 4**A). This is typically achieved with the instrument through the posterior portal while viewing from the anterosuperior portal. As posterior portal establishment is critical for the procedure, a spinal needle can be used to identify a path perpendicular to the center of the defect such that 2 anchors can be placed through 1 incision. It is critical that the 2 anchors are placed through separate piercings in the posterior capsule which creates the tissue bridge for the repair (**Fig. 4**B). The working limb from the posterior anchor is

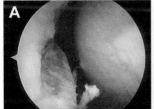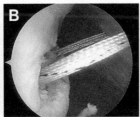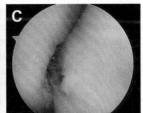

Fig. 4. (*A*) Arthroscopic view of left shoulder, viewing from anterosuperior portal of a Hill-Sachs lesion. (*B*) Arthroscopic view of a left shoulder of remplissage repair after anchors are placed but before tension is applied. Anchors are placed at anterior and posterior aspects of defect through separate piercings of the posterior capsule. (*C*) Arthroscopic view of a left shoulder of remplissage repair just before final tension demonstrating reduction of the capsule into the defect.

passed through the pulley of the anterior anchor and vice versa. Once accomplished, the suture limbs are tensioned until the capsule is reduced into the defect (**Fig. 4**C). This allows the remplissage procedure to be done without entering the subacromial space and without the need to pass sutures through tissue separate from the anchor placement.

REMPLISSAGE PATIENT SELECTION

As with other stabilization procedures, the outcomes of the remplissage depend on the appropriate selection of patients. Standard indications are evolving but thought to include patients with an engaging Hill-Sachs lesion with minimal or no glenoid bone loss.[26] Specifically, Di Giacomo and colleagues[24] recommend utilizing the remplissage for "off-track" Hill-Sachs lesions with less than 25% glenoid bone loss. Hill-Sachs lesions are considered "off-track" when they extend beyond the glenoid track, putting the patient at risk for lesion engagement and dislocation. Determining whether a Hill-Sachs lesion is on-track or off-track can be determined in several ways and involves measuring the size of the glenoid track and lesion. The width of the glenoid track can be measured arthroscopically with a probe by the Pico[27] method on radiographs or by measuring the glenoid width on computed topography scans.[28] The glenoid track and determination of on-track versus off-track nature of the Hill-Sachs lesion can be calculated as shown in Box 1.

REMPLISSAGE OUTCOMES

Outcomes of the remplissage procedure have generally been favorable in correctly chosen individuals. In 2016, Garcia and colleagues[29] reported a recurrence rate of 11.8% at 5 years follow-up and overall return to sport in 96% of 50 patients undergoing remplissage. A relatively low rate of recurrence and high rate of return to sport was also noted on a 2023 systematic review of 736 patients managed with arthroscopic Bankart with remplissage.[30] This review specifically showed a return to sport rate of 80% to 100% for contact athletes. Of note, both studies demonstrated inferior outcomes in terms of range of motion and return to sport in throwing athletes. Several series have also directly compared the outcomes between the remplissage and Bankart procedures. In a series of 123 patients by Horinek and colleagues[31], patients who underwent remplissage showed similar postoperative function to isolated arthroscopic Bankart repair despite worse preoperative pathology, leading investigators to suggest that the indications for remplissage should be widened. It has also been shown in a randomized controlled trial that the addition of remplissage to arthroscopic Bankart significantly reduces the rate of recurrent instability.[32] Further, while the reported failure rates of the Bankart procedure range between 9% and 35%, recurrence rate after the arthroscopic remplissage is reported to be as low as 4.4%.[33–36] Failure rates were also shown to be higher with isolated Bankart versus Bankart with remplissage in a systematic review of 694 patients, in which isolated Bankart failure ranged between 7% and 57% compared to the addition of remplissage which showed a failure rate between 0% and 20%.[37] The remplissage continues to demonstrate favorable results although future high-quality studies are warranted to inform the indications and expected results of the procedure, especially in the contact athlete.

BONY AUGMENTATION PROCEDURES

It is particularly important to evaluate for glenoid bone loss prior to proceeding with a soft tissue–based procedure such as arthroscopic Bankart repair with or without remplissage. Specific to contact athletes, it has been shown that recurrent instability occurs in up to 51% of adolescents who undergo arthroscopic labral repair alone.[38] Special attention is also warranted for the presence of a significant glenoid bony defect, as these lesions portend high rates of recurrent instability and worse functional outcomes.[17,39,40] Unfortunately, defects of the glenoid are common in patients with glenohumeral instability. They are found in an estimated 22% of first-time dislocators and in up to 73% of recurrent cases.[41,42] Several studies have quantified the amount of "critical" bone loss that predicts these worse outcomes. These estimates range between 21% and 26%; however, it has been demonstrated that "subcritical" bone loss as low as 13.5% predicts instability and decreased patient satisfaction.[40,43,44] Up to one-third of initial dislocations will cause subcritical bone loss, so it remains critical to evaluate for bone loss even in the primary setting.[45]

In addition to the amount of glenoid bone loss, special consideration should also be made for "bipolar" lesions, or concomitant lesions to the glenoid and humerus. As a result of the dynamic relationship between the glenoid and humerus, a posterolateral humeral head defect can cause recurrent instability as explained by the glenoid track concept.[24] A humeral head defect that is "off-track," or out of the physiologic glenoid track, has been shown to be a risk factor for instability. Further, these lesions have been proven to be risk factors for failure after bony instability procedures.[46,47] As a result, it is widely accepted that these bony defects should be addressed when managing instability, particular in the contact athlete. Several arthroscopic augmentation and grafting procedures exist to manage these cases involving instability and bony defects.

LATARJET BRISTOW

Of the various bone grafting procedures, coracoid transfer procedures have the longest term follow-up and track record. Latarjet[48] first proposed the coracoid transfer in 1954 and originally described a technique involving graft delivery to the anterior inferior glenoid and fixed with screws through a longitudinal split in the subscapularis. The Latarjet procedure is reported to increase stability through the so-called "triple blocking" effect. The majority of stability afforded by the procedure results from the conjoint tendon providing a sling to support the inferior capsule and subscapularis, thereby improving stability with the shoulder in the vulnerable position of abduction and external rotation.[49] Stability is also provided directly from the coracoid, which increases the anteroposterior diameter of the glenoid, increasing the excursion required for dislocation.[50] Lastly, additional restraint to instability is provided from supplementation of the capsule with the coracoacromial ligament. Although the terminology of Bristow was originally used to describe coracoid transfer through a vertical subscapularis split, it is more commonly used to describe techniques involving osteotomy of the tip, rather than the entire, coracoid.[51]

The Latarjet was originally described as an open technique involving graft passage through a subscapularis split and fixation with 2 bicortical screws (**Fig. 5**).[52] The all-arthroscopic Latarjet was first reported in 2010 as it was believed the success of the open Latarjet could be achieved arthroscopically to offer the benefits of minimally invasive surgery.[53] This technique involves releasing the soft tissues adjacent to the coracoid before the graft harvesting and eventual transfer through a subscapularis split. Specialized instruments are utilized to allow for arthroscopic drilling and graft fixation. Despite favorable outcomes overall, cost, complications, and technical difficulty remain drawbacks of the arthroscopic versus open procedure.[54]

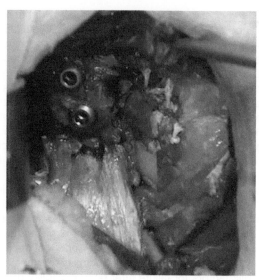

Fig. 5. Right shoulder demonstrating completed Latarjet procedure, with 2 screws through coracoid graft and coracoacromial (CA) ligament reattached to the anterior capsule.

DISTAL CLAVICLE AUTOGRAFT

The distal clavicle is a separate autograft option to manage glenoid bone loss. In 2014, the arthroscopic technique for distal clavicular autograft was reported with the use of suture anchor fixation.[55] Benefits of this technique are thought to include minimal harvest site morbidity, autograft availability, and low cost. Further, it has been shown to have a greater radius of glenoid reconstruction when compared to the Latarjet and glenoid restoration within 1 mm of non-degenerative shoulders.[56] Despite offering favorable glenohumeral contact pressure, inconsistency in graft size and density represent drawbacks.[57–59] Further studies are needed, particularly in the contact athlete population, to inform the indications and role of the distal clavicle autograft. It remains a reliable option for subcritical bone loss to replace smaller defects (**Fig. 6**).

DISTAL TIBIA ALLOGRAFT

In addition to autograft, various allograft options have been reported for use in glenoid reconstruction procedures. A prominent option, the distal tibia allograft, was first reported as a graft option in 2009.[60] The distal tibia offers excellent conformity to the native glenoid, a cartilaginous articular surface, and dense weight-bearing cortical bone.[60] Originally reported as an open technique, more recently an all-arthroscopic technique was developed that utilizes standard arthroscopic portals (**Fig. 7**).[61] Initial techniques involved screw fixation; however, subsequent modifications have included suture button and suture anchor fixation.[61,62] In terms of outcomes, the distal tibia allograft has demonstrated promising early results in both the primary as well as revision settings.[63] Specifically, it has shown outcomes similar to those of the Latarjet procedure in addition to minimal graft resorption at up to 2 years.[64–66] However, concerns exist regarding graft radius of curvature consistency, technical difficulty, and high cost.[67] Further, results of the distal tibial allograft in the contact athlete population remain unknown.

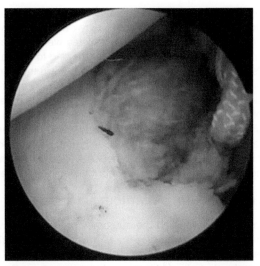

Fig. 6. Arthroscopic view of a left shoulder demonstrating a completed placement of a distal clavicle autograft. The graft has been marked in blue to delineate edge, and replacement of 20% bone defect was achieved.

LATARJET OUTCOMES

The Latarjet is supported by promising long-term outcomes. These studies have shown a satisfaction rate of 98% and only 5.9% recurrent instability at 20 years of follow-up.[68,69] Importantly, outcomes are different in the setting of significant glenoid defects. Although functional outcomes remain satisfactory, nearly 20% of patients have recurrent instability after the Latarjet when performed in shoulders with significant glenoid bone loss.[70] However, meta-analyses have consistently shown that the Latarjet still outperforms the Bankart in restoring glenohumeral instability.[71,72] Importantly, this remains true when glenoid bone loss in the contact athlete as the Latarjet has shown lower rates of recurrent instability as well as reoperation in this population.[73] Several studies have evaluated return to sport rates after the Latarjet procedure. Although return to sport

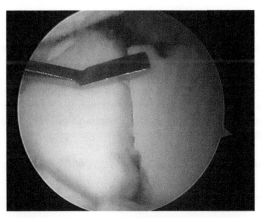

Fig. 7. Arthroscopic view of a left shoulder demonstrating a completed placement of a distal tibia allograft for anterior 25% bone defect.

rates have been reported as low as 50% in some series, a systematic review of over 2000 athletes demonstrated an overall return to play rate of 88%, with a 73% rate of returning to the same level.[70,74] When contact athletes were isolated in these series, overall return was reported to be 75%, with 49% returning to the same level of sport. The Latarjet has also demonstrated more favorable results in the elite over the recreational athlete, leading some to argue for the Latarjet for primary stabilization in athletes with high functional demands.[75] Despite these favorable outcomes, the Latarjet is limited by a complication rate as high as 25%, the most common of which include hardware-related issues, graft mal-positioning, graft resorption, osteolysis, and, in some cases, permanent neurovascular injury[76,77] Although these issues have prompted the use of different autograft options, the Latarjet continues to demonstrate the longest and most promising record for managing recurrent instability in athletes.[78]

LATARJET VERSUS BANKART WITH OR WITHOUT REMPLISSAGE

Several investigations have compared the outcomes of the Latarjet versus the arthroscopic Bankart. In a series of rugby players with less than 20% glenoid bone loss, both procedures led to excellent functional outcomes with nearly 90% in each group returning to pre-injury level of play.[73] However, the arthroscopic Bankart group had a recurrence rate that was 5 times that of the Latarjet group at 40 months follow-up. These results were corroborated in a systematic review of 3275 shoulders that showed significantly lower risk of recurrence at long-term follow-up in the Latarjet group when compared to the arthroscopic Bankart repair.[79] Although these investigations demonstrate that the Latarjet may outperform the Bankart in isolation, there are mixed results when compared to Bankart procedure with the addition of a remplissage. A retrospective series of 71 shoulders compared these 2 procedures and found similar patient-reported outcomes, clinical outcomes, and return to sport between the 2 groups, although they also reported less subjective instability in the Latarjet cohort.[80] This is contrasted by other studies that suggest the arthroscopic Bankart with remplissage is at least equal or better than the Latarjet in the primary setting, with higher return to sport for overhead or contact athletes, lower recurrence rates, and lower complication rates.[81,82] However, the body of evidence comparing these 2 procedures remains small and further high-quality investigations will guide the proper use of these interventions.[83]

SUMMARY

Anterior shoulder instability is a common and challenging problem in the contact athlete. Arthroscopic procedures such as the Bankart repair and remplissage continue to demonstrate favorable results in appropriately selected patients. Glenoid bone defects are well established as a risk factor for recurrent instability, especially in the high-level athlete. Although several bony augmentation procedures exist, the Latarjet procedure demonstrates the longest term follow-up and best track record in athletes. Further studies will assist in the understanding of the role of arthroscopic Bankart with remplissage versus the coracoid or other graft options for shoulder stabilization in the contact athlete with primary shoulder instability.

CLINICS CARE POINTS

Pearls:
- Perform a full evaluation of patient factors to indicate the best procedure for the patient. (Reference 18)

- Thorough bony preparation of the anterior glenoid prior to Bankart repair improves healing response and allows for an improved capsulolabral shift
- Use at least three anchors when performing a bankart repair
- Accurate measurement of bone loss is key to indicate the correct procedure

Pitalls:
- Revision arthroscopic Bankart after a primary failed Bankart usually leads to inferior outcomes
- Performing a soft tissue procedure alone when critical bone loss is present
- Not performing a remplissage in the setting of an engaging hill-sachs lesion

DISCLOSURE

The authors have nothing to disclose.

REFERENCES

1. Gibbs DB, Lynch TS, Nuber ED, et al. Common shoulder injuries in American Football Athletes. Curr Sports Med Rep 2015;14(5):413–9.
2. Owens BD, Agel J, Mountcastle SB, et al. Incidence of glenohumeral instability in collegiate athletics. Am J Sports Med 2009;37(9):1750–4.
3. Waterman B, Owens BD, Tokish JM. Anterior shoulder instability in the military athlete. Sports Health 2016;8(6):514–9.
4. De Martino I, Rodeo SA. The swimmer's shoulder: multi-directional instability. Curr Rev Musculoskelet Med 2018;11(2):167–71.
5. Owens BD, Duffey ML, Nelson BJ, et al. The incidence and characteristics of shoulder instability at the United States Military Academy. Am J Sports Med 2007;35(7):1168–73.
6. Arciero RA, Wheeler JH, Ryan JB, et al. Arthroscopic Bankart repair versus nonoperative treatment for acute, initial anterior shoulder dislocations. Am J Sports Med 1994;22(5):589–94.
7. Urayama M, Itoi E, Sashi R, et al. Capsular elongation in shoulders with recurrent anterior dislocation. Quantitative assessment with magnetic resonance arthrography. Am J Sports Med 2003;31(1):64–7.
8. Bankart AS. Recurrent or habitual dislocation of the shoulder-joint. Br Med J 1923; 2(3285):1132–3.
9. Lacheta L, Dekker TJ, Anderson N, et al. Arthroscopic knotless, tensionable all-suture anchor bankart repair. Arthrosc Tech 2019;8(6):e647–53.
10. Abdul-Rassoul H, Galvin JW, Curry EJ, et al. Return to sport after surgical treatment for anterior shoulder instability: a systematic review. Am J Sports Med 2019; 47(6):1507–15.
11. Memon M, Kay J, Cadet ER, et al. Return to sport following arthroscopic Bankart repair: a systematic review. J Shoulder Elbow Surg 2018;27(7):1342–7.
12. Chen AZ, Greaves KM, deMeireles AJ, et al. Clinical outcomes of arthroscopic bony bankart repair for anterior instability of the shoulder: a systematic review. Am J Sports Med 2022;24. 3635465221094832.
13. Kim M, Haratian A, Fathi A, et al. Can we identify why athletes fail to return to sports after arthroscopic bankart repair: a systematic review and meta-analysis. Am J Sports Med 2022. 3635465221089980.
14. Bauer A, Engel G, Huth J, et al. 14 years of follow up after first arthroscopic Bankart repair in athletes: functional outcomes and MRI findings. J Shoulder Elbow Surg 2022. S1058-2746(22)00769-8.

15. Yamamoto N, Kijima H, Nagamoto H, et al. Outcome of Bankart repair in contact versus non-contact athletes. Orthop Traumatol Surg Res 2015;101(4):415–9.
16. Levy BJ, Grimm NL, Arciero RA. When to abandon the arthroscopic bankart repair: a systematic review. Sports Health 2020;12(5):425–30.
17. Burkhart SS, De Beer JF. Traumatic glenohumeral bone defects and their relationship to failure of arthroscopic Bankart repairs: significance of the inverted-pear glenoid and the humeral engaging Hill-Sachs lesion. Arthroscopy 2000;16(7): 677–94.
18. Balg F, Boileau P. The instability severity index score. A simple pre-operative score to select patients for arthroscopic or open shoulder stabilisation. J Bone Joint Surg Br 2007;89(11):1470–7.
19. Provencher MT, Frank RM, Leclere LE, et al. The Hill-Sachs lesion: diagnosis, classification, and management. J Am Acad Orthop Surg 2012;20(4):242–52.
20. Connolly J. Humeral head defects associated with shoulder dislocation: their diagnostic and surgical significance. AAOS Instr Course Lect 1972;21:42–54.
21. Purchase RJ, Wolf EM, Hobgood ER, et al. Hill-sachs "remplissage": an arthroscopic solution for the engaging hill-sachs lesion. Arthroscopy 2008;24(6):723–6.
22. Koo SS, Burkhart SS, Ochoa E. Arthroscopic double-pulley remplissage technique for engaging Hill-Sachs lesions in anterior shoulder instability repairs. Arthroscopy 2009;25(11):1343–8.
23. Alexander TC, Beicker C, Tokish JM. Arthroscopic Remplissage for Moderate-Size Hill-Sachs Lesion. Arthrosc Tech 2016;5(5):e975–9.
24. Di Giacomo G, Itoi E, Burkhart SS. Evolving concept of bipolar bone loss and the Hill-Sachs lesion: from "engaging/non-engaging" lesion to "on-track/off-track" lesion. Arthroscopy 2014;30(1):90–8.
25. McQuivey KS, Brinkman JC, Tummala SV, et al. Arthroscopic remplissage using knotless, all-suture anchors. Arthrosc Tech 2022;11(4):e615–21.
26. Camp CL, Dahm DL, Krych AJ. Arthroscopic remplissage for engaging hill-sachs lesions in patients with anterior shoulder instability. Arthrosc Tech 2015;4(5): e499–502.
27. Magarelli N, Milano G, Sergio P, et al. Intra-observer and interobserver reliability of the "Pico" computed tomography method for quantification of glenoid bone defect in anterior shoulder instability. Skeletal Radiol 2009;38(11):1071–5.
28. Chuang TY, Adams CR, Burkhart SS. Use of preoperative three-dimensional computed tomography to quantify glenoid bone loss in shoulder instability. Arthroscopy 2008;24(4):376–82.
29. Garcia GH, Wu HH, Liu JN, et al. Outcomes of the Remplissage Procedure and Its Effects on Return to Sports: Average 5-Year Follow-up. Am J Sports Med 2016; 44(5):1124–30.
30. Gouveia K, Harbour E, Athwal GS, et al. Return to sport after arthroscopic bankart repair with remplissage: a systematic review. Arthroscopy 2023. S0749-8063(23) 00015-4.
31. Horinek JL, Menendez ME, Callegari JJ, et al. Consideration may be given to lowering the threshold for the addition of remplissage in patients with subcritical glenoid bone loss undergoing arthroscopic bankart repair. Arthrosc Sports Med Rehabil 2022;4(4):e1283–9.
32. MacDonald P, McRae S, Old J, et al. Arthroscopic Bankart repair with and without arthroscopic infraspinatus remplissage in anterior shoulder instability with a Hill-Sachs defect: a randomized controlled trial. J Shoulder Elbow Surg 2021;30(6): 1288–98.

33. Buza JA, Iyengar JJ, Anakwenze OA, et al. Arthroscopic Hill-Sachs remplissage: a systematic review. J Bone Joint Surg Am 2014;96(7):549–55.

34. Martinez-Catalan N, Kazum E, Zampeli F, et al. Long-term outcomes of arthroscopic Bankart repair and Hill-Sachs remplissage for bipolar bone defects. Eur J Orthop Surg Traumatol 2022;33(4):947–53.

35. Ono Y, Dávalos Herrera DA, Woodmass JM, et al. Long-term outcomes following isolated arthroscopic Bankart repair: a 9- to 12-year follow-up. JSES Open Access 2019;3(3):189–93.

36. Wolf EM, Arianjam A. Hill-Sachs remplissage, an arthroscopic solution for the engaging Hill-Sachs lesion: 2- to 10-year follow-up and incidence of recurrence. J Shoulder Elbow Surg 2014;23(6):814–20.

37. Liu JN, Gowd AK, Garcia GH, et al. Recurrence rate of instability after remplissage for treatment of traumatic anterior shoulder instability: a systematic review in treatment of subcritical glenoid bone loss. Arthroscopy 2018;34(10):2894–907.e2.

38. Torrance E, Clarke CJ, Monga P, et al. Recurrence after arthroscopic labral repair for traumatic anterior instability in adolescent rugby and contact athletes. Am J Sports Med 2018;46(12):2969–74.

39. Boileau P, Villalba M, Héry JY, et al. Risk factors for recurrence of shoulder instability after arthroscopic Bankart repair. J Bone Joint Surg Am 2006;88(8):1755–63.

40. Shaha JS, Cook JB, Song DJ, et al. Redefining "critical" bone loss in shoulder instability: functional outcomes worsen with "subcritical" bone loss. Am J Sports Med 2015;43(7):1719–25.

41. Bois AJ, Fening SD, Polster J, et al. Quantifying glenoid bone loss in anterior shoulder instability: reliability and accuracy of 2-dimensional and 3-dimensional computed tomography measurement techniques. Am J Sports Med 2012;40(11):2569–77.

42. Taylor DC, Arciero RA. Pathologic changes associated with shoulder dislocations. Arthroscopic and physical examination findings in first-time, traumatic anterior dislocations. Am J Sports Med 1997;25(3):306–11.

43. Itoi E, Yamamoto N, Kurokawa D, et al. Bone loss in anterior instability. Curr Rev Musculoskelet Med 2013;6(1):88–94.

44. Lo IKY, Parten PM, Burkhart SS. The inverted pear glenoid: an indicator of significant glenoid bone loss. Arthroscopy 2004;20(2):169–74.

45. Dickens JF, Slaven SE, Cameron KL, et al. Prospective evaluation of glenoid bone loss after first-time and recurrent anterior glenohumeral instability events. Am J Sports Med 2019;47(5):1082–9.

46. Calvo C, Calvo J, Rojas D, et al. Clinical relevance of persistent off-track Hill-Sachs lesion after arthroscopic latarjet procedure. Am J Sports Med 2021;49(8):2006–12.

47. Shaha JS, Cook JB, Rowles DJ, et al. Clinical validation of the glenoid track concept in anterior glenohumeral instability. J Bone Joint Surg Am 2016;98(22):1918–23.

48. Latarjet M. [Treatment of recurrent dislocation of the shoulder]. Lyon Chir 1954;49(8):994–7.

49. Yamamoto N, Muraki T, An KN, et al. The stabilizing mechanism of the Latarjet procedure: a cadaveric study. J Bone Joint Surg Am 2013;95(15):1390–7.

50. Moon SC, Cho NS, Rhee YG. Quantitative assessment of the latarjet procedure for large glenoid defects by computed tomography: a coracoid graft can sufficiently restore the glenoid arc. Am J Sports Med 2015;43(5):1099–107.

51. Giles JW, Degen RM, Johnson JA, et al. The Bristow and Latarjet procedures: why these techniques should not be considered synonymous. J Bone Joint Surg Am 2014;96(16):1340–8.

52. Young AA, Maia R, Berhouet J, et al. Open Latarjet procedure for management of bone loss in anterior instability of the glenohumeral joint. J Shoulder Elbow Surg 2011;20(2 Suppl):S61–9.

53. Lafosse L, Boyle S. Arthroscopic Latarjet procedure. J Shoulder Elbow Surg 2010;19(2 Suppl):2–12.

54. Willemot LB, Elhassan BT, Verborgt O. Bony reconstruction of the anterior Glenoid Rim. J Am Acad Orthop Surg 2018;26(10):e207–18.

55. Tokish JM, Fitzpatrick K, Cook JB, et al. Arthroscopic distal clavicular autograft for treating shoulder instability with glenoid bone loss. Arthrosc Tech 2014;3(4): e475–81.

56. Kwapisz A, Fitzpatrick K, Cook JB, et al. Distal clavicular osteochondral autograft augmentation for glenoid bone loss: a comparison of radius of restoration versus latarjet graft. Am J Sports Med 2018;46(5):1046–52.

57. Petersen SA, Bernard JA, Langdale ER, et al. Autologous distal clavicle versus autologous coracoid bone grafts for restoration of anterior-inferior glenoid bone loss: a biomechanical comparison. J Shoulder Elbow Surg 2016;25(6):960–6.

58. Hudson PW, Pinto MC, Brabston EW, et al. Distal clavicle autograft for anterior-inferior glenoid augmentation: A comparative cadaveric anatomic study. Shoulder Elbow 2020;12(6):404–13.

59. Rodriguez S, Mancini MR, Kakazu R, et al. Comparison of the coracoid, distal clavicle, and scapular spine for autograft augmentation of glenoid bone loss: a radiologic and cadaveric assessment. Am J Sports Med 2022;50(3):717–24.

60. Provencher MT, Ghodadra N, LeClere L, et al. Anatomic osteochondral glenoid reconstruction for recurrent glenohumeral instability with glenoid deficiency using a distal tibia allograft. Arthroscopy 2009;25(4):446–52.

61. Hassebrock JD, Starkweather JR, Tokish JM. Arthroscopic technique for bone augmentation with suture button fixation for anterior shoulder instability. Arthrosc Tech 2019;9(1):e97–102.

62. Tokish JM, Brinkman JC, Hassebrock JD. Arthroscopic technique for distal tibial allograft bone augmentation with suture anchor fixation for anterior shoulder instability. Arthrosc Tech 2022;11(5):e903–9.

63. Ruzbarsky JJ, Nolte PC, Elrick BP, et al. Complex revision glenoid reconstruction with use of a distal tibial allograft. JBJS Essent Surg Tech 2021;11(1). e20.00017.

64. Provencher MT, Frank RM, Golijanin P, et al. Distal tibia allograft glenoid reconstruction in recurrent anterior shoulder instability: clinical and radiographic outcomes. Arthroscopy 2017;33(5):891–7.

65. Wong I, John R, Ma J, et al. Arthroscopic anatomic glenoid reconstruction using distal tibial allograft for recurrent anterior shoulder instability: clinical and radiographic outcomes. Am J Sports Med 2020;48(13):3316–21.

66. Frank RM, Romeo AA, Richardson C, et al. Outcomes of latarjet versus distal tibia allograft for anterior shoulder instability repair: a matched cohort analysis. Am J Sports Med 2018;46(5):1030–8.

67. Decker MM, Strohmeyer GC, Wood JP, et al. Distal tibia allograft for glenohumeral instability: does radius of curvature match? J Shoulder Elbow Surg 2016;25(9): 1542–8.

68. Hovelius L, Sandström B, Sundgren K, et al. One hundred eighteen Bristow-Latarjet repairs for recurrent anterior dislocation of the shoulder prospectively

followed for fifteen years: study I--clinical results. J Shoulder Elbow Surg 2004; 13(5):509–16.

69. Mizuno N, Denard PJ, Raiss P, et al. Long-term results of the Latarjet procedure for anterior instability of the shoulder. J Shoulder Elbow Surg 2014;23(11):1691–9.

70. Yang JS, Mazzocca AD, Cote MP, et al. Recurrent anterior shoulder instability with combined bone loss: treatment and results with the modified Latarjet Procedure. Am J Sports Med 2016;44(4):922–32.

71. An VVG, Sivakumar BS, Phan K, et al. A systematic review and meta-analysis of clinical and patient-reported outcomes following two procedures for recurrent traumatic anterior instability of the shoulder: Latarjet procedure vs. Bankart repair. J Shoulder Elbow Surg 2016;25(5):853–63.

72. Bhatia S, Frank RM, Ghodadra NS, et al. The outcomes and surgical techniques of the latarjet procedure. Arthroscopy 2014;30(2):227–35.

73. Rossi LA, Tanoira I, Gorodischer T, et al. Recurrence and revision rates with arthroscopic bankart repair compared with the latarjet procedure in competitive rugby players with glenohumeral instability and a glenoid bone loss <20. Am J Sports Med 2021;49(4):866–72.

74. Hurley ET, Montgomery C, Jamal MS, et al. Return to play after the latarjet procedure for anterior shoulder instability: a systematic review. Am J Sports Med 2019;47(12):3002–8.

75. Baverel L, Colle PE, Saffarini M, et al. Open latarjet procedures produce better outcomes in competitive athletes compared with recreational athletes: a clinical comparative study of 106 athletes aged under 30 years. Am J Sports Med 2018;46(6):1408–15.

76. Shah AA, Butler RB, Romanowski J, et al. Short-term complications of the Latarjet procedure. J Bone Joint Surg Am 2012;94(6):495–501.

77. Woodmass JM, Welp KM, Chang MJ, et al. A reduction in the rate of nerve injury after Latarjet: a before-after study after neuromonitoring. J Shoulder Elbow Surg 2018;27(12):2153–8.

78. McHale KJ, Sanchez G, Lavery KP, et al. Latarjet technique for treatment of anterior shoulder instability with glenoid bone loss. Arthrosc Tech 2017;6(3):e791–9.

79. Imam MA, Shehata MSA, Martin A, et al. Bankart repair versus latarjet procedure for recurrent anterior shoulder instability: a systematic review and meta-analysis of 3275 shoulders. Am J Sports Med 2021;49(7):1945–53.

80. Paul RW, Reddy MP, Sonnier JH, et al. Increased rates of subjective shoulder instability after bankart repair with remplissage compared to latarjet surgery. J Shoulder Elbow Surg 2022. S1058-S2746(22)00873-00874.

81. Davis WH, DiPasquale JA, Patel RK, et al. Arthroscopic Remplissage Combined With Bankart Repair Results in a Higher Rate of Return to Sport in Athletes Compared With Bankart Repair Alone or the Latarjet Procedure: A Systematic Review and Meta-analysis. Am J Sports Med 2023. 3635465221138559.

82. Horinek JL, Menendez ME, Narbona P, et al. Remplissage yields similar 2-year outcomes, fewer complications, and low recurrence compared to latarjet across a wide range of preoperative glenoid bone loss. Arthroscopy 2022;38(10): 2798–805.

83. Haroun HK, Sobhy MH, Abdelrahman AA. Arthroscopic Bankart repair with remplissage versus Latarjet procedure for management of engaging Hill-Sachs lesions with subcritical glenoid bone loss in traumatic anterior shoulder instability: a systematic review and meta-analysis. J Shoulder Elbow Surg 2020;29(10): 2163–74.

Open Bankart Repair
Technique and Outcomes for the High-Level Athlete

Michael R. Mancini, MD*, Robert A. Arciero, MD

KEYWORDS

- Glenohumeral instability • Open Bankart repair • Capsular shift • High-level athlete
- Collision athlete

KEY POINTS

- The open Bankart repair has had a long-term history of more than 70 years of success for surgical management of anterior glenohumeral instability.
- Open Bankart repairs may reduce recurrent instability rates in collision athletes when compared with arthroscopic Bankart repairs.
- Our indications for open Bankart repair include high-risk or collision male athletes aged less than 25 years old with an intact subscapularis, revisions of well-done arthroscopic procedures with minor glenoid bone loss, 10% to 20% glenoid bone loss, and so-called intermediate or subcritical bone loss.

INTRODUCTION

The glenohumeral joint is the most dislocated joint in the human body because of its low constraint and high mobility.[1,2] Glenohumeral instability is a common shoulder pathology in the United States with a reported incidence of 0.08 per 1000 person-years.[3] The incidence increases from 0.08 to 1.69 per 1000 person-years in high-risk populations, such as young men, collision athletes, and military members.[3,4] Following a shoulder dislocation, injuries often occur at the anterior-inferior capsulolabral junction, known as a Bankart lesion. Additional injuries of the glenohumeral joint are possible and are influenced by the direction of force applied to the shoulder, the arm positioning during impact, and the function of the deltoid and rotator cuff muscles.[5] Injuries may involve the glenohumeral soft tissues or osseous deformities. Common soft tissue injuries include laxity/stretching of the inferior glenohumeral ligament and capsule,

Department of Orthopaedic Surgery, University of Connecticut Health Center, University of Connecticut Health Musculoskeletal Institute, 263 Farmington Avenue, Farmington, CT 06030, USA
* Corresponding author.
E-mail address: mancini.michaelr@gmail.com
Twitter: @MichaelRMancini (M.R.M.); @BobArciero (R.A.A.)

Clin Sports Med 43 (2024) 617–633
https://doi.org/10.1016/j.csm.2023.12.002
0278-5919/24/© 2023 Elsevier Inc. All rights reserved.

humeral avulsion of the glenohumeral ligaments, and complete capsular rupture. Common osseous injuries include fractures of the anterior glenoid, known as a bony Bankart, and humeral head impaction on the glenoid rim, known as a Hill-Sachs lesion.[6,7]

Treatment of glenohumeral instability may be operative or nonoperative. Nonoperative management includes intentional physical therapy exercises to strengthen the dynamic shoulder stabilizers to support humeral head compression within the glenoid. Rehabilitation has not been proven effective in managing traumatic anterior instability. Operative management attempts to restore the native anatomy and shoulder biomechanics to improve glenohumeral stability. Historically, the open Bankart repair has been the gold standard technique to manage anterior glenohumeral stability because it allows for primary repair of the capsulolabral injury via its excellent joint exposure and the option for a large capsular shift to tighten the loose capsule.[8-12] As surgical advancements have been made, minimally invasive options have been developed and the arthroscopic Bankart repair is now the most common technique used to repair Bankart lesions.[13,14] A recent study by Ahmed and colleagues[14] assessed the rates and trends in the treatment of glenohumeral instability over a 10-year period using the IBM Watson MarketScan national database. The authors concluded that the rate of arthroscopic Bankart repairs remained steady from 2009 to 2018 (89% to 93% of all cases) but the number of open Bankart repairs decreased by 65%.[14] Compared with the open Bankart repair, arthroscopic Bankart repairs allow for improved intra-articular diagnostic assessment and smaller incisions, which leads to decreased morbidity, operative times, and injury to the subscapularis muscle.[10,15-17]

Despite the advantages of arthroscopic Bankart repair, studies have demonstrated that high-risk patients continue to report suboptimal glenohumeral instability recurrence and reoperation rates along with persistent capsular laxity.[12,18,19] In the setting of glenoid or humeral bone loss, early failures rates are as high as 67%.[20] Given that glenoid and Hill-Sachs lesions are present in 75% and 88% of cases of recurrent glenohumeral instability,[21] an arthroscopic Bankart repair alone would be inadequate for patients with recurrent instability. Therefore, in the appropriate setting, it is our opinion that open Bankart repairs may have a larger implication in the surgical management of glenohumeral instability.

INDICATIONS

The senior author has more than 35 years of experience treating high-level collision athletes and military personnel with glenohumeral instability. Through the course of his career, he has developed several indications for open Bankart repair, which include

- High-risk or collision male athletes aged less than 25 years old with an intact subscapularis
- Revision surgeries of well-performed arthroscopic Bankart procedures with minor glenoid bone loss
- Instability events experienced during activities of daily living with intermediate glenoid bone loss (10%–20% of the glenoid diameter)

PROCEDURAL APPROACH

The steps of the open Bankart repair are as follows:

1. Formal examination under anesthesia
2. Skin incision

3. Identify the deltopectoral interval
4. Incise clavipectoral fascia, release falciform ligament
5. Subscapularis tenotomy: "L-shaped"
6. Capsulotomy: "T-shaped"
7. Bankart repair: horizontal mattress sutures
8. Capsular shift
9. Subscapularis repair
10. Closure

OUR TECHNIQUE

The patient is positioned supine as close to the operative side of the table as possible. Before the sterile preparation, a formal examination under anesthesia is performed to determine the load-shift grading, assess for concomitant posterior or multidirectional instability, and evaluate for an engaging Hill-Sachs lesion (**Fig. 1**). The patient is then placed in a modified beach-chair position, but closer to a supine position, with about 20° of back flexion and a bump beneath the medial scapula to retract the scapula and position the glenoid more parallel and less tilted in a forward position (**Fig. 2**). It is imperative that there is complete muscle relaxation to facilitate retraction particularly in large patients. Standard sterile preparation and draping is performed.

With the operative arm extended laterally on a padded mayo stand, a standard anterior axillary incision from just distal to the coracoid to the axilla is made along Langer lines (**Fig. 3**). A standard deltopectoral approach is performed using sharp and blunt dissection along with needle-tip electrocautery down to the deltopectoral fascia. It is helpful to use a lap pad here to separate the overlying fat from the muscles. Once the cephalic vein is identified, it is taken laterally to not disrupt feeder vessels from the deltoid. One key to open surgery is to make the dissection wider as the wound

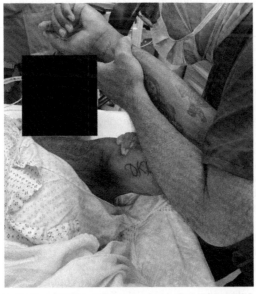

Fig. 1. Before the sterile preparation, a formal examination under anesthesia is performed to determine the load-shift grading, assess for concomitant posterior or multidirectional instability, and evaluate for an engaging Hill-Sachs lesion.

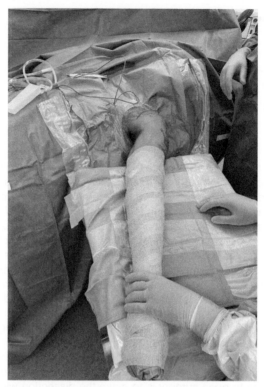

Fig. 2. The patient is then placed in a modified beach-chair position, but closer to a supine position, with about 20° of back flexion and a bump beneath the medial scapula to retract the scapula and position the glenoid more parallel and less tilted in a forward position.

gets deeper by spreading superiorly, inferiorly, medially, and laterally in a trapezoidal manner. A self-retaining or link retractor is used to retract the deltoid laterally and the pectoralis major muscle medially to expose the conjoint tendon (**Fig. 4**). There is often a pink stripe of muscle marking the lateral edge of the muscle of the short head of the biceps laterally. The clavipectoral fascia is released here to minimize bleeding (**Fig. 5**). This incision extends superiorly to the coracoacromial ligament and inferiorly to the falciform ligament to give a more extensile approach. Here, the anterior vessels and the coracoacromial ligament are visualized and the coracoacromial ligament is partially incised to retract the conjoint structures (**Fig. 6**) more easily. The retractors are then deepened to retract the deltoid laterally and the conjoint tendon medially to visualize the subscapularis muscle (**Fig. 7**).

The superior and inferior borders of the subscapularis tendon are then identified; the upper edge of the subscapularis muscle is often a very rolled, definitive structure. A sponge with a suture attached is then placed into the axilla to push the neurovasculature structures medially away from the surgical field. Three or four heavy, nonabsorbable tagging stitches are secured approximately 1.5 cm medial to the lesser tuberosity (**Fig. 8**). The senior author prefers a subscapularis takedown, in contrast to a subscapularis split technique, especially if the patient has features of hyperlaxity. Using electrocautery, an L-shaped subscapularis tenotomy is made with the vertical limb located just lateral to the tagging sutures extending from just proximal to the

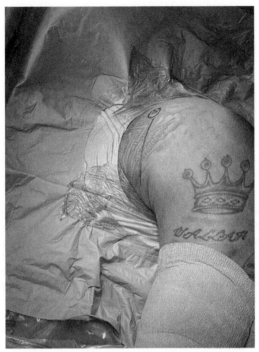

Fig. 3. The skin incision is made anteriorly from just distal to the coracoid to the axilla along Langer lines. The coracoid is marked with a circle.

anterior humeral circumflex vessels to the rotator interval and the horizontal limb is extended medially to avoid the axillary nerve (**Figs. 9** and **10**). One can typically palpate the axillary nerve inferior to the circumflex vessels and slightly medially. Meticulous blunt dissection is used to separate the subscapularis tendon from the

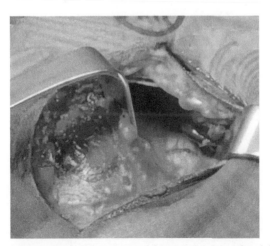

Fig. 4. A standard deltopectoral approach is performed down to the deltopectoral fascia. Once the cephalic vein is identified, it is taken laterally to not disrupt feeder vessels from the deltoid. A self-retaining or link retractor is used to retract the deltoid laterally and the pectoralis major muscle medially to expose the conjoint tendon.

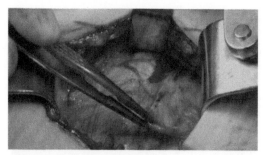

Fig. 5. The clavipectoral fascia is released lateral to the coracobrachialis and then the cora-coacromial ligament is released proximally.

underlying shoulder capsule. It is easiest to reflect the subscapularis when starting inferiorly and slightly medial to separate the muscle and expose the capsule. The interval between the subscapularis and the capsule is found along the inferomedial corner of the subscapularis, just above the circumflex vessels. After identifying the leading edge of the subscapularis, scissors are used to spread inferiorly and medially, again separating the muscle from the capsule (**Fig. 11**). The capsule becomes visible beneath the subscapularis and continues the dissection superiorly and then laterally and the tendon edge is more defined.

Once the subscapularis is reflected, the rotator interval becomes exposed. A suture is then placed laterally within the rotator interval for additional stability, especially if inferior laxity is present (**Fig. 12**). With the arm externally rotated at 45°, the lateral 1 to 1.5 cm of the rotator interval is closed using a nonabsorbable suture. Importantly, the rotator interval is closed laterally, not medially, to avoid restricting external

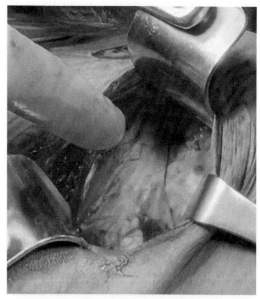

Fig. 6. After release of the clavipectoral fascia and coracoacromial ligament, the conjoint tendon is well visualized with the subscapularis beneath it.

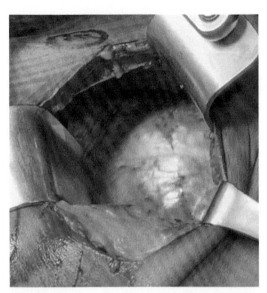

Fig. 7. The link retractor is placed deeper, and the conjoint tendon is retracted medially to visualize the subscapularis.

rotation. Next, with the patient's arm at 30° of external rotation, a T-shaped capsulotomy is performed using electrocautery. The vertical limb is made laterally at the level of the humeral neck and two tagging sutures are placed along the superior and inferior borders of the cut capsule. The horizontal limb is created at the midglenoid level and extended medially in between the two tagging sutures, which creates superior and inferior capsular leaflets (**Figs. 13** and **14**). To visualize the glenoid and Bankart

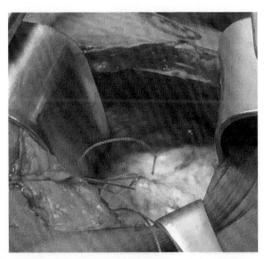

Fig. 8. Three or four heavy, nonabsorbable tagging stitches are secured approximately 1.5 cm medial to the lesser tuberosity.

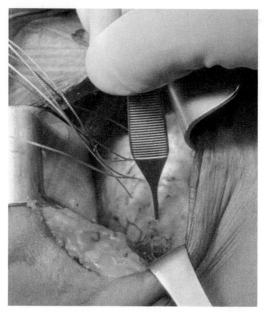

Fig. 9. Identification of the anterior humeral circumflex vessels just distal to the extent of the L-shaped vertical capsulotomy.

lesion, a Fukuda retractor is used to retract the humeral head, and a scapular neck ("Batman") retractor is placed along the medial scapular neck (**Fig. 15**).

 With adequate visualization to the anterior glenoid and Bankart lesion, the Bankart lesion is now addressed. A combination of rongeur and burr is then used to remove

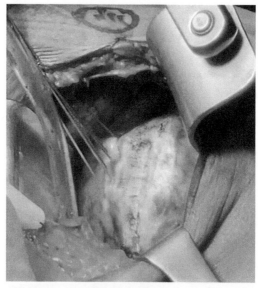

Fig. 10. Using electrocautery, an L-shaped subscapularis tenotomy is made with the vertical limb located just lateral to the tagging sutures from the anterior humeral circumflex vessels to the rotator interval.

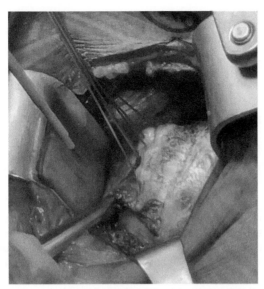

Fig. 11. A critical move to reflect the subscapularis is to start inferiorly at the interval between the subscapularis and the capsule along the inferomedial corner of the subscapularis, just above the circumflex vessels.

any fibrous tissue to create a bony bed for suture anchor placement. Anchors are placed at the 5-o'clock or 7-o'clock positions along the glenoid articular surface for right and left shoulders, respectively (**Fig. 16**). Typically, three to four double-loaded suture anchors are used and placed approximately 5 mm apart to reduce the risk of

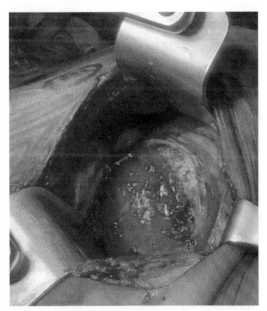

Fig. 12. With the rotator interval exposed, a suture is placed laterally within the rotator interval for additional stability, especially if inferior laxity is present.

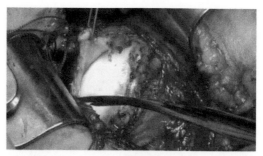

Fig. 13. A demonstration of the capsulotomy and creation of the inferior and superior capsular leaflets.

anchor pullout. For patients with larger Bankart lesions, a double-row repair is made medially on the glenoid neck, if necessary. With the anchors in place, the scapular neck retractor is removed from within the Bankart lesion, and the sutures are passed through the capsulolabral tissue in a horizontal mattress technique from inferior to superior. We believe this is a distinct advantage over arthroscopic repair. In the open technique described sutures are placed entirely through the capsulolabral complex and subsequently tied from inferior to superior (**Fig. 17**). This completely obliterates the false pouch created by the Bankart lesion and the footprint of reattachment is more robust than the arthroscopic method. If needed, it is helpful to place another retractor on the pectoralis major tendon because the muscle can advance superiorly into the working area. Adequate exposure is important here because the needles are being passed inferiorly and can injure the axillary nerve with improper visualization.

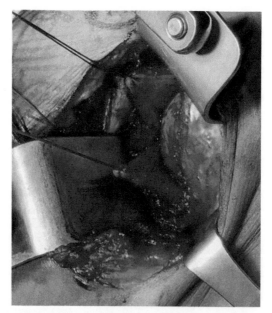

Fig. 14. A T-shaped capsulotomy is performed with the horizontal limb at the midglenoid level and extended medially between two tagging sutures, which creates superior and inferior capsular leaflets.

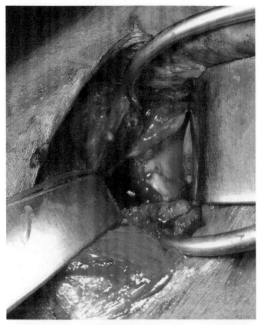

Fig. 15. To visualize the glenoid and Bankart lesion, a Fukuda retractor is used to retract the humeral head and a scapular neck ("Batman") retractor is placed along the medial scapular neck.

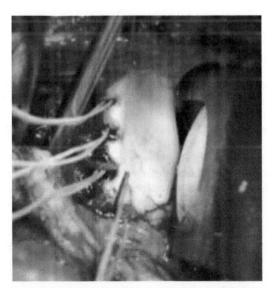

Fig. 16. Anchors are placed at the 5-o'clock or 7-o'clock positions along the glenoid articular surface for right and left shoulders, respectively, using three to four double-loaded suture anchors.

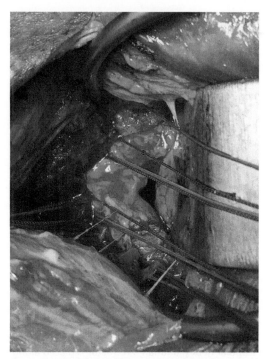

Fig. 17. The sutures from the double-loaded suture anchors are passed through the capsu-lolabral tissue in a horizontal mattress technique from inferior to superior.

Following the Bankart repair, the capsular shift is addressed. The horizontal limb of the capsulotomy is closed with a reefing stitch using a high-strength, nonabsorbable suture. It is placed, but not tied, until completion of the capsular shift. The leaflets are then tensioned using another high-strength, nonabsorbable suture via an outside-in, outside-in technique for the superior limb and inside-out, inside-out technique for the inferior limb.

Next, two double-loaded suture anchors are placed just medial to the subscapularis insertion site along the superolateral and inferolateral aspects of the lesser tuberosity. The inferior leaflet is tensioned superiorly toward the superolateral anchor and secured in place using the horizontal mattress sutures from the anchor (**Fig. 18**). With an adequate release, the inferior leaflet almost covers the entire joint itself. The inferior capsule is shifted superiorly until the inferior pouch is eliminated. The superior leaflet is tensioned inferiorly toward the inferolateral anchor and secured in place using the horizontal mattress sutures from the anchor to complete the capsular shift (**Fig. 19**). During capsulotomy closure, the arm is positioned in 30° abduction and external rotation. This repair is performed medial to where the subscapularis tendon will be reattached because it is important to have a separate layer for the subscapularis closure.

After the completion of the capsular shift, the subscapularis tendon is repaired. To repair the tendon, the previously placed sutures are passed into the remaining stump on the lesser tuberosity in a horizontal mattress fashion and tied from superior to inferior. Using a #1 Vicryl suture, the repair is then oversewn from superior to inferior (**Fig. 20**). To prevent future subscapularis failures and deficiencies, it is imperative that a meticulous closure of the subscapularis tendon is performed. The arm is taken

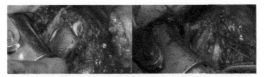

Fig. 18. The inferior leaflet is tensioned superiorly toward the superolateral anchor and secured in place using the horizontal mattress sutures from the anchor.

through range of motion and tested for stability. Lastly, closure of the deltopectoral interval and skin is performed at the discretion of the operating surgeons.

CLINICAL OUTCOMES

Return to sport and return to function are two important outcomes to consider when weighing surgical treatment options for glenohumeral instability. The impact of open Bankart repairs on return to sport has been well-studied. Over a 30-year period, Rowe and colleagues[22] investigated 162 shoulders following open Bankart repairs and found that athletes demonstrated early return of motion and early return to sport, with 98% reporting good-to-excellent outcomes, 69% demonstrating full range of motion, and only a 2% recurrent dislocation rate. Pelet and colleagues[23] followed 30 patients who underwent open Bankart repair for a mean of 29 years and concluded that 100% returned to their previous level of sporting and only 10% had an episode of redislocation. In their study of 60 patients who underwent open Bankart repair over a 7-year period, Monk and colleagues[24] concluded that 92% of athletes returned to sport. Likewise, Hickey and colleagues[25] reported high satisfaction rates, functional outcomes, and return to sport rates after open Bankart repairs in the medium-term among young collision athletes aged 18 years or less. A recent systematic review by AlSomali and coworkers[26] assessed outcomes after open Bankart repair in high-demand populations. Eleven articles composed of 563 patients with a mean age of 27.4 years at the time of surgery and a mean follow-up of 11.5 years were included in this study.[26] The authors found good-to-excellent results using Rowe scores, an overall recurrent instability rate of 8.5%, and 87% of patients were able to return to sport and work postoperatively.[26]

Glenohumeral instability is a challenging problem to manage in the athletic population because of the risk of recurrent dislocation.[27] The instability severity index score was developed to preoperatively identify patients at increased risk for recurrent instability and differentiate those who may benefit from a Bristow-Latarjet procedure rather than a Bankart procedure.[28] In their study, Balg and Boileau[28] found that risk factors for recurrent glenohumeral instability include age less than 20 years old at the time of surgery, involvement in collision sports or forced overhead activity, presence of a Hill-

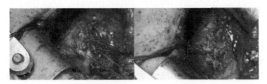

Fig. 19. The superior leaflet is tensioned inferiorly toward the inferolateral anchor and secured in place using the horizontal mattress sutures from the anchor to complete the capsular shift.

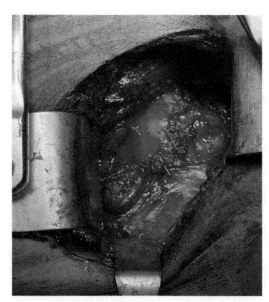

Fig. 20. Subscapularis is repaired by passing the sutures into the remaining stump on the lesser tuberosity in a horizontal mattress fashion and tied from superior to inferior. The repair is then oversewn using a #1 Vicryl suture.

Sachs lesion, and shoulder hyperlaxity. Collision athletes are at a particularly high risk of recurrent instability following Bankart repair, with rates of recurrent instability between 11% and 16.5% within 3 years postoperatively.[27]

Compared with arthroscopic Bankart repair, open Bankart repairs may reduce the risk of recurrent glenohumeral instability in collision athletes. Rhee and colleagues[27] compared 48 shoulders from collision athletes and found that only 12.5% of athletes had evidence of recurrent instability after open Bankart repair compared with 25% of athletes after arthroscopic Bankart repair. Similarly, in a review of 60 collision athletes who underwent open Bankart repair, Monk and colleagues[24] demonstrated a redislocation rate of 13%. Other studies have demonstrated even lower rates of recurrent instability after open Bankart repair. Pagnani[29] investigated 119 patients, with approximately 70% involved in collision sports, and found only a 2% rate of recurrence after open Bankart repair. Additionally, Hatch and Hennrikus[30] found a 0% recurrence rate following open Bankart repair at 2 years postoperatively in teenage athletes with a mean age of 16 years old. These recurrence rates are remarkably lower than the rates reported following arthroscopic Bankart repair. In a study of 115 competitive athletes, Nakagawa and colleagues[31] found a 20.4% recurrence rate within 2 years postoperatively after arthroscopic Bankart repair. Analogously, McLeod and Delaney[32] reported a recurrent dislocation rate of 21% after arthroscopic Bankart repair in a study of Irish collision sport athletes with a mean follow-up of 24 months. In studies of arthroscopic Bankart procedures, male sex and younger age at the time of first dislocation have been shown to be independent risk factors for recurrent instability; however, these have not been shown to be independent risk factors associated with open Bankart procedures.[33–35] In addition to decreased recurrent instability rates, the time to recurrent instability is significantly prolonged following open Bankart repair when compared with arthroscopic Bankart repairs.[8] In a cohort study with 82 shoulders from 80 patients evaluated at a mean of 39 months postoperatively, Virk and colleagues[8] found the average time to recurrence after arthroscopic Bankart repair was 12.6 months and 34.2 months after open Bankart repairs.

CLINICS CARE POINTS

- The open Bankart repair has historically been a proven long-term approach for surgical management of anterior glenohumeral instability.
- Arthroscopic Bankart repair is now the most common technique to perform a Bankart repair.
- Arthroscopic Bankart repairs have high recurrent instability rates and capsular laxity, particularly in high-risk collision athletes.
- Open Bankart repair may reduce recurrent instability rates in high-risk collision athletes.
- Based on the senior author's experience with military personnel and high-level athletes, his indications for open Bankart repair include high-risk or collision male athletes aged less than 25 years old with an intact subscapularis, revisions of well-done arthroscopic procedures with minor glenoid bone loss, 10% to 20% glenoid bone loss, and so-called intermediate or subcritical bone loss.
- Further investigations are needed to identify the indications for arthroscopic versus open Bankart repair and compare their outcomes in high-level athletes.

DISCLOSURE

M.R. Mancini has nothing to disclose. R.A. Arciero has received speaking fees from Arthrex, Inc and consulting fees from Smith & Nephew, Inc.

REFERENCES

1. Hindle P, Davidson EK, Biant LC, et al. Appendicular joint dislocations. Injury 2013;44(8):1022–7.
2. Yang N, Chen H, Phan D, et al. Epidemiological survey of orthopedic joint dislocations based on nationwide insurance data in Taiwan, 2000-2005. BMC Muscoskel Disord 2011;12:253.
3. Waterman B, Owens BD, Tokish JM. Anterior shoulder instability in the military athlete. Sports Health 2016;8(6):514–9.
4. Galvin JW, Ernat JJ, Waterman BR, et al. The epidemiology and natural history of anterior shoulder instability. Curr Rev Musculoskelet Med 2017;10(4):411–24.
5. DePalma AF. The classic. Recurrent dislocation of the shoulder joint. Ann Surg 1950;132:1052–65. Clin Orthop Relat Res. 2008;466(3):520-530.
6. Wintzell G, Haglund-Akerlind Y, Tengvar M, et al. MRI examination of the glenohumeral joint after traumatic primary anterior dislocation. A descriptive evaluation of the acute lesion and at 6-month follow-up. Knee Surg Sports Traumatol Arthrosc 1996;4(4):232–6.
7. Verma N, Chahar D, Chawla A, et al. Recurrent anterior instability of the shoulder associated with coracoid fracture: an unusual presentation. J Clin Orthop Trauma 2016;7(Suppl 1):99–102.
8. Virk MS, Manzo RL, Cote M, et al. Comparison of time to recurrence of instability after open and arthroscopic Bankart repair techniques. Orthop J Sports Med 2016;4(6). 2325967116654114.

9. Mohtadi NGH, Bitar IJ, Sasyniuk TM, et al. Arthroscopic versus open repair for traumatic anterior shoulder instability: a meta-analysis. Arthroscopy 2005;21(6): 652–8.

10. Coughlin RP, Crapser A, Coughlin K, et al. Open Bankart revisited. Arthrosc Tech 2017;6(1):e233–7.

11. Chen L, Xu Z, Peng J, et al. Effectiveness and safety of arthroscopic versus open Bankart repair for recurrent anterior shoulder dislocation: a meta-analysis of clinical trial data. Arch Orthop Trauma Surg 2015;135(4):529–38.

12. Boileau P, Villalba M, Hery J, et al. Risk factors for recurrence of shoulder instability after arthroscopic Bankart repair. J Bone Joint Surg Am 2006;88(8): 1755–63.

13. Haskoor J, Wang KY, Best MJ, et al. Trends in utilization and patient demographics for shoulder instability procedures from 2010 to 2019. J Shoulder Elbow Surg 2022;31(6S):S13–7.

14. Ahmed AS, Gabig AM, Dawes A, et al. Trends and projections in surgical stabilization of glenohumeral instability in the United States from 2009 to 2030: rise of the Latarjet procedure and fall of open Bankart repair. J Shoulder Elbow Surg 2023;32(8):e387–95.

15. Zhang AL, Montgomery SR, Ngo SS, et al. Arthroscopic versus open shoulder stabilization: current practice patterns in the United States. Arthroscopy 2014; 30(4):436–43.

16. Berthold DP, LeVasseur MR, Muench LN, et al. Minimum 10-year clinical outcomes after arthroscopic 270 degrees labral repair in traumatic shoulder instability involving anterior, inferior, and posterior labral injury. Am J Sports Med 2021;49(14):3937–44.

17. van der Linde JA, van Kampen DA, Terwee CB, et al. Long-term results after arthroscopic shoulder stabilization using suture anchors: an 8- to 10-year follow-up. Am J Sports Med 2011;39(11):2396–403.

18. Lenters TR, Franta AK, Wolf FM, et al. Arthroscopic compared with open repairs for recurrent anterior shoulder instability. A systematic review and meta-analysis of the literature. J Bone Joint Surg Am 2007;89(2):244–54.

19. Kim S, Ha K, Cho Y, et al. Arthroscopic anterior stabilization of the shoulder: two to six-year follow-up. J Bone Joint Surg Am 2003;85(8):1511–8.

20. Burkhart SS, De Beer JF. Traumatic glenohumeral bone defects and their relationship to failure of arthroscopic Bankart repairs: significance of the inverted-pear glenoid and the humeral engaging Hill-Sachs lesion. Arthroscopy 2000;16(7): 677–94.

21. Nakagawa S, Iuchi R, Hanai H, et al. The development process of bipolar bone defects from primary to recurrent instability in shoulders with traumatic anterior instability. Am J Sports Med 2019;47(3):695–703.

22. Rowe CR, Patel D, Southmayd WW. The Bankart procedure: a long-term end-result study. J Bone Joint Surg Am 1978;60(1):1–16.

23. Pelet S, Jolles BM, Farron A. Bankart repair for recurrent anterior glenohumeral instability: results at twenty-nine years' follow-up. J Shoulder Elbow Surg 2006; 15(2):203–7.

24. Monk AP, Crua E, Gatenby GC, et al. Clinical outcomes following open anterior shoulder stabilization for glenohumeral instability in the young collision athlete. J Shoulder Elbow Surg 2022;31(7):1474–8.

25. Hickey IPM, Davey MS, Hurley ET, et al. Return to play following open Bankart repair in collision athletes aged 18 years or less. J Shoulder Elbow Surg 2022; 31(6S):S8–12.

26. AlSomali K, Kholinne E, Van Nguyen T, et al. Outcomes and return to sport and work after open Bankart repair for recurrent shoulder instability: a systematic review. Orthop J Sports Med 2021;9(10). 23259671211026907.

27. Rhee YG, Ha JH, Cho NS. Anterior shoulder stabilization in collision athletes: arthroscopic versus open Bankart repair. Am J Sports Med 2006;34(6):979–85.

28. Balg F, Boileau P. The instability severity index score. A simple pre-operative score to select patients for arthroscopic or open shoulder stabilisation. J Bone Joint Surg Br 2007;89(11):1470–7.

29. Pagnani MJ. Open capsular repair without bone block for recurrent anterior shoulder instability in patients with and without bony defects of the glenoid and/or humeral head. Am J Sports Med 2008;36(9):1805–12.

30. Hatch MD, Hennrikus WL. The open Bankart repair for traumatic anterior shoulder instability in teenage athletes. J Pediatr Orthop 2018;38(1):27–31.

31. Nakagawa S, Mae T, Sato S, et al. Risk factors for the postoperative recurrence of instability after arthroscopic Bankart repair in athletes. Orthop J Sports Med 2017;5(9). 2325967117726494.

32. McLeod A, Delaney R. Outcomes of the arthroscopic Bankart procedure in Irish collision sport athletes. Ir J Med Sci 2022;191(1):239–45.

33. Aboalata M, Plath JE, Seppel G, et al. Results of arthroscopic Bankart repair for anterior-inferior shoulder instability at 13-year follow-up. Am J Sports Med 2017; 45(4):782–7.

34. Goodrich E, Wolf M, Vopat M, et al. Sex-specific differences in outcomes after anterior shoulder surgical stabilization: a meta-analysis and systematic review of literature. JSES Int 2021;6(1):123–31.

35. Shymon SJ, Roocroft J, Edmonds EW. Traumatic anterior instability of the pediatric shoulder: a comparison of arthroscopic and open Bankart repairs. J Pediatr Orthop 2015;35(1):1–6.

The Latarjet Procedure for Recurrent Anterior Shoulder Instability in the Contact Athlete

Giovanni Di Giacomo, MD[a],*, Luigi Piscitelli, MD[a], Gianmarco Marcello, MD[b,1]

KEYWORDS

- Shoulder anterior instability • Glenoid bone loss • Hill–Sachs lesion
- Bipolar bone loss • Glenoid track • Latarjet procedure

KEY POINTS

- Bipolar bone loss evaluation is critical in the management of recurrent anterior shoulder instability, as it has an essential role in predicting outcomes.
- Determining whether or not the Hill–Sachs lesion engages the anterior rim is crucial because it helps predict postoperative stability, as "off-track" lesions show high failure rates if treated with a Bankart repair.
- Patients treated with the Latarjet procedure show a lower rate of recurrence, lower complication rates, lower failure rates, better range of motion (ROM), and postoperative stability, and they can return to full competition at a faster rate compared with the Bankart repair.

INTRODUCTION

In young athletes, anterior shoulder instability is a prevalent disease.

The incidence of glenohumeral instability in collegiate athletes is thought to be as high as 0.12 per 1000 athlete exposures, with a higher prevalence in collision and contact sports. Furthermore, young athletes who play contact sports have a low return-to-competition rate and are highly vulnerable to recurrent instability if treated nonoperatively.[1,2]

Ages 15 to 29 years account for the majority of cases of anterior glenohumeral instability, with younger people suffering from recurring episodes at a rate of 72% compared to older people at 27%.[1,2]

[a] Orthopedics and Traumatology Unit, Concordia Hospital, 90 Sette Chiese Street, 00145 Rome, Italy; [b] Orthopedics and Traumatology Unit, Campus Bio-Medico University Hospital, 200 Álvaro del Portillo Street, 00128, Rome, Italy
[1] Present address: Concordia Hospital, 90 Sette Chiese Street, 00145 Rome, Italy
* Corresponding author.
E-mail address: concordia@iol.it

Clin Sports Med 43 (2024) 635–648
https://doi.org/10.1016/j.csm.2024.03.021
0278-5919/24/© 2024 Elsevier Inc. All rights reserved.

Contact sports with a high risk of injury include boxing, rugby, soccer, basketball, volleyball, handball, martial arts, and many others. In these sports, the damage typically takes place with the arm in external rotation and abduction, leading to an anteroinferior humeral head dislocation.

The physical demands of the sport and the athletes' increased speed and muscle strength are the causes of the recent rise in high-energy trauma incidence.[1]

Owing to these high-energy injuries, contact athletes are more likely to develop bone loss, along with a higher redislocation rate, as for rugby players or goalkeepers. In addition to decreased performance and extended recovery, staying away from sports practice can have a disastrous impact on an athlete's career.

The management of glenoid and humeral bone loss (bipolar defects) in patients with recurrent anterior shoulder instability has received greater emphasis over the past 10 years. A significant amount of attention has been focused on evidence-based treatment algorithms based on the patient's activity level and/or sport, the amount and location of bone loss, and the glenoid track (contact area between the posterior humeral articular surface and the glenoid as the arm moves in abduction and external rotation).[3]

It is crucial to ascertain how surgery influences return-to-competition rates and career length in professional athletes, especially contact athletes, since for them these are two of the most crucial indicators of success after surgical therapy.

DISCUSSION

The most recent research demonstrates that anterior shoulder instability in contact sports has a high recurrence among elite athletes. Around 20.4% of the athletes who underwent Bankart repair (BR) failed in the Nakagawa and colleagues' study.[4] Ten percent of the new dislocations, according to Bacilla and colleagues' research, occurred after just 18 months of follow-up.[5] In a different research, Rossi and colleagues[6] observed that patients treated with the Latarjet method had a 4% rate of recurrence, compared to a 20% recurrence with arthroscopic surgery in 80 rugby players with less than 20% of glenoid bone loss. Additionally, there were differences in the 2 groups' reoperation rates (4% vs 16%, respectively).

In a comparison study comparing the Latarjet and BR on 185 shoulders, Hovelius and colleagues[7] discovered that patients who underwent the Latarjet operation had greater postoperative stability and reduced complication rates. The Latarjet treatment has reduced failure rates and offers superior external rotation compared to the BR, according to An and colleagues' meta-analysis.[8] According to Cerciello and colleagues and Beranger and colleagues, the Latarjet method leads to improved clinical outcomes, decreased dislocation and subluxation rates, and higher safety for athletes to start over their activities.[9,10]

A careful examination of the reasons that caused the recurrence is necessary for the athlete's therapy following a failed instability operation.

In a comprehensive review that combined information from 26 studies that concentrated on contact and collision athletes, Leroux and colleagues[11] reported rates of failure and recurring instability of 18% after soft tissue treatments. However, in cases without considerable bone loss where the surgeon utilized at least 3 anchors, this rate fell to 8%, which is comparable to the observed rate of 5% following the Latarjet operation.[6]

In patients with an "inverted pear" glenoid (with a bone loss of at least 25% of the width of the inferior glenoid) who solely underwent a soft tissue treatment, Burkhart and De Beer and Burkhart,[12] Burkhart and colleagues[13] noted a 67% recurrence rate. With an open Latarjet technique, these patients had a 4.9% recurrence rate.

Some experts advocated a bony procedure for recurrent anterior shoulder instability associated to bone loss as a result of this evidence.

In the studies of Sugaya and colleagues[14] and Edwards and colleagues,[15] glenoid and/or humeral bone lesions have been demonstrated to be present in 90% to 95% of shoulders with recurrent instability. Bipolar bone loss assessment is critical in the management of recurrent anterior shoulder instability, as it has a critical role in predicting outcomes (**Fig. 1**).

Bipolar Bone Loss

Approximately 40% of patients with a single dislocation and 85% of patients with recurrent dislocation experience glenoid bone loss,[16] which alone is responsible for mid-range instability because the stability of the joint is primarily provided by bone congruency in the mid-range of motion, whereas at the end range the capsule tightens and prevents translation. In this way, the Hill–Sachs lesion (HSL) has no effect on the risk of glenoid bone loss.[17]

The HSL is prevalent in 65% to 67% of cases following initial dislocation and 84% to 93% of cases following recurrent dislocation[18,19] In the posterior end range of movement, the HSL cannot produce any instability if it is completely covered by the glenoid. Otherwise, it can collide with the glenoid's front rim and dislocate the joint. Thus, the risk given by the HSL is related to the end-range instability. Therefore, the risk of engagement or dislocation relies on the size and placement of the HSL in relation to the glenoid, as well as the amount of bone loss in the glenoid.[17]

There are 2 ways to evaluate the risk posed by an HSL. One method is to perform a dynamic examination during arthroscopic surgery. However, it should be performed after the BR, with the risk of damaging the repair. The second approach is to use the "glenoid track" concept.[20,21] The portion of the posterior humeral articular surface that comes into contact with the glenoid when the arm moves through the posterior end range of motion is known as the glenoid track (**Fig. 2**).

The width of the glenoid track was calculated as 83% of the glenoid width (usually obtained with the best-fit circle method on the "en face" view of a 3D computed tomography [CT]).[21] If there is a bony defect of the glenoid, the defect width needs to be subtracted from the previously calculated value to obtain the true width of the glenoid track.

It is necessary to measure also the Hill–Sachs interval (distance from the rotator cuff attachments to the medial rim of the HSL) on the axial images at the point with the largest medial extent of the HSL. If the glenoid track width is bigger than the Hill–Sachs interval,

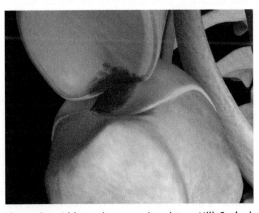

Fig. 1. Bipolar bone loss: glenoid bone loss associated to a Hill–Sachs lesion.

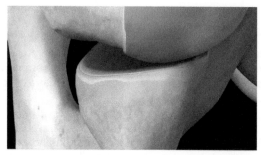

Fig. 2. The glenoid track (blue area).

then the HSL will not engage with the anterior rim of the glenoid after the BR (on-track HSL). Otherwise, the engagement is possible, and we have an off-track HSL (**Fig. 3**). One should also consider that the range of motion varies in different patients (eg, in lax vs stiff patients) and it influences the glenoid track (lax patients will have a smaller glenoid track, while stiff patients will have a bigger one).

The BR has been demonstrated to have a high failure rate when used to address "off-track" lesions, therefore knowing whether the HSL engages the anterior rim is crucial for predicting postoperative stability.[22] In contrast to 27% for on-track HSLs, Schwihla and colleagues observed a rate of recurrent instability of 74% for off-track HSLs ($P < .001$).[23]

Several investigators tried to biomechanically define the "critical limit" at which glenoid bone loss effectively destabilizes the glenohumeral joint.[24] Bigliani and colleagues[25] proposed a 25% decrease in glenoid width as a reasonable cutoff to denote the critical entity of the bone defect, which has been indicated also in other investigations as critical glenoid bone loss.[17,20,26]

Historically, the Latarjet procedure has only been used to treat shoulder instability in patients with more than 25% of glenoid bone loss, which has been shown to cause instability by inducing a lack of glenohumeral articular conformity.[20,27]

However, there is a gray area known as subcritical bone loss between the "safe zone" and the "critical zone" of the amount of glenoid bone loss, and its description differs in literature studies.

Shaha and colleagues' recent clinical report[28] demonstrated that even though patients did not experience recurrent instability, bone loss of 13.5% to 20% resulted in a clinically significant decline in their quality of life, which is consistent with an undesirable outcome. According to a more recent clinical study,[29] the crucial amount that could lead to recurrent instability following surgery is a bone loss of 17.3% or

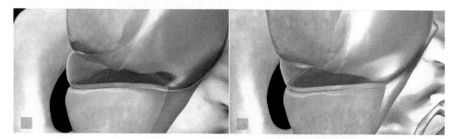

Fig. 3. Off-track HSL (to the left) and on-track HSL (to the right) in shoulders without glenoid bone loss, shown after a BR has been performed. If a glenoid bone loss is present, it reduces the glenoid track, thus possibly turning an on-track HSL into an off-track one.

higher. According to a study by Yamamoto and colleagues, patients with glenoid bone loss greater than 17% had significantly lower Western Ontario Shoulder Instability Index (WOSI) scores.[30]

Additionally, there is subcritical humeral bone loss. The Hill–Sachs occupancy ratio, which is equal to the Hill–Sachs interval divided by the glenoid track, is an important index to quantify the risk of an HSL. When assessing the risk of an on-track HSL, it was found that those with the Hill–Sachs occupancy ratio ≥75% (peripheral-track lesion) showed significantly worse WOSI score without recurrent instability events than those with the ratio less than 75% (central-track lesion).[31]

If a patient with an on-track lesion has a subcritical glenoid bone loss or a peripheral track lesion, the lesion must be treated as an off-track lesion if the patient has multiple risk factors of instability. In fact, an augmentation procedure such as remplissage or Latarjet should be considered also in case of a peripheral-track lesion if the patient is a contact athlete.[31]

Remplissage Versus Latarjet

Among the several surgical procedures described to treat the engaging Hill–Sachs bone defect, emphasis has also been placed on the remplissage, the posterior soft tissue filling of the HSL hill-sachs remplissage (HSR), since it represents a minimally invasive approach to treat engaging HSLs. According to preliminary findings, the association of an HSR may lower the redislocation rate following isolated BR in case of engaging HSL.[32,33] However, remplissage is not an anatomic reconstruction and might compromise glenohumeral range of motion (decreased external rotation, with subsequent early onset of osteoarthritis).[34]

Haroun and colleagues,[35] in a systematic review and meta-analysis on arthroscopic BR with remplissage versus Latarjet procedure in case of engaging HSLs with subcritical glenoid bone loss, discovered that both techniques produce similar clinical results. However, because of fewer postoperative complications, the first may be safer.

In a research by Yang and colleagues,[36] complications were more frequent after the Latarjet (12.1% vs 1%, $P = .002$). This technique resulted in a reduced recurrence rate (6.06% vs 28.6%, $P = .034$) and lower revision rate (3.03% vs 21.4%, $P = .041$) in patients with greater than 10% glenoid bone loss. Among collision and contact athletes, the procedure exhibited improved WOSI scores and a decreased recurrence rate (30% vs 0%, $P = .005$).

The Latarjet procedure, according to these authors, seems to be a better option in revision instability surgery, for collision and contact athletes, and in those with greater than 10% glenoid bone loss.

While the Latarjet procedure is commonly accepted as the procedure of choice in cases of multiple dislocations with critical or subcritical glenoid bone loss, today the debate focuses on the management of patients with multiple dislocations and an off-track HSL with a glenoid bone loss less than 10%, as in these cases there is not a significant glenoid bone loss which needs to be fixed with the Latarjet technique. In these cases, a BR plus remplissage may also be indicated.

We prefer to perform the Latarjet procedure in patients with multiple dislocations and an off-track HSL and in contact athletes with a peripheral-track HSL.

Instability Severity Index Score and Glenoid Track Instability Management Score

The instability severity index score (ISIS), developed by Balg and Boileau,[37] can be used to identify patients who will benefit from an open bony reconstruction. In order to determine which patients are most at risk for recurrent instability following an arthroscopic BR, the ISIS ranks patients on a 10 point scale based on preoperative risk variables (**Table 1**). The authors reported that patients who score greater than 6 had a 70% risk of recurrent instability after arthroscopic BR, and therefore, a Latarjet procedure has been recommended in these patients.

However, Phadnis and colleagues[38] observed a 70% recurrence of instability after arthroscopic BR in patients scoring 4.

Additionally, Verweij and colleagues[39] found the following risk factors for recurrence after an arthroscopic BR in a meta-analysis of 4584 shoulders: age 20 years or lesser, involvement in competitive sports, off-track HSL, glenoid bone loss, anterior labral periosteal sleeve avulsion (ALPSA) lesion, greater than 1 preoperative dislocations, greater than 6 months surgical delay from a first-time dislocation to surgery, and ISIS greater than 3.

Di Giacomo[40] and colleagues introduced a new treatment algorithm, the "Glenoid Track Instability Management Score" (GTIMS), incorporating the glenoid track concept into ISIS (**Table 2**). The authors compared treatment decision-making using either GTIMS or ISIS in patients with recurrent anterior instability and found that significantly fewer patients underwent a Latarjet procedure using GTIMS than would have if surgical decision-making was based on ISIS alone ($P < .001$).

Although additional clinical studies are needed to validate GTIMS, the current literature on the glenoid track concept[12,22,41] suggests that GTIMS may more accurately predict failure after arthroscopic BR and therefore more accurately identify patients who should undergo a Latarjet.

Latarjet-Patte Procedure

In 1954, Michel Latarjet published a description of his method for stabilizing the shoulder, which involved transposing the horizontal limb of the coracoid process to the

Table 1 Instability severity index score	
ISIS Prognostic Factors	**Score**
Age at surgery (years)	
$\leq$20	2
>20	0
Type of sport	
Contact or forced overhead	1
Other	0
Level of competition in sport	
Competitive	2
Recreational or none	0
Shoulder hyperlaxity	
Confirmed anterior or inferior hyperlaxity	1
Normal laxity	0
Loss of sclerotic line of the glenoid on AP radiograph	
Yes	2
No	0
Hill–Sachs lesion visible in external rotation on AP radiograph	
Yes	2
No	0
Total ISIS	10

Table 2	
Glenoid track instability management score	
GTIMS Prognostic Factors	**Score**
Age at surgery (years)	
≤20	2
>20	0
Type of sport	
Contact or forced overhead	1
Other	0
Level of competition in sport	
Competitive	2
Recreational or none	0
Shoulder hyperlaxity	
Confirmed anterior or inferior hyperlaxity	1
Normal laxity	0
Evaluation of bone loss on 3D CT	
"On-track"	0
"Off-track"	4
Total GTIMS	10

anteroinferior glenoid rim through a window in the subscapularis and fixing it with a single screw. A variation of this that uses 2 screws and repairs the anterior capsule to the coracoacromial ligament stump is the Latarjet-Patte technique.[42]

The lateral margin of the acromion level is at the edge of the surgical table while the patient is in a beach chair position. After a limited deltopectoral approach is performed, in order to keep exposure a self-retaining retractor is placed between the deltoid and pectoralis major. A Hohmann retractor is positioned over the coracoid, and the coracoacromial ligament is cut 1 cm laterally to its coracoid insertion. The pectoralis minor is detached from the coracoid with electrocautery by ablating directly off the bone, so that the surgeon can safely avoid injury to the brachial plexus. Without harming the coracoclavicular ligaments, a coracoid graft longer than 25 mm can be usually obtained. Two central drill holes are produced in the coracoid using a particular tool, spaced about 1 cm apart.

At the intersection of its superior two-thirds and inferior one-third, the subscapularis is split. A horizontal incision is performed in the capsule at the level of the joint line. The anterior labrum and periosteum are removed. In the right shoulder, the inferior hole in the glenoid is made between 4 and 5 o'clock, and in the left shoulder, between 7 and 8 o'clock (**Fig. 4**). The hole must be medial enough to avoid lateral coracoid overhang, and the right distance is usually 7 mm from the glenoid margin. An offset guide can be used to create the holes at the right distance from the articular surface.

A second hole is made in the glenoid using the same tool used for coracoid holes which serves to respect the correct distance between the screws. The holes must be drilled with a cannulated drill in a direction parallel to the glenoid surface in order to avoid lateral overhang. The offset guide helps to follow the right direction (**Fig. 5**). The coracoid graft is fixed with two 32 mm long 4.5 mm partially threaded cannulated malleolar screws. It is possible to implant a medial wedge mini-plate of Arthrex to simplify the procedure as explained hereafter.

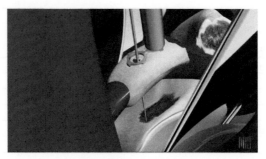

Fig. 4. Left shoulder. Placing the most vascularized portion of the coracoid (the one close to the tendon attachment) adjacent to the location of the bone loss optimizes mechanotransduction leading to optimal osteointegration.

The graft must be 1 mm medial to the front edge of the glenoid. If any lateral overhang is noticed, it should be adjusted with bone rongeurs or a high-speed burr.

The coracoacromial residual on the coracoid is sutured to the capsule with the shoulder in full external rotation to enable immediate postoperative full range of motion and prevent stiffness. Finally, we repair the split in the subscapularis tendon with one stitch.

The coracoid graft provides a "bony effect" re-establishing the anteroposterior diameter of the glenoid, thus increasing stability and preventing the engagement of an HSL on a deficient anteroinferior glenoid rim. The most important stabilizing effect of the Latarjet-Patte procedure is anyway the interaction between the conjoint tendon and lower subscapularis with the arm in abduction and external rotation. In this

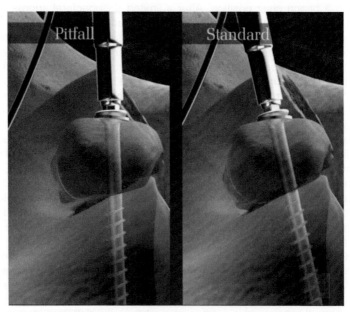

Fig. 5. Incorrect (left) and correct (right) screw positioning during coracoid graft fixation to the glenoid. Inserting screws parallel to the articular surface reduces the risk of lateral overhang and nonunion of the graft.

position, the conjoint tendon reinforces the inferior subscapularis fibers and the capsule through a tensioning effect ("sling effect").[43] The further the arm moves into the at-risk position of abduction and external rotation, the tighter become these soft tissues. Lastly, the "triple blocking" effect is achieved with the repair of the anterior capsule to the residual of the coracoacromial ligament on the graft.

Coracoid Complications

In our experience,[43] coracoid fracture, nonunion, and osteointegration represent 3 different scenarios. Unless pre-existing, graft fractures are a technical error. They can be the result of an excessive compression, particularly if the coracoid is small and the screw holes are not drilled at the proper distance.

Pseudoarthrosis of the coracoid–glenoid interface can result from an inappropriate local biology, an incomplete match between both surfaces or inadequate compression. In our opinion, these are technical errors that can be prevented.

It is very interesting to analyze the third scenario: the "bone reabsorption." In our opinion, unlike certain literature that deems it a complication, it represents a normal biological evolution (**Fig. 6**[44]). One of our reports has clearly shown that a coracoid reabsorption, even as high as 70%, does not necessarily lead to a worse clinical result, but it is a natural phenomenon, an evident expression of Wolff's law.[43] Wolff's law states that healthy bone will undergo adaptive changes relative to the loads under which it is placed, so if loading on a particular bone increases, the bone will remodel itself over time to become stronger to resist that loading and vice versa. The internal architecture of the trabeculae undergoes adaptive changes, followed by secondary changes to the external cortical portion of the bone, becoming thicker as a result. The most important part of the graft is the distal one, closest to the tendon, which is the most vascularized by branches of the thoracoacromial artery. This will allow the osteointegration to recreate "the pear-shaped glenoid"; the rest of the graft will naturally be reabsorbed because it does not experience compressive loading.

The use of the wedged mini-plate is interesting because it allows "safe compression" through a uniformly distributed force on the coracoid, reducing the risk of intraoperative fracture. Thanks to a 20° medial wedge, it also permits to tilt the coracoid (rotation of the coracoid on its longitudinal axis) while tightening the screws, in order to correctly compress the medial portion of the graft on the glenoid neck even if the screws are not positioned perpendicular to the contact surface of the glenoid, thus lowering the risk of violating the articular surface, which would be higher in case of

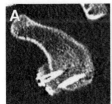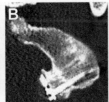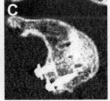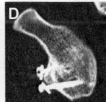

Fig. 6. Classification of postoperative bone resorption of the coracoid on computed tomography images with multiplanar reconstruction. (*A*) None: no bone resorption. (*B*) Mild: slight bone resorption, but it did not reach the screw head. (*C*) Moderate: bone resorption reached the screw head. (*D*) Severe: severe bone resorption with exposure of the screw shaft and loosening of the washer. (*From:* Tanaka M, Hanai H, Kotani Y, et al. Open Bristow vs Open Latarjet for Anterior Shoulder Instability in Rugby Players: Radiological and Clinical Outcomes. Orthop J Sports Med. 2022;10(5):23259671221095094.)

screws positioned as closest as possible to being perpendicular to the glenoid surface. In this way, it is possible to easily achieve the right contact between the 2 surfaces for a better integration of the graft. This tilt of the coracoid is needed especially in case of a subcritical glenoid bone loss, where the glenoid neck surface is much more steep (**Fig. 7**), while in case of critical bone loss the flatter glenoid neck surface makes this step easier.

Latarjet in Contact Athletes

In their study, Privitera and colleagues[45] reported that 8% of contact or collision athletes experienced a dislocation after the procedure. Forty-nine percent of the patients returned to their preoperative sports level, 14% decreased their activity level in the same sport, 12% changed sports, and 25% decreased their level of activity and changed sports or stopped participating in sports altogether. Patients with ≥ 2 stabilization procedures prior to the Latarjet procedure demonstrated a lower likelihood of returning to their original sport ($P = .019$).

In a study by Rossi and colleagues[46] on competitive athletes with anterior instability and glenoid bone loss less than 20%, the recurrence rate was 4.6% and the revision rate was 1.5%. Ninety-four percent were able to return to sports and 84% returned at the same level. No significant difference in shoulder ROM was found between preoperative and postoperative results, nor between primary and revision cases. The bone block healed in 95% of the cases.

The Latarjet procedure also allows contact athletes to return to full competition at a faster rate compared with arthroscopic and open Bankart procedures.[42]

In a study by Neyton and colleagues on professional level rugby players treated with the Latarjet procedure, some patients even returned to full competition by 4 months. Mean return to full training was 6 months, and mean return to full competition was 7 months. The technique allowed to return to rugby practice in almost all cases if desired. Only one player of 34 did not return to playing rugby because of the operated shoulder.[47]

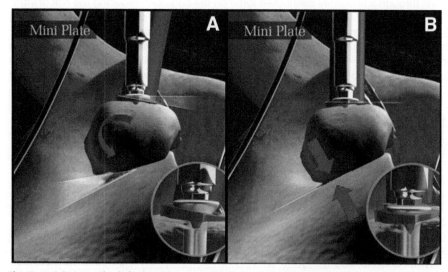

Fig. 7. Axial view of a left shoulder: in subcritical glenoid bone loss, the use of a wedged plate results in a counterclockwise tilt of the coracoid (*A*), thus increasing the contact surface between the deep medial surface of the coracoid and the glenoid neck (*B*).

In addition to this, complications with the Latarjet-Patte procedure are rare with a meticulous surgical technique. Although a 62% glenohumeral arthritis rate has previously been reported with the Latarjet procedure,[48] only 30% of the rugby players in the authors' study showed arthritis at 12 year follow-up.[47] All these patients had mild arthritis, which has been shown to have no effect on shoulder function.[48]

Hovelius and colleagues[49] suggest that degenerative joint disease may be related to pre-existing factors, since no significant difference in postoperative arthritis is seen following soft tissue and bony stabilization procedures.[50] The authors thought the main avoidable factor at the time of the Latarjet procedure surgery is lateral coracoid overhang.

A higher loss of external rotation was observed following subscapularis tenotomy for glenoid exposure.[48]

In conclusion, the Latarjet procedure resulted in excellent functional outcomes, with most of the patients returning to sports at the preinjury level with a low rate of recurrences.

SUMMARY

Shoulder instability is a condition frequently affecting young and active population, especially professional contact athletes, and therefore often needs surgical treatment. Bone loss is an almost constant finding after a major episode of anterior shoulder dislocation, both on the humeral and glenoid side, thus defined as bipolar, and it must be evaluated together with other factors such as age, sport practiced, and number of dislocation episodes to decide the best management for each patient.

The effectiveness of the Latarjet procedure relies not only in lower rates of recurrence and early functional improvement, but also in allowing athletes to return early to high performance levels in their professional activities.

CLINICS CARE POINTS

- Seventy-two percent of individuals younger than 22 years suffer from recurrent instability episodes compared with 27% of those aged 30 years or more.
- Glenoid and/or humeral bone lesions are present in 90% to 95% of shoulders with recurrent instability.
- A subcritical glenoid and/or humeral bone loss leads to a clinically significant decrease in the quality of life, even though the patients do not sustain a recurrent instability.
- The Latarjet procedure appears to be a better choice in recurrent instability, revision instability surgery, collision and contact athletes, and those with greater than 10% glenoid bone loss.

DISCLOSURE

The authors declare no conflict of interest.

REFERENCES

1. Dickens JF, Owens BD, Cameron KL, et al. Return to play and recurrent instability after in-season anterior shoulder instability: a prospective multicenter study. Am J Sports Med 2014.

2. Owens BD, Agel J, Mountcastle SB, et al. Incidence of glenohumeral instability in collegiate athletics. Am J Sports Med 2009;37(9):1750–4.

3. Uhorchak J, Arciero RA, Huggard D, et al. Recurrent shoulder instability after open reconstruction in athletes involved in collision and contact sports. Am J Sports Med 2000;28(6):794–9.

4. Nakagawa S, Mae T, Sato S, et al. Risk factors for the postoperative recurrence of instability after arthroscopic bankart repair in athletes. Orthop J Sports Med 2017; 5(9). 2325967117726494.

5. Bacilla P, Field LD, Savoie FH III. Arthroscopic bankart repair in a high demand patient population 2009;13(1):202–7.

6. Rossi LA, Tanoira I, Gorodischer T, et al. Recurrence and revision rates with arthroscopic bankart repair compared with the latarjet procedure in competitive rugby players with glenohumeral instability and a glenoid bone loss <20. Am J Sports Med 2021;49(4):866–72.

7. Hovelius L, Vikerfors O, Olofsson A, et al. Bristow-Latarjet and Bankart: a comparative study of shoulder stabilization in 185 shoulders during a seventeen-year follow-up. J Shoulder Elbow Surg 2011;20(7):1095–101.

8. An VVG, Sivakumar BS, Phan K, et al. A systematic review and meta-analysis of clinical and patient-reported outcomes following two procedures for recurrent traumatic anterior instability of the shoulder: Latarjet procedure vs. Bankart repair. J Shoulder Elbow Surg 2016;25(5):853–63.

9. Cerciello S, Edwards TB, Walch G. Chronic anterior glenohumeral instability in soccer players: results for a series of 28 shoulders treated with the Latarjet procedure. J Orthop Traumatol 2012;13(4):197–202.

10. Beranger JS, Klouche S, Bauer T, et al. Anterior shoulder stabilization by Bristow–Latarjet procedure in athletes: return-to-sport and functional outcomes at minimum 2-year follow-up. Eur J Orthop Surg Traumatol 2016;26(3):277–82.

11. Leroux TS, Saltzman BM, Meyer M, et al. The Influence of evidence-based surgical indications and techniques on failure rates after arthroscopic shoulder stabilization in the contact or collision athlete with anterior shoulder instability. Am J Sports Med 2017;45(5):1218–25.

12. Burkhart S, De Beer J. Traumatic glenohumeral bone defects and their relationship to failure of arthroscopic Bankart repairs: significance of the inverted-pear glenoid and the humeral engaging Hill-Sachs lesion. Arthroscopy 2000;16(7): 677–94.

13. Burkhart S, De Beer J, Barth J, et al. Results of modified Latarjet reconstruction in patients with anteroinferior instability and significant bone loss. Arthroscopy 2007;23(10):1033–41.

14. Sugaya H, Moriishi J, Dohi M, et al. Glenoid rim morphology in recurrent anterior glenohumeral instability. J Bone Joint Surg Am 2003;85(5):878–84.

15. Edwards TB, Boulahia A, Walch G. Radiographic analysis of bone defects in chronic anterior shoulder instability. Arthroscopy 2003;19(7):732–9.

16. Griffith JF. Measuring glenoid and humeral bone loss in shoulder dislocation. Quant Imaging Med Surg 2019;9(2):134–43.

17. Itoi E. 'On-track' and 'off-track' shoulder lesions. EFORT Open Rev 2017;2(8): 343–51.

18. Spatschil A, Landsiedl F, Anderl W, et al. Posttraumatic anterior-inferior instability of the shoulder: arthroscopic findings and clinical correlations. Arch Orthop Trauma Surg 2006;12.

19. Yiannakopoulos CK, Mataragas E, Antonogiannakis E. A comparison of the spectrum of intra-articular lesions in acute and chronic anterior shoulder instability. Arthroscopy 2007;23(9):985–90.

20. Yamamoto N, Itoi E, Abe H, et al. Effect of an anterior glenoid defect on anterior shoulder stability: a cadaveric study. Am J Sports Med 2009;37(5):949–54.

21. Omori Y, Yamamoto N, Koishi H, et al. Measurement of the Glenoid Track In Vivo as Investigated by 3-Dimensional Motion Analysis Using Open MRI. Am J Sports Med 2014;42(6):1290–5.

22. Shaha JS, Cook JB, Rowles DJ, et al. Clinical Validation of the Glenoid Track Concept in Anterior Glenohumeral Instability. J Bone Joint Surg Am 2016; 98(22):1918–23.

23. Schwihla I, Wieser K, Grubhofer F, et al. Long-term recurrence rate in anterior shoulder instability after Bankart repair based on the on- and off-track concept. J Shoulder Elbow Surg 2023;32(2):269–75.

24. Piasecki DP, Verma NN, Romeo AA, et al. Glenoid bone deficiency in recurrent anterior shoulder instability: diagnosis and management. J Am Acad Orthop Surg 2009;17(8):482–93.

25. Bigliani LU, Newton PM, Steinmann SP, et al. Glenoid rim lesions associated with recurrent anterior dislocation of the shoulder. Am J Sports Med 1998;26:41–5.

26. Yamamoto N, Muraki T, Sperling JW, et al. Stabilizing mechanism in bone-grafting of a large glenoid defect. J Bone Joint Surg Am 2010;92(11):2059–66.

27. Burkhart SS, Danaceau SM. Articular arc length mismatch as a cause of failed bankart repair. Arthroscopy 2000;16(7):740–4.

28. Shaha JS, Cook JB, Song DJ, et al. Redefining "critical" bone loss in shoulder instability: functional out- comes worsen with "subcritical" bone loss. Am J Sports Med 2015;43:1719–25.

29. Shin SJ, Kim RG, Jeon YS, et al. Critical value of anterior glenoid bone loss that leads to recurrent glenohumeral instability after arthroscopic bankart repair. Am J Sports Med 2017;45:1975–81.

30. Yamamoto N, Kawakami J, Hatta T, et al. Effect of subcritical glenoid bone loss on activities of daily living in patients with anterior shoulder instability. Orthop Traumatol Surg Res 2019;105(8):1467–70.

31. Yamamoto N, Shinagawa K, Hatta T, et al. Peripheral-Track and Central-Track Hill-Sachs Lesions: A New Concept of Assessing an On-Track Lesion. Am J Sports Med 2020;48(1):33–8.

32. Cho NS, Yoo JH, Juh HS, et al. Anterior shoulder instability with engaging Hill-Sachs defects: a comparison of arthroscopic Bankart repair with and without posterior capsulodesis. Knee Surg Sports Traumatol Arthrosc 2016;24(12):3801–8.

33. Garcia GH, Park MJ, Zhang C, et al. Large Hill-Sachs Lesion: a Comparative Study of Patients Treated with Arthroscopic Bankart Repair with or without Remplissage. HSS J 2015;11(2):98–103.

34. Elkinson I, Giles JW, Faber KJ, et al. The effect of the remplissage procedure on shoulder stability and range of motion: an in vitro biomechanical assessment. J Bone Joint Surg Am 2012;94(11):1003–12.

35. Haroun HK, Sobhy MH, Abdelrahman AA. Arthroscopic Bankart repair with remplissage versus Latarjet procedure for management of engaging Hill-Sachs lesions with subcritical glenoid bone loss in traumatic anterior shoulder instability: a systematic review and meta-analysis. J Shoulder Elbow Surg 2020;29(10): 2163–74.

36. Yang JS, Mehran N, Mazzocca AD, et al. Remplissage versus modified latarjet for off-track hill-sachs lesions with subcritical glenoid bone loss. Am J Sports Med 2018;46(8):1885–91.
37. Balg F, Boileau P. The instability severity index score. A simple pre-operative score to select patients for arthroscopic or open shoulder stabilisation. J Bone Joint Surg Br 2007;89(11):1470–7.
38. Phadnis J, Arnold C, Elmorsy A, et al. Utility of the instability severity index score in predicting failure after arthroscopic anterior stabilization of the shoulder. Am J Sports Med 2015;43:1983–8.
39. Verweij LPE, van Spanning SH, Grillo A, et al. Age, participation in competitive sports, bony lesions, ALPSA lesions, > 1 preoperative dislocations, surgical delay and ISIS score > 3 are risk factors for recurrence following arthroscopic Bankart repair: a systematic review and meta-analysis of 4584. Verweij, et al. Knee Surg Sports Traumatol Arthrosc 2021;29(12):4004–14.
40. Di Giacomo G, Peebles LA, Pugliese M, et al. Glenoid Track Instability Management Score: Radiographic Modification of the Instability Severity Index Score. Arthroscopy 2020;36(1):56–67.
41. Trivedi S, Pomerantz ML, Gross D, et al. Shoulder instability in the setting of bipolar (glenoid and humeral head) bone loss: the gle- noid track concept. Clin Orthop Relat Res 2014;472:2352–62.
42. Joshi MA, Young AA, Balestro JC, et al. The Latarjet-Patte procedure for recurrent anterior shoulder instability in contact athletes. Orthop Clin North Am 2015;46(1):105–11.
43. Di Giacomo G. Editorial Commentary: Latarjet Mechanics and Biology: Thinking in Biodynamic Fashion. Arthroscopy 2020;36(3):696–700.
44. Tanaka M, Hanai H, Kotani Y, et al. Open bristow versus open latarjet for anterior shoulder instability in rugby players: radiological and clinical outcomes. Orthop J Sports Med 2022;10(5). 23259671221095094.
45. Privitera DM, Sinz NJ, Miller LR, et al. Clinical outcomes following the latarjet procedure in contact and collision athletes. J Bone Joint Surg Am 2018;100(6):459–65.
46. Rossi LA, Gorodischer T, Brandariz R, et al. High rate of return to sports and low recurrences with the latarjet procedure in high-risk competitive athletes with glenohumeral instability and a glenoid bone loss <20. Arthrosc Sports Med Rehabil 2020;2(6):e735–42.
47. Neyton L, Young A, Dawidziak B, et al. Surgical treatment of anterior instability in rugby union players: clinical and radiographic results of the Latarjet-Patte procedure with minimum 5-year follow-up. J Shoulder Elbow Surg 2012;21(12):1721–7.
48. Allain J, Goutallier D, Glorion C. Long-term results of the Latarjet procedure for the treatment of anterior instability of the shoulder. J Bone Joint Surg Am 1998;80(6):841–52.
49. Hovelius L, Saebo M. Neer Award 2008: arthropathy after primary anterior shoulder dislocation- 223 shoulders prospectively followed up for twenty-five years. J Shoulder Elbow Surg 2009;18(3):339–47.
50. Buscayret F, Edwards TB, Szabo I, et al. Glenohumeral arthrosis in anterior instability before and after surgical treatment: incidence and contributing factors. Am J Sports Med 2004;32(5):1165–72.

Open Bone Augmentation Solutions for the Failed Shoulder Stabilization

Ryan J. Whalen, BS, CSCS[a], Marco Adriani, MD[a,b,1],
Phob Ganokroj, MD[c,2],
Matthew T. Provencher, MD, MBA, MC, USNR (Ret)[a,d,*]

KEYWORDS

- Glenohumeral instability • Distal tibia allograft • Anterior shoulder stabilization
- Glenoid bone loss • Failed Latarjet

KEY POINTS

- Many patients who have had a failed anterior shoulder stabilization procedure (eg, Bankart repair and Latarjet) have glenoid bone loss that needs to be properly addressed to restore glenohumeral stability.
- Augmentation with a distal tibia allograft (DTA) can restore glenohumeral stability while offering a dense, weight-bearing bone-cartilage surface, lack of donor site morbidity, and favorable clinical outcomes.
- Biomechanical studies of the DTA have shown it to have excellent congruity with the humeral head, as well as contact pressures, contact areas, and peak forces that are all comparable to the native glenoid.
- The DTA is indicated in patients with greater than 15% to 25% glenoid bone loss, a prior failed stabilization procedure, and/or bipolar bone loss. It is contraindicated in patients without significant bone loss, infections, and/or prior nerve issues.
- Preoperative planning and intraoperative measurements are crucial to accurately visualize the defect and to properly size the graft.

[a] Steadman Philippon Research Insitute, 181 W Meadow Drive, Suite 400, Vail, CO 81657, USA;
[b] Department of Medical and Surgical Specialties, Radiological Sciences, and Public Health, University of Brescia, Viale Europa, 11-25123, Brescia, Italy; [c] Faculty of Medicine, Department of Orthopaedic Surgery, Siriraj Hospital, Mahidol University, 2 Thanon Wang Lang, Siriraj, Bangkok Noi, Bangkok 10700, Thailand; [d] The Steadman Clinic, 181 W Meadow Drive, Suite 400, Vail, CO 81657, USA
[1] Present address: Via Stresa 22, Milano (MI) 20125, Italia.
[2] Present address: 531/892 Ideo Mobi Charan Interchange, Charan Sanit Wong Road, Khwaeng Bang Khun Si, khet Bangkok Noi, Bangkok 10700.
* Corresponding author. 181 W Meadow Drive, Suite 400, Vail, CO 81657.
E-mail addresses: mprovencher@thesteadmanclinic.com; mtpresearch@sprivail.org

Clin Sports Med 43 (2024) 649–660
https://doi.org/10.1016/j.csm.2024.03.022
0278-5919/24/© 2024 Elsevier Inc. All rights reserved.

sportsmed.theclinics.com

INTRODUCTION
Background

Anterior shoulder stabilization procedures have the ability to restore glenohumeral (GH) stability and function but are not without complications. Recurrent instability is one of the main concerns following a stabilization procedure, with GH bone loss being an important risk factor for recurrence.[1-3] The current literature estimates glenoid bone loss (GBL) to be present in 56% to 89% of patients who underwent an anterior Bankart repair that had failed.[4,5] Bone block procedures are an important treatment for patients with significant GBL. Common procedures include the Latarjet procedure, iliac crest bone graft, distal clavicle autograft, scapular spine autograft, and the distal tibia allograft (DTA).[1,2,6,7] More recently, the DTA has been gaining popularity due to the many advantages it offers, including dense weight-bearing bone, lack of donor-site morbidity, a similar radius of curvature (ROC) to the native glenoid, and a cartilage surface, as well as the favorable clinical results in the literature.[8-10] Moreover, the DTA has been shown to be a viable option in the setting of a prior failed stabilization procedure, such as the Latarjet.[11]

Anatomy of the Distal Tibia Allograft

The anatomy of the DTA allows for the restoration of large glenoid defects while providing a dense bone with a cartilaginous structure that has great articular congruency with the humeral head and restores GH biomechanics.[10,11] The lateral aspect of the DTA has a curvature and concavity that has been shown to be comparable to the native glenoid, based on the biomechanical studies.[10]

The variability in DTA characteristics can be attributed to a range of factors, including the age, height, weight, gender, and body mass index of the donor. These factors can potentially impact the distal tibial dimensions and the ROC of individuals considered as potential donors for anterior glenoid augmentation. In a retrospective analysis of ankle MRIs conducted by Parada and colleagues, individuals who did not have any bony trauma of the ankle were examined. The findings indicated that individuals with a height of approximately 67 ± 5 inches are suitable candidates for a standard DTA, that is, 10 ± 22 mm in length. This standard DTA measurement is crucial for the reconstruction of a 25% to 30% glenoid defect and holds significant importance in the process of ordering and procuring allografts.[12]

Biomechanics

In a controlled laboratory investigation conducted by Bhatia and colleagues, GH contact pressures and contact areas after glenoid reconstruction using either the Latarjet or DTA procedure were examined. The outcomes of this study revealed that DTA reconstruction exhibited superior outcomes in terms of normalizing GH contact area, contact pressures, and peak forces across various abduction angles and loading conditions. The team highlighted that the utilization of the DTA for reconstructing the anterior glenoid bone defects yielded enhanced joint congruity and reduced peak forces within the GH joint when compared to Latarjet reconstruction, particularly at an abduction angle of 60°, and in the abduction and external rotation position.[8]

Indications

The DTA is one of the possible graft choices for reconstructing anterior glenoid defects. The indications for the DTA procedure include

1. GBL greater than 15 to 25% (or greater);

2. A prior failed stabilization procedure (**Fig. 1**A–C; ie, Bankart repair, postsurgical GH anchor arthropathy, and Latarjet procedure); and
3. Bipolar bone loss.

Contraindications for the DTA include

1. Patients without significant GBL;
2. Infections; and
3. Prior nerve issues.[9,13,14]

SURGICAL TECHNIQUE

The authors have described their preferred DTA graft preparation and fixation previously in the literature.[10,15–17]

Patient Setup and Operative Approach

Following the administration of appropriate anesthesia, which may include regional blocks when feasible and general anesthesia for muscle relaxation in the shoulder joint, the patient is positioned in the beach chair position, with the head elevated at approximately 45° angle. To maintain the stability of the glenoid and scapula and prevent anterior rotation, 2 blue towels are strategically positioned between the patient and the bed, behind the medial border of the scapula.

In order to properly assess the pathology and confirm the diagnosis, an examination under anesthesia (EUA) is performed. A modified deltopectoral approach is used to gain access to the anterior glenoid. The incision begins at the inferior tip of the coracoid process and continues down approximately 6 cm to the axillary fold. The deltopectoral interval is identified, the cephalic vein is retracted laterally, and the subfascial plane of the deltoid is mobilized. The lateral border of the conjoint tendon is then located, incised, and gently retracted medially. It is imperative to exercise caution to avoid excessive medial retraction in order to prevent damage to the musculocutaneous nerve and other important neurovascular structures. A Kolbel retractor is then positioned beneath the deltoid muscle and gently retracted underneath the conjoint tendon.

The next step involves the identification of the subscapularis (SSc) tendon, which is achieved by carefully releasing any adhesions both superiorly and inferiorly to the SSc

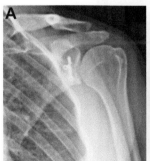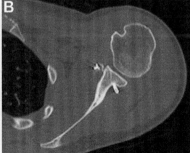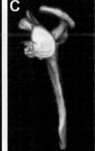

Fig. 1. Postoperative imaging of a failed Latarjet procedure. (*A*) Radiograph of a left shoulder in the anteroposterior view. (*B*) Axial 2 dimensional computed tomography (CT) scan of a left shoulder with a prior failed Latarjet procedure. (*C*) 3 dimensional CT scan of a left shoulder with a prior failed Latarjet.

using Metzenbaum scissors. An SSc split is then performed. This cut is carried out by using a 15 blade and incising in line with the fibers of the SSc. This split is positioned between the upper two-thirds and lower one-third of the SSc, extending medially to the level of the musculotendinous junction. It is crucial to exercise caution and avoid excessive medialization of the split, as this can increase the risk of iatrogenic nerve injury. However, performing an SSc split might be challenging in certain revision cases, so the surgeon can opt to convert to an SSc tenotomy at the superior half in order to achieve adequate exposure (**Fig. 2**).

To access the capsule, a pointed retractor is inserted within the SSc split. An inverse L-capsulotomy is carried out using a 15 blade, with the apex of the "L" positioned in the superomedial direction. The medial limb of the capsulotomy measures approximately 1 cm in length and extends to the glenoid neck. The lateral limb of the capsulotomy is extended laterally to the point where the fibers insert into the humeral head. To assist with capsular retraction and mobilization, a stay suture is placed in the superomedial corner of the capsule. This ensures that the anterior aspects of the GH joint and glenoid are fully exposed, with attention paid to palpating and safeguarding the axillary nerve, particularly in the inferior region.

A Fukuda retractor is carefully positioned within the GH joint to gently retract the humeral head laterally. A cobb is used to lift the adhered capsule away from the anterior glenoid. To facilitate optimal placement of the inferior graft, elevating the capsule as far inferior as possible is beneficial. If hardware is present from a prior surgery, the combination of an osteotome and rongeur is used to remove prior implants and debride scar tissue.

The anterior glenoid is then prepared for the graft by utilizing a high-speed burr and shaping it until the cortical layer exhibits signs of bleeding. Following this, a graft template block (7 or 10 mm sizes and angles of 5° or 15° [Arthrex, Naples, Florida]) is positioned onto the glenoid surface to verify complete exposure and confirm that the glenoid has been adequately prepared.

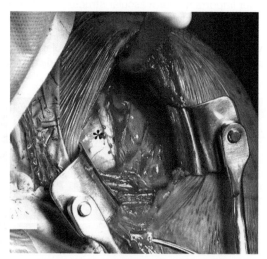

Fig. 2. Intraoperative image of a left shoulder in the beach chair position. A modified deltopectoral approach is used to visualize and access the GH joint. The lateral border of the conjoint tendon is then located, incised, and gently retracted medially. Asterisk denotes conjoint tendon.

Distal Tibia Allograft Preparation

On a preparation table, the fresh DTA should be precisely tailored to the necessary size, a determination made based on the preoperative CT scan planning and intraoperative measurements. The authors preferred method involves using the Distal Tibial Allograft Workstation (Arthrex, Naples, FL).[16]

The initial step entails placing the intramedullary section of the DTA over the cutting jig post of the DTA workstation, which firmly secures the allograft and simplifies the graft preparation process. To ensure optimal graft height and alignment, the deepest part of the lateral sulcus of the DTA should be aligned with the post (**Fig. 3**). The graft is fastened using 2 Kirshner wires (K-wires) through the graft post. Following this, the sizing template block, which has been selected as part of the glenoid preparation process, is positioned along the lateral surface of the DTA. This block is marked to indicate the center point, as well as the superior and inferior borders of the final graft placement. The graft is adjusted to align precisely with the center point indicated by the marker. This adjustment is done by loosening the black knobs and shifting the graft post accordingly.

The next step involves selecting the first cutting block assembly (CUT #1 and #2) to align with the desired angle and width indicated by the previously chosen sizing template. It is necessary to irrigate with normal saline in any steps that require the use of a sagittal saw or drill in order to ensure the viability of the cells and graft. Position the cutter stop securely into the "CUT #1" slot, ensuring a flush fit against the block. With this first cutting block, a sagittal saw with a 1 mm blade is used for the initial cut "CUT #1" slot, which removes the peroneal tubercle. It is essential to achieve an optimal graft cut with a flat surface before proceeding to the next step. Following this, an angled cut is performed using the "CUT #2" slot. Attention should be paid to ensure alignment between the blade's angle and the cutting guide.

The CUT #3 guide (graft thickness block) is positioned on top of the DTA. The height of the CUT #3 guide is adjusted to achieve a surface level similar to that of the articular surface and the sizing template. CUT #3 is carried out using an oscillating saw, with care taken to ensure that the saw blade maintains parallel alignment with the cutting guide and avoids any interference with the previously created drill holes (**Fig. 4**).

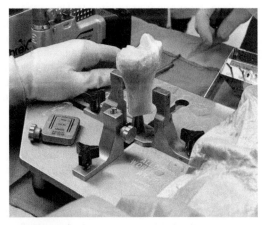

Fig. 3. On a back table, DTA graft preparation begins by placing the intramedullary portion of the DTA over the cutting jig post. It is important that the deepest part of the lateral sulcus of the DTA is aligned with the post.

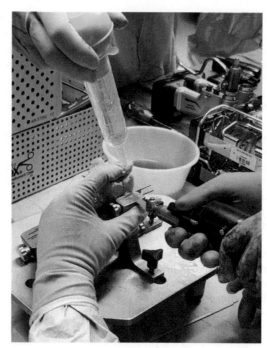

Fig. 4. DTA graft preparation on the back table. Cutting guide #3 (CUT #3) is in position, and its height is adjusted to achieve a surface level similar to that of the articular surface and the sizing template. It is important to provide copious irrigation to avoid overheating of the graft.

Vibrations from the saw can lead to loosening, thus, it is imperative to tighten all knobs periodically.

The final cut guide, CUT #4 (length cutter block), is firmly secured onto the post, ensuring it sits flush on top of the graft. This cutting block provides flexibility to produce grafts of varying sizes, from superior to inferior. Using the innermost slots, an 18 mm graft in length can be created. Using the outer slots will result in a 23 mm graft length, while using 1 inner slot and 1 outer slot will yield a 21.5 mm graft.

Next, a parallel guide with a finger projection is positioned directly over the graft, ensuring that the guide is precisely centered on the graft and is flush with the articular surface. Through this parallel drill guide, 2 K-wires are inserted (**Fig. 5**). A 4 mm cannulated drill is used to create 2 pilot holes, and then the K-wires are removed.

The graft is then carefully removed using the parallel drill guide, which is also used to position the graft against the glenoid. To verify the prepared graft's compatibility, the free graft guide can be used for comparison with the sizing template. Before fixation, it is advisable to use a sagittal saw to bevel the anterior edges of the graft using a free-hand technique. This step ensures that the graft is sized properly and will be fixated flush to the glenoid. The size of the distal tibia allows for another graft to be created, if necessary.

It is useful to use pulse lavage on the graft to eliminate any residual bone marrow components and reduce the potential for cross-reactivity and inflammatory reactions following graft fixation. The authors prefer to immerse the graft in an orthobiologic material, such as platelet-rich plasma, in order to facilitate and enhance the healing

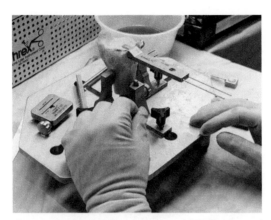

Fig. 5. DTA preparation on the back table. A guide with a finger projection is positioned directly over the graft, ensuring that the guide is precisely centered on the graft and is flush with the articular surface. Through this parallel drill guide, 2 K-wires are inserted and are used as a guide for drilling 2 pilot 4 mm holes.

process. In preparation for fixation, 2 K-wires are inserted into the graft at a 25° angle relative to the articular surface, thereby facilitating the graft's proper placement.

Graft Fixation

The graft is carefully positioned on the native glenoid to assess its conformity, size-match, and its angle relative to the articular surface, all guided by the finger guide and careful palpation. If necessary, further adjustments can be made to the graft to enhance its conformity. Once both the graft and the glenoid positions are deemed acceptable, 2 or 3 K-wires are used to provisionally secure the graft. It is crucial to ensure that there are no gaps along the glenoid articular surface.

Using a 2.5 mm drill, the glenoid screw holes are created at the predrilled graft holes. Following, two 3.75 mm fully threaded, noncannulated screws, equipped with suture washers (suture washer, titanium, with #2 FiberWire and curved needle, Arthrex, Naples, FL), are loaded with high tensile sutures, inserted through the graft, and then anchored into the glenoid (**Fig. 6**). The position, mobility, and stability of the graft are evaluated prior to the capsular closure.

The preloaded suture washers are used to secure the anterior capsule and labrum to the DTA, and the washers increase the peak torque allowed during screw insertion and allow for an increase in the load to failure.[18] In some instances, suture anchors may be used on the native glenoid, particularly at the inferior and superior margins of the graft, in order to facilitate the capsulolabral repair. The remaining portions of the capsule are repaired using permanent high tensile sutures. Following this, the repair of the SSc split uses standard techniques, utilizing high-strength, nonabsorbable sutures, and the remaining closure is performed.

Postoperative Rehabilitation

During the initial 2 weeks following the surgery, patients can engage in pendulum exercises and passive range of motion (ROM) exercises within the scapular plane and then progress to progressive passive ROM exercises. For the first 3 weeks postoperative, passive external rotation is restricted to a maximum of 30°. Starting at 4 weeks postoperative, patients are encouraged to progress to active-assisted ROM

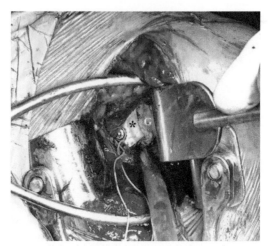

Fig. 6. Intraoperative picture after graft fixation. Two 3.75 mm fully threaded, noncannulated screws with a suture washer, loaded with a high tensile suture, are inserted through the graft and into the glenoid. G, glenoid articular surface; *, DTA graft.

exercises, which are then followed by progressing to active ROM exercises between weeks 6 and 8. Around weeks 6 to 8, a strengthening program is introduced. At 4 to 6 months postoperatively, patients can typically return to their regular duties and activities, so long as the patient is achieving satisfactory progress in terms of functional ROM, strength recovery, and successful graft incorporation. Obtaining a CT scan is the preferred method of assessing graft incorporation, but plain radiographs can also be utilized.

DISCUSSION

Several studies reported data on clinical outcomes of anterior glenoid reconstruction using DTA. Provencher and colleagues[9] conducted a retrospective review involving 27 patients, all of whom exhibited a minimum of 15% anterior GBL and had undergone anterior glenoid reconstruction using fresh DTA. Their findings revealed significant improvements in preoperative to postoperative functional outcomes, including the American Shoulder and Elbow Society Score (ASES; 63–91, $P < .01$), the Western Ontario Shoulder Instability Index (WOSI; 46% to 11% of normal, $P < .01$), Single Numerical Assessment Evaluation score (SANE; 50–90.5, $P < .01$), with an average follow-up duration of 45 months. Moreover, their study displayed a high allograft healing rate (89%, range, 80%–100%) at 1.4 years postoperatively through CT scan assessments (**Fig. 7**). The incidence of graft resorption remained low (3%, range, 0%–25%), and no instances of recurrent instability were observed within this study cohort.[9]

Wong and colleagues[19] studied an all-arthroscopic anatomic glenoid reconstruction using frozen DTA. They demonstrated excellent functional outcomes in the short-term to mid-term follow-up (mean follow-up, 4.7 ± 1.1 years), without any recurrence and a high union rate (100%). This arthroscopic approach to glenoid reconstruction with DTA augmentation showed excellent clinical and radiologic outcomes at the 2 year follow-up. This procedure has advantages, such as minimal invasiveness and anatomic reconstruction, effectively addressing both bone and soft tissue defects.[19]

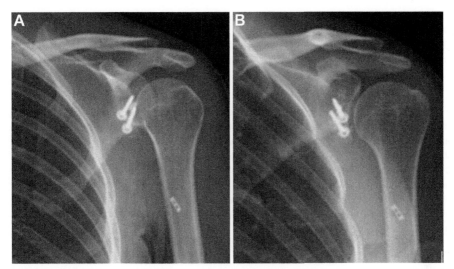

Fig. 7. Postoperative radiographs of a left shoulder that underwent DTA augmentation after a prior failed Latarjet procedure. (*A*) Anteroposterior (AP) view. (*B*) AP Grashey view.

Frank and colleagues[20] performed a matched cohort analysis of patients with a minimum of 15% anterior GBL, who had undergone either the DTA or Latarjet procedure for shoulder stabilization with a minimum of 2 years follow-up. The study revealed significant improvements in all postoperative outcome scores ($P < .05$ for all). No statistically significant differences were observed in the postoperative scores when comparing the Latarjet and DTA groups. Specifically, the scores for visual analog scale (VAS) (0.67 ± 0.97 vs 1.83 ± 2.31), ASES (91.06 ± 8.78 vs 89.74 ± 12.66), WOSI (74.30 ± 21.84 vs 89.69 ± 5.50), and SANE (80.68 ± 7.21 vs 90.08 ± 13.39) did not exhibit significant differences between the two groups ($P > .05$ for all). The overall complication rate for the entire cohort was 10%, comprised 5 cases in the Latarjet group (3 of which underwent reoperation) and 5 cases in the DTA group (3 of which underwent reoperation). The rate of recurrent instability was only 1% ($n = 1$). From these findings, it was concluded that anterior glenoid reconstruction using a fresh DTA leads to a clinically stable joint, yielding outcomes on par with the Latarjet procedure.[20]

While the Latarjet procedure has been performed since around 1954, there is a scarcity of literature that comprehensively outlines the optimal surgical techniques or the clinical outcomes following the revision of a failed Latarjet procedure. The use of DTA has been proposed as an alternative graft choice for anterior glenoid reconstruction in patients experiencing recurrent shoulder instability after a failed Latarjet procedure.

Provencher and colleagues[11] conducted a study investigating the clinical outcomes of 31 patients who underwent revision surgery using the DTA after a failed Latarjet procedure with an average follow-up of 47 months. There was a significant improvement in patient-reported outcomes from preoperative to postoperative assessments, as evidenced by improvements in the ASES (40–92, $P = .001$), SANE (44–91, $P = .001$), and WOSI (1300–310, $P = .001$). Preoperative CT scans revealed that 78% (range, 37%–100%) of the Latarjet coracoid graft had experienced resorption, with high rates of graft resorption and hardware complications. After undergoing the revision DTA procedure, there were no instances of recurrence, and final CT scans displayed complete union in 92% of the cases within the series.[11]

While patients with recurrent anterior shoulder instability following a failed Latarjet procedure present a challenging scenario, anterior glenoid reconstruction using fresh DTA emerges as a viable and highly effective revision procedure for addressing this patient population.

SUMMARY

The use of fresh DTA for anterior glenoid reconstruction proves to be a highly favorable choice for addressing cases of failed anterior shoulder stabilization with GBL. This approach offers numerous advantages, which include the lack of donor-site morbidity, the ability to effectively restore large glenoid defects, the reestablishment of articular congruency with the humeral head, restoration of glenoid biomechanics, and the addition of cartilage to the glenoid. Moreover, it is a robust and reliable option for managing failed stabilization procedures. Furthermore, it is associated with improvements in clinical outcomes and has an overall high rate of graft healing rate, all while maintaining a low incidence of recurrent instability.

CLINICS CARE POINTS

Pearls and pitfalls of anterior glenoid reconstruction using fresh DTA for failed shoulder stabilization.

Pearls	Pitfalls
• CT scans, especially 3 dimensional CT scans, are necessary to obtain preoperatively to accurately assess the amount of glenoid and humeral bone loss, and plan for graft size and position	• Inadequate preoperative imaging, planning, and templating can result in improper graft size and angulation
• Pathology and diagnosis are confirmed via EUA	
• Releasing any adhesions from the SSc allows for tendon excursion and to properly visualize the anterior glenoid	• Inadequate release of adhesions may prevent musculocutaneous nerve mobilization and may cause a traction injury to the nerve
• Make the SSc split medially at the level of the musculotendinous junction while avoiding over-medialization to decrease the risk of iatrogenic nerve injury	• The axillary nerve is protected and the area inferior to the SSc and the inferior aspect of the glenoid is avoided during the case
	• SSc split may have to be converted to an SSc tenotomy in the revision setting in order to have adequate exposure
• While making the cuts on the DTA, it is important to provide copious irrigation to avoid overheating the graft	
• A fixed, direct repair of the anterior capsule to the bone graft can be achieved by using a suture washer loaded with a permanent suture	
• Use of a powered rasp can help to provide a uniformly flat anterior glenoid surface	
• The graft is submersed in an orthobiologic (the authors prefer Platelet Rich Plasma) in order to enhance graft-to-bone healing prior to implantation	

DISCLOSURE

The authors declare that there are no relevant or material financial interests that directly relate to this work. Outside of this work, Matthew T. Provencher declares royalties from Arthrex, Inc. Arthrosurface, Responsive Arthroscopy (2020), and Anika Therapeutics, Inc.; Consulting fees from Arthrex, Inc., Joint Restoration Foundation (JRF), Zimmer Biomet Holdings, and Arthrosurface; received grants from the Department of Defense, United States (DoD), the National Institutes of Health, United States, (NIH), and the DJO (2020); Honoria from Flexion Therapeutics; is an editorial board or governing board member for SLACK, Inc.; Board or committee member for Arthoscopy Association of North America (AANA), American Academy of Orthopaedic Surgeons (AAOS), American Orthopaedic Society for Sports Medicine (AOSSM), ASES, San Diego Shoulder Institute (SDSI), and Society of Military Orthopaedic Surgeons (SOMOs); serves on the medical board of trustees for the Musculoskeletal Transplant Foundation (through 2018).

REFERENCES

1. Mauro CS, Voos JE, Hammoud S, et al. Failed anterior shoulder stabilization. J Shoulder Elbow Surg 2011;20(8):1340–50.
2. Provencher MT, Ferrari MB, Sanchez G, et al. Current treatment options for glenohumeral instability and bone loss: a critical analysis review. JBJS Rev 2017; 5(7):e6.
3. Provencher MT, Frank RM, Leclere LE, et al. The Hill-Sachs lesion: diagnosis, classification, and management. J Am Acad Orthop Surg 2012;20(4):242–52.
4. Burkhart SS, De Beer JF. Traumatic glenohumeral bone defects and their relationship to failure of arthroscopic Bankart repairs: significance of the inverted-pear glenoid and the humeral engaging Hill-Sachs lesion. Arthroscopy 2000;16(7): 677–94.
5. Tauber M, Resch H, Forstner R, et al. Reasons for failure after surgical repair of anterior shoulder instability. J Shoulder Elbow Surg 2004;13(3):279–85.
6. Menendez ME, Wong I, Tokish JM, et al. Free bone block procedures for glenoid reconstruction in anterior shoulder instability. J Am Acad Orthop Surg 2023; 31(21):1103–11.
7. Provencher MT, Midtgaard KS, Owens BD, et al. Diagnosis and management of traumatic anterior shoulder instability. J Am Acad Orthop Surg 2021;29(2): e51–61.
8. Bhatia S, Van Thiel GS, Gupta D, et al. Comparison of glenohumeral contact pressures and contact areas after glenoid reconstruction with latarjet or distal tibial osteochondral allografts. Am J Sports Med 2013;41(8):1900–8.
9. Provencher MT, Frank RM, Golijanin P, et al. Distal tibia allograft glenoid reconstruction in recurrent anterior shoulder instability: clinical and radiographic outcomes. Arthroscopy 2017;33(5):891–7.
10. Provencher MT, Ghodadra N, LeClere L, et al. Anatomic osteochondral glenoid reconstruction for recurrent glenohumeral instability with glenoid deficiency using a distal tibia allograft. Arthroscopy 2009;25(4):446–52.
11. Provencher MT, Peebles LA, Aman ZS, et al. Management of the failed latarjet procedure: outcomes of revision surgery with fresh distal tibial allograft. Am J Sports Med 2019;47(12):2795–802.
12. Parada SA, Griffith MS, Shaw KA, et al. Demographics and distal tibial dimensions of suitable distal tibial allografts for glenoid reconstruction. Arthroscopy 2019;35(10):2788–94.

13. Haber DB, Sanchez A, Sanchez G, et al. Bipolar bone loss of the shoulder joint due to recurrent instability: use of fresh osteochondral distal tibia and humeral head allografts. Arthrosc Tech 2017;6(3):e893–9.
14. Peebles LA, Aman ZS, Preuss FR, et al. Multidirectional shoulder instability with bone loss and prior failed latarjet procedure: treatment with fresh distal tibial allograft and modified t-plasty open capsular shift. Arthrosc Tech 2019;8(5):e459–64.
15. Liles JL, Ganokroj P, Peebles AM, et al. Primary distal tibia allograft for restoration of glenohumeral stability with anterior glenoid bone loss. Arthrosc Tech 2022; 11(6):e1039–43.
16. Liles JL, Ganokroj P, Peebles AM, et al. Fresh distal tibial allograft: an updated graft preparation technique for anterior shoulder instability. Arthrosc Tech 2022; 11(6):e1027–31.
17. Sanchez A, Ferrari MB, Akamefula RA, et al. Anatomical glenoid reconstruction using fresh osteochondral distal tibia allograft after failed latarjet procedure. Arthrosc Tech 2017;6(2):e477–82.
18. Parada SA, Shaw KA, McGee-Lawrence ME, et al. Anterior glenoid reconstruction with distal tibial allograft: biomechanical impact of fixation and presence of a retained lateral cortex. Orthop J Sports Med 2021;9(11). 23259671211050435.
19. Wong I, John R, Ma J, et al. Arthroscopic anatomic glenoid reconstruction using distal tibial allograft for recurrent anterior shoulder instability: clinical and radiographic outcomes. Am J Sports Med 2020;48(13):3316–21.
20. Frank RM, Romeo AA, Richardson C, et al. Outcomes of latarjet versus distal tibia allograft for anterior shoulder instability repair: a matched cohort analysis. Am J Sports Med 2018;46(5):1030–8.

Current Evidence and Techniques for Arthroscopic Bone Augmentation

Jillian Karpyshyn, MD, FRCSC, Jie Ma, MES,
Ivan Wong, MD, FRCSC, MAcM, Dip Sports Med, FAANA*

KEYWORDS

- Shoulder instability • Glenoid bone loss
- Arthroscopic anatomic glenoid reconstruction • Distal tibial allografts • Outcomes

KEY POINTS

- Clinical outcomes and rates of instability recurrence reported in arthroscopic anatomic glenoid reconstruction (AAGR) are similar to results following open bone block procedures and arthroscopic Latarjet.
- The most important factors to consider when planning surgery for recurrent anterior shoulder instability are the amount of glenoid bone loss, status of the capsulolabral complex, presence of off-track Hill–Sachs lesions, young male individuals, contact or overhead sport participation, and a high number of instability events preoperatively.
- Utilization of the Halifax portal allows proper trajectory of screws and prevents malreduction of the graft after final fixation.
- Repair of the capsulolabral complex over the graft is essential; therefore, in patients with insignificant capsulolabral complex remaining, a Latarjet procedure is recommended.
- Further evidence is needed regarding optimal bone graft type in AAGR.

INTRODUCTION

Traumatic anterior shoulder instability is a commonly encountered injury in young and active patients.[1] Approximately 2% of the population experience a shoulder dislocation in their lifetime and up to 70% of patients who dislocate once will experience a subsequent dislocation.[2] A resulting glenoid rim defect is reported in as high as 22% and 90% for initial and recurrent dislocations, respectively,[3,4] and can lead to an unacceptably high failure rate of soft tissue stabilization procedures.[5–7] Historically, a glenoid defect of greater than 20% was considered an indication for bone augmentation surgery; however, recently, more attention has been drawn to functional bone

Division of Orthopaedics, Department of Surgery, Dalhousie University, Halifax, Nova Scotia, Canada
* Corresponding author. 2106 - 5955 Veterans Memorial Lane, Halifax, NS B3H 2E1.
E-mail address: iw@drivanwong.com

Clin Sports Med 43 (2024) 661–682
https://doi.org/10.1016/j.csm.2024.03.023
0278-5919/24/© 2024 Elsevier Inc. All rights reserved.

loss with the introduction of the glenoid track concept. As a result, the indications for bone augmentation procedures have widened to include patients with less pronounced glenoid defects and have increased interest in determining the optimal bone augmentation procedure.

Several procedures have been described to augment the glenoid rim, which include open and arthroscopic techniques. The Latarjet procedure has been considered the gold standard for management of bone loss. Although this procedure has reported satisfying long-term results with low recurrence rate,[6,8] it has been associated with significant complication rates of up to 30%. The arthroscopic Latarjet has been described[9,10]; however, the procedure has gained limited popularity in North America because of the difficult surgical technique, steep learning curve, and similar rates of complication to the open Latarjet.[11] In cases of failure, the revision surgery becomes even more challenging due to the altered normal anatomy.

Free bone reconstruction with autograft or allograft is considered an alternative surgical option to the Latarjet procedure. Free bone blocks not only achieve anatomic reconstruction of the glenoid but are also the main revision strategy for a failed Latarjet. Free bone reconstruction has shown similar functional scores, complications, and recurrent instability rates when compared to Latarjet.[12] Furthermore, the importance of the sling effect achieved in coracoid transfer procedures via the conjoint tendon has been called into question recently.[13] Open anatomic glenoid reconstruction with free bone grafts was initially described with iliac crest autograft by Eden and Hybinette[14] and subsequently with distal tibial allograft (DTA) by Provencher and colleagues,[15] which have shown similar excellent clinical outcomes and recurrence rates to Latarjet.[16] However, violation of the subscapularis muscle in open techniques can lead to functional deficits and has been shown to cause weakness in isometric subscapularis muscle strength.[17]

Arthroscopic anatomic glenoid reconstruction (AAGR) has been described as the use of a bone block graft to restore glenoid shape, depth, and width while preserving the native coracoid.[18] It was developed to avoid damage to the subscapularis musculotendinous unit seen with open techniques through shuttling of the graft through the rotator interval.[17,19,20] Multiple grafts have been described for use in AAGR, including iliac crest bone autograft/allograft (ICBG), DTA, clavicle autograft, and scapular spine autograft. AAGR decreases the risk of severe neurovascular compromise, allows concomitant pathologies to be addressed, and patients have been shown to have less pain[21] and stiffness[10] in the early postoperative period. It has been associated with good results, low recurrence rates, minimal complications, and a relatively easy learning curve with the ability to teach the technique virtually. Additionally, a recent systematic review and meta-analysis by Wei and colleagues[22] found that arthroscopic bone block surgery had a lower incidence of recurrent instability compared to open surgery (2.3% vs 4.1%) as well as a lower incidence of noninstability-related complications (3.9% vs 7.2%). This review focuses on the biomechanics, patient workup, current evidence, and the authors' preferred surgical technique for AAGR.

CRITICAL/SUBCRITICAL BONE LOSS

Anterior glenoid bone loss is one of the most important risk factors for recurrent dislocation. "Critical" bone loss, or the amount of bone loss associated with recurrent instability, is often defined as a glenoid defect of 20% to 25% and is an indication for a bone block augmentation.[4,23–28] Cadaveric testing showed that forces required for dislocation were significantly reduced with a loss of 19% of the glenoid rim.[29]

Similar results have been found in clinical studies. Glenoid bone loss greater than 25% is an independent predictor of failure and was associated with a 75% failure rate of arthroscopic soft tissue stabilization in one series.[30,31]

Recently, increased understanding of the importance of the location and size of bony lesions through concepts such as the glenoid track theory have improved algorithms of bipolar lesions and glenoid bone loss in the "subcritical" zone. Studies have shown increased failure rates and worsened functional outcomes after soft tissue stabilization procedures with bone loss in subcritical ranges of 13.5% to 17.3%.[32–35] Garcia and colleagues[36] showed that in cases with large Hill–Sachs lesions and minimal glenoid bone loss of 5.3%, the failure rate of Bankart repair alone was 50%. Further, a cadaveric study[2] showed that even small Hill–Sachs defects involving less than 19% of the articular surface in the presence of a glenoid defect of 10% to 20% may contribute to clinical instability.

GRAFT BIOMECHANICS

The radius of curvature of a selected graft in relation to the native glenohumeral articulation is an important consideration when performing bony augmentation of the glenoid. In comparison to the lateral coracoid and iliac crest grafts, DTA and the inferior coracoid have been found to have the most similar radius of curvature to the glenoid.[37] Provencher and colleagues[15] and Willemot and colleagues[38] examined DTAs and found nearly identical radius of curvature to the glenoid and good conformation to the humeral head. Furthermore, reconstruction with DTA has shown significantly greater glenohumeral contact areas and lower contact pressure and peak force compared with coracoid bone block in a cadaveric model.[39] Clavicular autograft is a relatively new graft option; however. it has encouraging results in initial biomechanic studies. A recent cadaveric study found that although the articular cartilage of the glenoid was significantly thicker than the distal clavicle cartilage, the clavicle graft was able to reconstruct 44% of the glenoid diameter compared to 33% using a coracoid graft.[40]

PATIENT EVALUATION
History

Evaluation of the patient's history, physical examination, and imaging allows the clinician to make an appropriate diagnosis when a patient presents with shoulder instability as a primary complaint. A detailed patient history should include preinjury level, age at the time of first dislocation, mechanism of injury, generalized ligamentous laxity, total number of dislocations, previous treatment, activity level, and expectations for the treatment. Several findings on history may increase the likelihood of having associated bone loss.

1. Dislocations that occur with lower energy events and with simple activities of daily living.
2. Initial high-energy traumatic event, typically involving a mechanism that axially loads the glenoid.[5]
3. Progressive ease of subluxation.
4. Symptoms for greater than 5 months.[41]

Physical Examination

The physical examination for an unstable shoulder should be comprehensive and systematic. Both shoulders should be assessed for deformity, scapular dyskinesis, and rotator cuff atrophy. A thorough neurovascular examination should be performed, as well as active and passive range of motion (ROM) and rotator cuff strength, with special attention to subscapularis function. Special tests for glenohumeral instability include apprehension test, relocation test, sulcus sign, surprise test, load and shift test, and anterior drawer and posterior drawer test.[42] These should be compared to the contralateral shoulder. Of note, when performing the apprehension test, a greater relative degree of early and midrange (20–60°) apprehension is more likely seen with bony involvement.[43] The Beighton score can be used to assess for joint hypermobility. Additionally, attention should be paid to differentiate between unidirectional and multidirectional instability. A sulcus sign is characteristic of multidirectional instability and a posterior jerk test or push–pull test can be indicative of posterior or combined instability.[42]

Imaging

Routine anteroposterior (AP) shoulder radiographs with the shoulder in external rotation and a true AP radiograph is recommended. The loss of contour or irregularities of the sclerotic line on the anteroinferior glenoid can be assessed on the true AP, which can raise suspicion for glenoid rim defect. The lateral Y view can assess translation in the sagittal plane and help to confirm whether the dislocation is anterior or posterior. The apical oblique and west point views are additional radiographs that can assess for glenoid bone defects.

Advanced imaging such as MRI and CT are often obtained, especially if there is a concern for glenoid bone loss. Accurate determination of the degree and location of glenoid and humeral bone loss is essential to guide treatment. Multiple validated techniques have been described to quantify the amount of glenoid bone loss on CT, which have been summarized in **Table 1**. Measurements of Hill–Sachs lesions, however, are highly variable within the literature with no agreement in terms of technique.

Intraoperative Assessment

A thorough examination of the amount of bone loss is critical prior to performing a bony reconstruction. The anteroposterior width of the defect at the level of the bare spot is measured and compared to measurements obtained from the preoperative

Table 1 Methods to quantify the amount of glenoid bone loss	
The circle method[44]	A best fit circle is drawn on the inferior two-thirds of the glenoid on a three-dimensional CT (3D CT). The amount of missing bone from the circle is then quantified as a percentage of the total surface area of the glenoid. This method has also been shown to be accurate in MRI studies.[45]
Flat anterior glenoid[46]	An easily recognizable pattern of a flat anterior glenoid on 3D CT corresponds to a 13% glenoid bone loss.
Measurements based on contralateral CT	
Assessment based on ipsilateral glenoid height[47]	The height (H) of the glenoid is measured from the superior pole of the glenoid at the level of the base of the coracoid (12 o'clock position) to the inferior pole (6 o'clock position) of the glenoid. The width is then measured perpendicular to this line. The expected width (W) of the glenoid is calculated as $W = 2.53 \text{ mm} + 0.71 \text{ H}$

CT scan. This will determine the size of bone block required for accurate reconstruction of the glenoid. Additionally, assessment of the capsulolabral complex should be performed, and if there is inadequate capsulolabral tissue remaining, reconstruction with a free bone block may not be indicated due to the inability to perform a capsulolabral repair over the graft.

INDICATIONS AND CONTRAINDICATIONS

Although indications for AAGR have not been clearly established, the following indications and contraindications can be suggested in **Box 1** based on the literature, including a recent international consensus statement and the authors' experience:[48,49]

Algorithm

The most important factors to take into consideration when choosing the optimal surgical procedure for a patient with recurrent shoulder instability are:

1. Amount of glenoid bone loss
2. Presence or absence of a Hill–Sachs lesion and whether it is on track or off track
3. The status of the capsulolabral tissue.

For smaller glenoid lesions (<13.5%), Bankart repair with or without remplissage still remains an excellent option with good outcomes. However, for patients with bone loss in the subcritical range (13.5%–20%), patients with risk factors such as an off-track Hill–Sachs lesion, young men, contact or overhead sport participation, or a high number of instability events preoperatively would benefit from a bony procedure. If the patient has no additional risk factor, surgeon preference is warranted. For larger defects, the Latarjet procedure or AAGR is indicated; however, in higher ranges of bone loss, free bone block reconstruction is recommended due to the limit in size that can be obtained from a coracoid autograft. When arthroscopic free bone grafting is performed, it

---

Box 1
Indications and contraindications for arthroscopic anatomic glenoid reconstruction.

Indications
1. Anterior glenoid bone loss >20%
2. Bone loss 13.5% to 20% with bipolar off-track Hill–Sachs lesion
3. Bone loss greater than can be treated with a coracoid transfer
4. Surgeon preference
5. Failed prior Latarjet or bone grafting procedure
6. Epilepsy[48,50]
7. Primary episode of shoulder instability in high-risk patient (young men playing contact and overhead sports)
8. Recurrent instability following Bankart repair

Contraindications
1. Minimal bone loss
2. Infection
3. Axial nerve injury
4. Multidirectional instability
5. Voluntary dislocators
6. Uncontrolled epilepsy
7. Irreparable rotator cuff (RC) tear
8. Shoulder contractures
9. Severe osteoarthritis (OA)
10. Poor quality of capsulolabral tissue

is essential to perform a capsulolabral complex reconstruction. This creates a capsular effect which is similar to the sling effect described in the Latarjet procedure. Therefore, when patients with poor and fragile capsules are encountered, AAGR is contraindicated and the Latarjet procedure should be performed instead.[51] The authors' current algorithm for shoulder instability is depicted in **Fig. 1.**

AUTHORS' PREFERRED SURGICAL TECHNIQUE

Multiple techniques for AAGR exist in the literature with considerable heterogeneity in positioning, number and location of portals, avoidance of subscapularis, and graft type.[18,49,52] The authors' preferred surgical technique for AAGR for patients with critical or subcritical bone loss is described with DTA utilizing the Halifax portal and a capsulolabral repair in the following.

Preoperatively, a 3D CT scan is evaluated to determine the amount of glenoid bone loss. The height (H) of the glenoid is measured from the superior pole of the glenoid at the level of the base of the coracoid (12 o'clock position) to the inferior pole (6 o'clock position) of the glenoid. The width is then measured perpendicular to this line as depicted in **Fig. 2**. The expected width (W) of the glenoid is calculated as $W = 2.53$ mm $+ 0.71H$[47] and used to determine the size of graft harvested. A 3D printed model of the patient's scapula is then examined to determine the optimal location and trajectory of the posterior portal in order to be parallel with the face of the glenoid.

The patient is placed under general anesthetic and is given tranexamic acid and cefazolin intravenously. Examination under anesthesia is performed, evaluating the amount of anterior, posterior, and inferior translation, as well as the spontaneity of reduction once over the glenoid rim.

The patient is placed in the semilateral decubitus position with a slight posterior body tilt at 30° from vertical with a bean bag positioner. The arm is placed in a pneumatic arm holder and is abducted 60° in balanced suspension. Patient

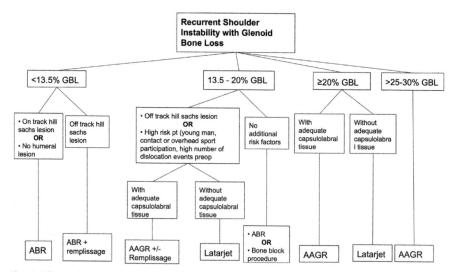

Fig. 1. The authors' suggested algorithm for treatment of recurrent anterior shoulder instability with glenoid bone loss. ABR, arthroscopic Bankart repair; AAGR, arthroscopic anatomic glenoid reconstruction; GBL, glenoid bone loss.

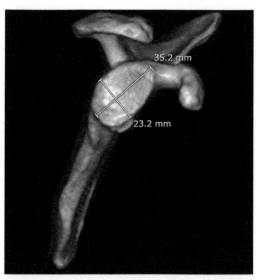

Fig. 2. Preoperative measurement of glenoid bone loss. The height of the glenoid is measured from the superior pole of the glenoid at the level of the base of the coracoid (12 o'clock position) to the inferior pole (6 o'clock position) of the glenoid. The width is then measured perpendicular to this line.

positioning in slight posterior body tilt is an exceedingly important step to ensure adequate arthroscopic visualization. Standard skin landmarks are drawn on the patient and a posterior portal is established first based on the preoperative evaluation of the 3D printed scapula. A diagnostic arthroscopy is performed with evaluation of all intra-articular structures. The integrity of the articular cartilage, biceps anchor, and labrum are assessed, and arthroscopic photographs are taken to document the injury.

An anteroinferior portal is landmarked with a spinal needle, entering the joint at the intersection of the biceps tendon and lateral subscapularis border. The spinal needle is used to ensure that the anteroinferior glenoid (6 o'clock position) can be reached prior to making an incision and insertion of a cannula. The rotator interval is then opened using a shaver and cautery until the CA ligament and conjoint tendon are visualized (**Fig. 3**). An anterosuperior portal is then created and becomes the main viewing portal. The location and trajectory of the posterior portal is then examined to ensure that it is parallel to the glenoid face, and adjustments are made if necessary. Assessment of the degree of glenoid bone loss is performed by visualizing the shape of the glenoid, looking for the inverted pear morphology described by Lo and colleagues,[25] as well as by direct measurement with a probe inserted from the posterior portal. The presence of a Hill–Sachs lesion is documented and measured as the distance from the cuff insertion to intact cartilage.

A spectrum is used to pass a traction suture through the labral and capsular tissue at the 3 o'clock position. Following this, an episiotomy of the labrum is performed between the biceps anchor and the traction suture. The suture is shuttled out of the cannula and a snap is placed against the skin to provide traction.

The labral and capsular tissue are then elevated from the anterior glenoid rim toward the 6 o'clock position and burr is used to flatten the anterior–inferior surface of the glenoid and expose bleeding bone. The glenoid is marked at the 3 o'clock position, which denotes where the center of the graft should line up.

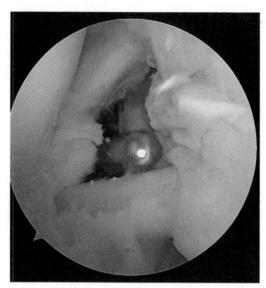

Fig. 3. Arthroscopic view from the posterior portal showing the CA ligament and conjoint tendon following opening of the rotator interval.

A fresh-frozen, nonirradiated DTA from the opposite sided limb is used for this arthroscopic reconstruction. Typically, a graft measuring 1.5 cm in height, 2 cm in thickness, and 1 cm in width is measured and harvested from the anterolateral surface of the distal tibia; however, preoperative and intraoperative measurements of bone loss should guide the width of the harvested graft (**Fig. 4**). A small bevel can be added to the graft on the glenoid side in order to maximize bony contact. Two Kirschner wires are then inserted through a guide into the graft, parallel to the cartilage. This is then over drilled and tapped prior to 2 top hat washers being inserted into the tapped holes.

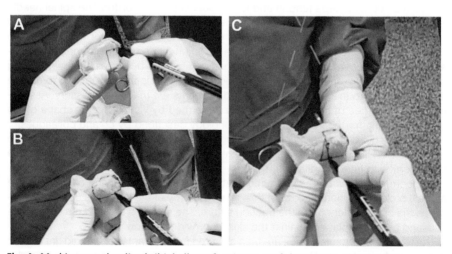

Fig. 4. Markings on the distal tibial allograft prior to graft harvest (*A-C*). A graft measuring 1.5 cm in height, 2 cm in thickness, and 1 cm in width is typically harvested; however, intra-operative measurements of bone loss should guide the final width of the graft.

The DTA graft is loaded onto a double-barrel cannula and then irrigated with normal saline solution and saturated in gentamicin solution.

Once graft preparation is complete, the Halifax portal is made. A switching stick is inserted into the posterior portal parallel to the glenoid. The arm is internally rotated and adducted to reduce subscapularis tension. The switching stick is used to pass superior to the subscapularis tendon (retracting it inferiorly), lateral to the conjoint tendon, and toward the anterior axilla. An approximately 4 cm skin incision is made over the switching stick. Two half-pipe cannulas are inserted into the Halifax portal over the switching stick, which is subsequently removed. The graft is then advanced through the 2 half pipes and advanced toward the anterior inferior glenoid. A switching stick is used to help position the graft and make sure it stays level to the glenoid cartilage.

Two K-wires are used to drill through the double-barrel cannula. First, attention should be taken to ensure the graft is as inferior as possible on the glenoid. Small adjustments in rotation can be made following this to ensure that the graft is flush with the glenoid cartilage. Alternating insertion and removal of each K-wire can be done in order to adjust the final position of the graft into the correct position. A calibrated drill bit is used to drill through the graft and native glenoid and measure screw length. Two 4.0 mm cannulated cortical screws are inserted over the K-wires until flush to the top hats, compressing the graft to the native glenoid (**Fig. 5**).

The capsulolabral tissue is then reduced over the graft. Anchors are placed in the 6 and 3 o'clock position and sequentially tied over the capsulolabral tissue using a spectrum. The traction suture is then shifted from the 3 o'clock position and inserted in a knotless anchor, just anterior to the biceps anchor. The reconstruction and repair are then assessed to ensure:

1. The humeral head is balanced onto the glenoid.
2. The Bankart repair completely covers the graft.
3. The graft is compressed to the glenoid without any gapping.

Postoperatively, the patient is placed in an external rotation brace with passive ROM initiated by a physiotherapist immediately. Active ROM starts at 4 weeks, and a strengthening program and scapular training are started at 6 weeks.

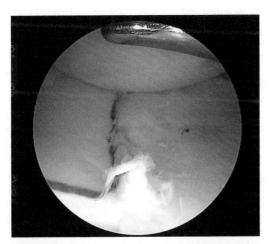

Fig. 5. View from the anterosuperior portal of the distal tibial allograft following insertion of 2 cannulated screws. The graft is placed as inferior as possible on the glenoid and flush with the glenoid surface.

Clinics care points

1. A DTA from the opposite side as the shoulder undergoing surgery should be used.
2. A 30° posterior tilt is essential to allow adequate visualization of the anterior inferior glenoid. Any anterior tilting will make visualization difficult.
3. A lateral jack and an assistant to pull the humerus posteriorly and lateral will further increase view of the anteroinferior glenoid.
4. Draping medial to the nipple line and inferior to the axilla is essential in order to develop the Halifax portal.
5. Opening of the rotator interval and visualization of the CA ligament and conjoint tendon is an essential step to allow visualization of critical structures and to facilitate insertion of the graft.
6. The traction suture is key for viewing, exposing the anterior glenoid, and shifting the capsule superiorly from the 3 to 12 o'clock position.
7. The anterior glenoid surface must be flat, and a small bevel can be added to the graft on the glenoid side to maximize bony contact.

OUTCOMES/DISCUSSION

Clinical outcomes after AAGR are successful in treating shoulder instability, as shown in **Table 2**. A recent systematic review and meta-analysis on clinical and radiographic outcomes of AAGR for recurrent anterior instability analyzed 15 studies and included 165 patients.[53] Although the majority of the studies were level 3 or 4 evidence, the mean length of follow-up was 30.4 months with validated clinical outcomes. There was a significant improvement in functional and instability scores, with similar scores previously reported in open and arthroscopic Latarjet procedures.[54,55] Recurrent instability was reported as 6.6% of the pooled population with 7 dislocations and 10 persistent subluxations and graft union was greater than 90% in the majority of the studies. Since this systematic review, 5 studies have been completed examining AAGR and have shown failure rates ranging from 0% to 11%.[7,51,56–58]

Although the majority of studies on AAGR have reported on short-term outcomes, there have been 2 authors to report midterm results with a minimum follow-up of 5 years.[51,72] Boehm and colleagues[72] evaluated 14 patients undergoing AAGR with ICBG autograft and reported satisfactory clinical and radiologic outcomes with a mean follow-up of 6.5 years (78.7 months) and a reported dislocation rate of 7% (1 of 14). Ueda and colleagues[51] evaluated 24 shoulders with ICBG autograft augmentation with a mean follow-up of 8 years. Although they found excessive graft resorption in 13%, they only had one recurrent dislocation (4%). The mechanism of dislocation in both of these studies was reported as due to highly traumatic events. In comparison, the rate of recurrence reported in the literature is 1.9% to 3.4% for arthroscopic Latarjet, 1.4% to 8.5% for open Latarjet, and up to 9.8% for open iliac bone block techniques.[6,21,74] The remainder of this discussion will focus on comparative studies and current evidence for different graft choices in AAGR, including union rate, amount of resorption, arthritic progression, and different techniques for fixation of the graft.

Comparative Studies

Three comparative studies between the AAGR and Latarjet procedure have been published to this date. Wong and colleagues[65] and Moga and colleagues.[66] assessed arthroscopic DTA compared to arthroscopic Latarjet. Although DTA did show a higher rate of resorption (83%) compared to coracoid (42%), there was no significant difference in graft union and the anteroposterior dimensions of the reconstructed glenoid, with 2 patients experiencing subluxations in the coracoid group (16%) as well as 2

Table 2
Outcomes of arthroscopic anatomic glenoid reconstruction

Study	Level of Evidence	Number of Subjects	Mean Age (Years)	Surgical Technique	Length of Follow-up (Months)	Outcomes
Kraus et al,[59] 2014	4	15	41.4	ICBG autograft	20.6	No dislocations. 1 patient described shoulder as unstable Mean graft resorption: 14.7% Graft union in all patients
Zhao et al,[60] 2014	4	52	26.3	ICBG autograft	39	Failure rate of 5.8% (1 redislocation and 2 patients with sense of instability without dislocation) 100% union rate Mean graft resorption: 32.3%
Anderl et al,[61] 2016	4	15	30	ICBG autograft	25.9	No dislocations Mean graft resorption of 10% No progression of GH arthritis
Nebelung et al,[62] 2016	5	24	29	ICBG autograft	19	No dislocations 100% union rate
Giannakos et al,[63] 2017	4	12	37.5	ICBG autograft	28.8	No dislocations. 2 patients (17%) with persistent subluxations, 5 with persistent apprehension Union rate of 58.3% Complete resorption in 1 patient (8%) Progression of arthritis in 2 patients
Amar et al,[64] 2018	4	36	26.73	DTA	16	No dislocations. 1 patient with positive shoulder apprehension test 100% union rate No graft resorption in 42%, 50% graft resorption in 42%, >50% resorption in 16%

(continued on next page)

Table 2
(continued)

Study	Level of Evidence	Number of Subjects	Mean Age (Years)	Surgical Technique	Length of Follow-up (Months)	Outcomes
Wong et al,[65] 2018	3	36	29.7	DTA	26.12	No dislocations, 2 subluxations (5.5%) 94% union rate No graft resorption in 42%, 50% graft resorption in 42%, >50% resorption in 16%
Moga et al,[66] 2018	3	27	29	DTA	24	AAGR significantly faster to perform than arthroscopic Latarjet (AL) Desired position of graft on glenoid identified more often in AAGR than AL
Taverna et al,[67] 2018	4	26	25.5	DTA	29.6	1 posterior redislocation 92.30% union rate Complete graft resorption in 1 patient (4%) Post-op arthritis in 1 patient (4%)
Bockman et al,[68] 2018	4	32	32	ICBG autograft	42	3 post-traumatic dislocations
Bockman et al,[69] 2019	3	9	31	ICBG autograft	34	No redislocations Thickness of graft cartilage/scar tissue comparable to native cartilage on contralateral side
Boileau et al,[70] 2019	4	7	30.7	ICBG autograft	18	No redislocations 100% union rate Arthritic changes in 2 patients (29%)
Boehm et al,[71] 2020	4	10	31.9	ICBG autograft	23.2	No redislocations, 1 persistent subluxation, 3 positive apprehension tests Mean graft resorption 31.8%
Boehm et al,[72] 2020	4	14	31.1	ICBG autograft	78.7	1 post-traumatic dislocation 100% graft union Mean graft resorption 16.2% Arthritic changes in 8 patients (57%)

Study				Graft		Outcomes
Malik et al,[73] 2020	4	22	27.7	ICBG autograft (12) or allograft (10)	26.6	ICBG allograft: 1 dislocation and 1 subluxation ICBG autograft: 1 dislocation and 1 subluxation Union rate: 37.5% in allograft and 84% in autograft Resorption: 75% partial resorption in allograft, 40% partial resorption in autograft
Ueda et al,[51] 2021	4	25	30	ICBG autograft	96	1 traumatic shoulder dislocation (4%) 54% graft remodeling 13% with excessive resorption Arthritic changes in 50%
Russo et al,[57] 2021	4	19	27.5	ICBG autograft	34.6	2 traumatic dislocations (11%) Graft resorption seen in all patients (partial in 9 and complete in 10) No arthritic changes
Tucker et al,[7] 2022	3	174	23.4 in ABR 29.37 in AAGR	DTA (67) or ABR (107)	24	No redislocations in AAGR group, 25 redislocations in ABR group Noninstability complication rate: 12% in AAGR and 11% in ABR
Mahmoud et al,[56] 2022	2	50	27.7	ICBG autograft (25), Coracoid (25)	50.1	No dislocations in ICBG group, 1 dislocation in Latarjet group 92% union in ICBG, 100% union in Latarjet Partial graft resorption in 2 ICBG patents, none in Latarjet Overall complication rate: 24% in ICBG, 4% in Latarjet

Abbreviation: ABR, arthroscopic Bankart repair. GH, glenohumeral.

patients in the DTA group (6%). Additionally, arthroscopic Latarjet was associated with a higher incidence of articular step compared to AAGR with DTA. AAGR with bone block took less time in all phases of the learning curve and achieved desired graft positioning with more consistency (89% vs 70%). Mahmoud and colleagues[56] compared arthroscopic ICBG autograft to mini open Latarjet procedure among 50 patients. They reported no difference in patient-reported outcomes and ROM between the groups; however, they noted a higher complication rate in the ICBG group (24%) compared to Latarjet group (4%). The ICBG group had no dislocations, whereas 1 dislocation was noted in the Latarjet group (4%). The 6 complications in the ICBG group were all noninstability-related complications, with 2 partial graft resorptions, 3 bone graft morbidities, and 1 hardware prominence. These results are inconsistent with the literature which find a much higher rate of complications with the Latarjet procedure and suggest that further comparative studies are needed.

Graft Choice: Allograft or Autograft

Graft choice in AAGR is highly debated. Several factors go into consideration when determining the optimal graft. Autograft has the benefit of being readily available, low cost, and has no risk of disease transmission. Kraus and colleagues[59] and Taverna and colleagues[75] described an arthroscopic technique utilizing an intra-articular autologous tricortical iliac crest graft with satisfying results. Limitations of this technique involve the high donor site morbidity and concerns for long-term osteoarthritis due to the lack of articular cartilage on the iliac crest graft.[76] Fortun and colleagues[77] described a variation of this technique with the addition of a Bankart repair, making the graft extra-articular, and sparing of the subscapularis muscle. The safety of this technique was studied showing no intraoperative complications, no dislocations post-op, and complete graft union in 11 of 12 patients.[78] Tokish and colleagues[79] recently described an arthroscopic technique utilizing distal clavicular osteochondral autograft in order to decrease the chance of osteoarthritis related to a graft without articular cartilage. This has been shown to provide excellent reconstruction of the glenoid surface area in a cadaveric study[40]; however, no clinical studies have been conducted using this technique thus far. Similarly, scapular autograft has been described,[80] with promising short-term clinical results and radiographic healing at 1 year,[58] but no mid-term to long-term results.

Allografts offer certain advantages such as avoidance of donor site morbidity and potentially decreasing the risk of osteoarthritis progression with certain allografts by recreating a cartilage-lined concave surface for humeral head articulation. Tricortical iliac crest allograft has shown excellent results with a 2% redislocation and 100% graft integration rate at a mean of 39 months in one study.[60] Wong and Urquhart[52] described a subscapularis-sparing AAGR technique with DTA through the Halifax portal with an additional inferior to superior capsular shift of the capsulolabral complex.[81] This technique has shown excellent short-term and mid-term clinical outcomes, with good graft positioning and healing rate on CT, with a recurrence rate of 3%.[64,82,83] Additionally, the safety profile of the Halifax portal has been established, showing it to be a safe distance from neurovascular structures with no intraoperative complications in one series.[64,84]

In a recent systematic review and meta-analysis including both open and arthroscopic bone block procedures, Wei and colleagues[22] found that autograft had a higher incidence of recurrent instability than allograft (4.4% vs 1.5%), which is inconsistent with previous findings that reported equivalent recurrence rates between autograft and allograft.[73,85] Autograft also had a higher rate of noninstability-related complications (8.1% vs 3.4%), where the primary complications related to autograft were high incidence of pain, hematoma, and nerve sensation at donor site. Additionally, they found that DTA and coracoid grafts had a lower recurrence rate than surgery with iliac crest grafts. Malik and colleagues[73] compared outcomes of AAGR in 10 patients with allograft ICBG to 12 patients with autograft ICBG. They found no difference in recurrent instability with 2 failures in each group; however, clinical outcome scores were higher in the autograft group. Boehm and colleagues noticed complete graft resorption and a recurrence rate of 10% with allograft ICBG and subsequently switched to ICBG autograft and later reported a failure rate of 7%.[71,72] The current literature reports a failure rate of 4% to 17% for autograft ICBG, 3.5% to 11% for allograft ICBG, and 1.4% to 5.6% for DTA (see **Table 2**). Caution should be employed when interpreting these numbers, as there is heterogeneity in the definition of recurrence, complexity of instability, and amount of bone loss among studies. This highlights the need for a randomized control trial directly comparing the different graft options in AAGR.

Graft Union

Graft union has been a common concern associated with the use of allograft bone blocks but is also seen in autograft transfers. Tahir and colleagues[53] found union rates to be high (>90%) in 8 of 10 studies in their systematic review, regardless of graft type. In contrast, Malik and colleagues[73] reported a much lower union rate of 37.5% in ICBG allograft versus 42% in ICBG autograft group. However, they noted partial union in an additional 42% of autograft compared to none in allograft. Differences in the way studies assess union and different allograft preservation techniques could be a possible explanation for the disparities in union rates seen. Additionally, proper positioning of the graft on the glenoid may affect union rates, which is sparsely reported in the AAGR literature. Provencher and colleagues[86] found that DTA grafts with lesser allograft angles (<15°) were better opposed to the glenoid and showed superior healing and graft incorporation; thus, type of graft is not the only consideration when assessing union.

Graft Resorption

Graft resorption is well documented in the literature, with consistently higher graft resorption in allografts being reported when directly compared to autograft.[56,65,73] Malik and colleagues[73] reported on 12 patients with autograft ICBG and 10 patients with allograft ICBG. They found partial resorption in 75% of allograft and 40% of autograft. However, despite excessive graft resorption, these patients did not experience recurrence of instability symptoms, which is consistently reported in the literature.[57,60,65,71] Russo and colleagues[57] reported on 19 patients with iliac crest allograft. They found resorption in all patients; however, excellent clinical results occurred in 17 patients and there was no correlation between bone graft resorption and recurrent dislocation. Additionally, graft resorption is not an issue exclusive to allografts. Di Giacomo[87] found complete coracoid osteolysis in 59.5% of his patient population with partial resorption in 93.4%. Therefore, the use of allograft may be advantageous, as it offers the ability to create a larger graft in anticipation of resorption. A hypothesis for the maintained glenohumeral stability regardless of graft resorption is that the bone graft may improve the inferior capsule healing in the first several months postoperatively, creating a robust capsulolabral structure on the anterior glenoid rim and enlarging the footprint of the repaired anterior capsule.[53,57]

Articular Congruity and Osteoarthritis

Articular congruency and osteoarthritis progression are important considerations that can contribute to failure of bone grafting procedures. The overall risk of osteoarthritis progression after open or arthroscopic free bone block reconstruction has been reported as 10.9% in one meta-analysis.[22] However, only mild-to-moderate arthritic changes and progression of arthritis by only stage have been noted in multiple studies examining AAGR.[9,51,59,63]

Precise positioning of the free bone block is essential to avoid excessive arthritic changes. An ideal graft position should restore stability while preserving the centered position of the humeral head in the glenoid fossa. Montgomery and colleagues[88] reported the effectiveness of a graft is related to both the height and extent of contouring of the graft. A nonanatomically, non-contoured, or too laterally positioned graft can cause the undesired posterior displacement of the humeral head. There is a consensus that the graft should not be placed above the 3 o'clock position or below the 5 o'clock position or outside the glenoid circle in regard to vertical positioning.[89] In the horizontal plane, the graft should not protrude outward to prevent early osteoarthritis and should not be placed more than 5 mm inside to prevent an empty glenoid position leading to failure.[8,89–92] AAGR has shown highly consistent graft positioning,[66] which is an advantage to the technique, however, requires a few important considerations intraoperatively. The arm should be positioned in adduction and slight forward flexion when shuttling the graft through the rotator interval to reduce tension on the conjoint tendon and subscapularis muscle. This allows the safe passage of the graft between these anatomic structures and facilitates proper positioning of the graft. We advocate for rigid fixation of the graft through the Halifax portal to achieve proper trajectory of the screws and prevent malreduction after final fixation.

Graft Fixation

Previous reports on AAGR show heterogeneity in the type of fixation of the free bone block. Metal screws, bioabsorbable screws, suture buttons, and suture anchor techniques have been described. Metal screws are supported by clinical and biomechanical studies,[93,94] however, may lead to hardware prominence and irritation.[63,68] Advocates for bioabsorbable screws postulate that metal screws adversely affect the development of postoperative arthritis and graft resorption.[51] The use of bioabsorbable screws have also been hypothesized to lead to increased osteolysis; however, neither of these statements has been confirmed in the literature. Nebelung and colleagues[62] examined 15 patients with metal screws and 9 patients with bioabsorbable screws. At a mean follow-up of 19 months, there was no difference in recurrence or healing of the graft.

Suture button fixation has been gaining popularity due to ease of insertion and low risk of hardware irritation and has been found to have similar biomechanical strength to screw fixation.[95] However, a recent study by Sparavalo and colleagues[96] retrospectively reviewed 38 patients undergoing AAGR with screw fixation versus button fixation. The group with button fixation had significantly worse Western Ontario Shoulder Instability (WOSI) scores at 2 years and a significantly higher failure rate, with 6 dislocations in the button group and 0 in the screw group. These results may be due to graft resorption prior to complete union of the graft, resulting in detensioning of the suture button configuration and eventual failure of the graft. Further studies, however, are needed to confirm the long-term outcomes and risk factors for failure to determine which fixation type is superior.

SUMMARY

This review has demonstrated that AAGR is associated with excellent patient-reported outcomes with an acceptably low rate of recurrent instability and complications. There is still further investigation that is needed regarding long-term outcomes, graft selection, and fixation method. Additionally, direct comparison between the different methods of AAGR is indicated to determine the optimal procedure for shoulder instability with glenoid bone loss.

DISCLOSURE

There are no commercial or financial conflicts of interest to disclose. There are no funding sources for any of the authors.

REFERENCES

1. Leroux T, Wasserstein D, Veillette C, et al. Epidemiology of primary anterior shoulder dislocation requiring closed reduction in Ontario, Canada. Am J Sports Med 2014;42(2):442–50.
2. Gottschalk LJ 4th, Walia P, Patel RM, et al. Stability of the glenohumeral joint with combined humeral head and glenoid defects: a cadaveric study. Am J Sports Med 2016;44(4):933–40.
3. Edwards TB, Boulahia A, Walch G. Radiographic analysis of bone defects in chronic anterior shoulder instability. Arthroscopy 2003;19(7):732–9.
4. Itoi E, Lee SB, Berglund LJ, et al. The effect of a glenoid defect on anteroinferior stability of the shoulder after Bankart repair: a cadaveric study. J Bone Joint Surg Am 2000;82(1):35–46.
5. Burkhart SS, De Beer JF. Traumatic glenohumeral bone defects and their relationship to failure of arthroscopic Bankart repairs: significance of the inverted-pear glenoid and the humeral engaging Hill-Sachs lesion. Arthroscopy 2000;16(7): 677–94.
6. Longo UG, Loppini M, Rizzello G, et al. Latarjet, Bristow, and Eden-Hybinette procedures for anterior shoulder dislocation: systematic review and quantitative synthesis of the literature. Arthroscopy 2014;30(9):1184–211.
7. Tucker A, Ma J, Sparavalo S, et al. Arthroscopic anatomic glenoid reconstruction has a lower rate of recurrent instability compared to arthroscopic Bankart repair while otherwise maintaining a similar complication and safety profile [published online ahead of print, 2022 May 29]. J ISAKOS 2022;S2059-7754(22):00066-9.
8. Hovelius L, Sandström B, Olofsson A, et al. The effect of capsular repair, bone block healing, and position on the results of the Bristow-Latarjet procedure (study III): long-term follow-up in 319 shoulders. J Shoulder Elbow Surg 2012;21(5): 647–60.
9. Boileau P, Mercier N, Roussanne Y, et al. Arthroscopic bankart-bristow-latarjet procedure: the development and early results of a safe and reproducible technique. Arthroscopy 2010;26(11):1434–50.
10. Lafosse L, Lejeune E, Bouchard A, et al. The arthroscopic Latarjet procedure for the treatment of anterior shoulder instability. Arthroscopy 2007;23(11):1242.e1-5.
11. Tibone J. Editorial commentary: not for the faint of heart: the arthroscopic latarjet procedure, a north american experience. Arthroscopy 2016;32(10):1971–2.
12. Gilat R, Haunschild ED, Lavoie-Gagne OZ, et al. Outcomes of the latarjet procedure versus free bone block procedures for anterior shoulder instability: a systematic review and meta-analysis. Am J Sports Med 2021;49(3):805–16.
13. Moroder P, Schulz E, Wierer G, et al. Neer Award 2019: Latarjet procedure vs. iliac crest bone graft transfer for treatment of anterior shoulder instability with glenoid bone loss: a prospective randomized trial. J Shoulder Elbow Surg 2019; 28(7):1298–307.

14. LAVIK K. Habitual shoulder luxation: Eden-Hybinette's operation. Acta Orthop Scand 1961;30:251–64.
15. Provencher MT, Ghodadra N, LeClere L, et al. Anatomic osteochondral glenoid reconstruction for recurrent glenohumeral instability with glenoid deficiency using a distal tibia allograft. Arthroscopy 2009;25(4):446–52.
16. Frank RM, Kim J, O'Donnell PJ, et al. Outcomes of latarjet versus distal tibial allograft for anterior shoulder instability repair: a prospective matched cohort analysis. Orthop. J. Sports Med 2017;5(7_suppl6). 2325967117S00275.
17. Paladini P, Merolla G, De Santis E, et al. Long-term subscapularis strength assessment after Bristow-Latarjet procedure: isometric study. J Shoulder Elbow Surg 2012;21(1):42–7.
18. McNeil D, Coady C, Wong IH. Arthroscopic anatomic glenoid reconstruction in lateral decubitus position using allograft with nonrigid fixation. Arthrosc Tech 2018;7(11):e1115–21.
19. Skendzel JG, Sekiya JK. Arthroscopic glenoid osteochondral allograft reconstruction without subscapularis takedown: technique and literature review. Arthroscopy 2011;27(1):129–35.
20. Valencia M, Fernández-Bermejo G, Martín-Ríos MD, et al. Subscapularis structural integrity and function after arthroscopic Latarjet procedure at a minimum 2-year follow-up. J Shoulder Elbow Surg 2020;29(1):104–12.
21. Horner NS, Moroz PA, Bhullar R, et al. Open versus arthroscopic Latarjet procedures for the treatment of shoulder instability: a systematic review of comparative studies. BMC Musculoskelet Disord 2018;19(1):255.
22. Wei J, Lu M, Zhao L, et al. Free bone grafting improves clinical outcomes in anterior shoulder instability with bone defect: a systematic review and meta-analysis of studies with a minimum of 1-year follow-up. J Shoulder Elbow Surg 2022;31(4): e190–208.
23. Bigliani LU, Newton PM, Steinmann SP, et al. Glenoid rim lesions associated with recurrent anterior dislocation of the shoulder. Am J Sports Med 1998;26(1):41–5.
24. Chen AL, Hunt SA, Hawkins RJ, et al. Management of bone loss associated with recurrent anterior glenohumeral instability. Am J Sports Med 2005;33(6):912–25.
25. Lo IK, Parten PM, Burkhart SS. The inverted pear glenoid: an indicator of significant glenoid bone loss. Arthroscopy 2004;20(2):169–74.
26. Lynch JR, Clinton JM, Dewing CB, et al. Treatment of osseous defects associated with anterior shoulder instability. J Shoulder Elbow Surg 2009;18(2):317–28.
27. Willemot LB, Elhassan BT, Verborgt O. Bony reconstruction of the anterior glenoid rim. J Am Acad Orthop Surg 2018;26(10):e207–18.
28. Yamamoto N, Itoi E, Abe H, et al. Effect of an anterior glenoid defect on anterior shoulder stability: a cadaveric study. Am J Sports Med 2009;37(5):949–54.
29. Yamamoto N, Muraki T, Sperling JW, et al. Stabilizing mechanism in bone-grafting of a large glenoid defect. J Bone Joint Surg Am 2010;92(11):2059–66.
30. Ahmed I, Ashton F, Robinson CM. Arthroscopic Bankart repair and capsular shift for recurrent anterior shoulder instability: functional outcomes and identification of risk factors for recurrence. J Bone Joint Surg Am 2012;94(14):1308–15.
31. Boileau P, Villalba M, Héry JY, et al. Risk factors for recurrence of shoulder instability after arthroscopic Bankart repair. J Bone Joint Surg Am 2006;88(8): 1755–63.
32. Dickens JF, Owens BD, Cameron KL, et al. The effect of subcritical bone loss and exposure on recurrent instability after arthroscopic bankart repair in intercollegiate american football. Am J Sports Med 2017;45(8):1769–75.

33. Shaha JS, Cook JB, Song DJ, et al. Redefining "critical" bone loss in shoulder instability: functional outcomes worsen with "subcritical" bone loss. Am J Sports Med 2015;43(7):1719–25.

34. Shin SJ, Koh YW, Bui C, et al. What is the critical value of glenoid bone loss at which soft tissue bankart repair does not restore glenohumeral translation, restricts range of motion, and leads to abnormal humeral head position? Am J Sports Med 2016;44(11):2784–91.

35. Shin SJ, Kim RG, Jeon YS, et al. Critical value of anterior glenoid bone loss that leads to recurrent glenohumeral instability after arthroscopic bankart repair. Am J Sports Med 2017;45(9):1975–81.

36. Garcia GH, Park MJ, Zhang C, et al. Large hill-sachs lesion: a comparative study of patients treated with arthroscopic bankart repair with or without remplissage. HSS J 2015;11(2):98–103.

37. Dehaan A, Munch J, Durkan M, et al. Reconstruction of a bony bankart lesion: best fit based on radius of curvature. Am J Sports Med 2013;41(5):1140–5.

38. Willemot LB, Akbari-Shandiz M, Sanchez-Sotelo J, et al. Restoration of articular geometry using current graft options for large glenoid bone defects in anterior shoulder instability. Arthroscopy 2017;33(9):1661–9.

39. Bhatia S, Van Thiel GS, Gupta D, et al. Comparison of glenohumeral contact pressures and contact areas after glenoid reconstruction with latarjet or distal tibial osteochondral allografts. Am J Sports Med 2013;41(8):1900–8.

40. Kwapisz A, Fitzpatrick K, Cook JB, et al. Distal clavicular osteochondral autograft augmentation for glenoid bone loss: a comparison of radius of restoration versus latarjet graft. Am J Sports Med 2018;46(5):1046–52.

41. Dekker TJ, Peebles LA, Bernhardson AS, et al. Risk factors for recurrence after arthroscopic instability repair-the importance of glenoid bone loss >15%, patient age, and duration of symptoms: a matched cohort analysis. Am J Sports Med 2020;48(12):3036–41.

42. Provencher MT, Midtgaard KS, Owens BD, et al. Diagnosis and management of traumatic anterior shoulder instability. J Am Acad Orthop Surg 2021;29(2): e51–61.

43. Warner JJ, Gill TJ, O'hollerhan JD, et al. Anatomical glenoid reconstruction for recurrent anterior glenohumeral instability with glenoid deficiency using an autogenous tricortical iliac crest bone graft. Am J Sports Med 2006;34(2):205–12.

44. Piasecki DP, Verma NN, Romeo AA, et al. Glenoid bone deficiency in recurrent anterior shoulder instability: diagnosis and management. J Am Acad Orthop Surg 2009;17(8):482–93.

45. Huijsmans PE, Haen PS, Kidd M, et al. Quantification of a glenoid defect with three-dimensional computed tomography and magnetic resonance imaging: a cadaveric study. J Shoulder Elbow Surg 2007;16(6):803–9.

46. Lansdown DA, Wang K, Yanke AB, et al. A flat anterior glenoid corresponds to subcritical glenoid bone loss. Arthroscopy 2019;35(6):1788–93.

47. Rayes J, Xu J, Sparavalo S, et al. Calculating glenoid bone loss based on glenoid height using ipsilateral three-dimensional computed tomography [published correction appears in Knee Surg Sports Traumatol Arthrosc. 2022 Jul 6. Knee Surg Sports Traumatol Arthrosc 2023;31(1):169–76.

48. Hurley ET, Matache BA, Wong I, et al. Anterior shoulder instability part ii-latarjet, remplissage, and glenoid bone-grafting-an international consensus statement. Arthroscopy 2022;38(2):224–33.e6.

49. Joannette-Bourguignon M, Wong I. Arthroscopic anatomic glenoid reconstruction in the unstable shoulder: technique, pearls, and pitfalls. VJSM 2023;3(1). https://doi.org/10.1177/26350254221141906. 26350254221141906.
50. Raiss P, Lin A, Mizuno N, et al. Results of the Latarjet procedure for recurrent anterior dislocation of the shoulder in patients with epilepsy. J Bone Joint Surg Br 2012;94(9):1260–4.
51. Ueda Y, Sugaya H, Takahashi N, et al. Arthroscopic iliac bone grafting for traumatic anterior shoulder instability with significant glenoid bone loss yields low recurrence and good outcome at a minimum of five-year follow-up. Arthroscopy 2021;37(8):2399–408.
52. Wong IH, Urquhart N. Arthroscopic anatomic glenoid reconstruction without subscapularis split. Arthrosc Tech 2015;4(5):e449–56.
53. Tahir M, Malik S, Jordan R, et al. Arthroscopic bone block stabilisation procedures for glenoid bone loss in anterior glenohumeral instability: A systematic review of clinical and radiological outcomes. Orthop Traumatol Surg Res 2021; 107(5):102949.
54. Castricini R, Longo UG, Petrillo S, et al. Arthroscopic Latarjet for Recurrent Shoulder Instability. Medicina (Kaunas) 2019;55(9):582.
55. Chillemi C, Guerrisi M, Paglialunga C, et al. Latarjet procedure for anterior shoulder instability: a 24-year follow-up study. Arch Orthop Trauma Surg 2021;141(2): 189–96.
56. Mahmoud HF, Farhan AH, Fahmy FS. Satisfactory functional results and complication rates after anterior glenoid bone block reconstruction in recurrent shoulder dislocation: a mean 4-year follow-up comparative study. J ISAKOS 2022;7(4): 47–53.
57. Russo R, Maiotti M, Cozzolino A, et al. Arthroscopic iliac crest bone allograft combined with subscapularis upper-third tenodesis shows a low recurrence rate in the treatment of recurrent anterior shoulder instability associated with critical bone loss. Arthroscopy 2021;37(3):824–33.
58. Xiang M, Yang J, Chen H, et al. Arthroscopic autologous scapular spine bone graft combined with bankart repair for anterior shoulder instability with subcritical (10%-15%) glenoid bone loss. Arthroscopy 2021;37(7):2065–74.
59. Kraus N, Amphansap T, Gerhardt C, et al. Arthroscopic anatomic glenoid reconstruction using an autologous iliac crest bone grafting technique. J Shoulder Elbow Surg 2014;23(11):1700–8.
60. Zhao J, Huangfu X, Yang X, et al. Arthroscopic glenoid bone grafting with nonrigid fixation for anterior shoulder instability: 52 patients with 2- to 5-year follow-up. Am J Sports Med 2014;42(4):831–9.
61. Anderl W, Pauzenberger L, Laky B, et al. Arthroscopic implant-free bone grafting for shoulder instability with glenoid bone loss: clinical and radiological outcome at a minimum 2-year follow-up. Am J Sports Med 2016;44(5):1137–45.
62. Nebelung W, Reichwein F, Nebelung S. A simplified arthroscopic bone graft transfer technique in chronic glenoid bone deficiency. Knee Surg Sports Traumatol Arthrosc 2016;24(6):1884–7.
63. Giannakos A, Vezeridis PS, Schwartz DG, et al. All-arthroscopic revision eden-hybinette procedure for failed instability surgery: technique and preliminary results. Arthroscopy 2017;33(1):39–48.
64. Amar E, Konstantinidis G, Coady C, et al. Arthroscopic treatment of shoulder instability with glenoid bone loss using distal tibial allograft augmentation: safety profile and short-term radiological outcomes. Orthop J Sports Med 2018;6(5). https://doi.org/10.1177/2325967118774507. 2325967118774507.

65. Wong IH, King JP, Boyd G, et al. Radiographic analysis of glenoid size and shape after arthroscopic coracoid autograft versus distal tibial allograft in the treatment of anterior shoulder instability. Am J Sports Med 2018;46(11):2717–24.

66. Moga I, Konstantinidis G, Coady C, et al. Arthroscopic Anatomic Glenoid Reconstruction: Analysis of the Learning Curve. Orthop J Sports Med 2018;6(11). https://doi.org/10.1177/2325967118807906. :2325967118807906.

67. Taverna E, Garavaglia G, Perfetti C, et al. An arthroscopic bone block procedure is effective in restoring stability, allowing return to sports in cases of glenohumeral instability with glenoid bone deficiency. Knee Surg Sports Traumatol Arthrosc 2018;26(12):3780–7.

68. Bockmann B, Venjakob AJ, Reichwein F, et al. Mid-term clinical results of an arthroscopic glenoid rim reconstruction technique for recurrent anterior shoulder instability. Arch Orthop Trauma Surg 2018;138(11):1557–62.

69. Bockmann B, Venjakob AJ, Gebing R, et al. Bone grafts used for arthroscopic glenoid reconstruction restore the native glenoid anatomy. Knee Surg Sports Traumatol Arthrosc 2018;26(1):299–305.

70. Boileau P, Duysens C, Saliken D, et al. All-arthroscopic, guided Eden-Hybbinette procedure using suture-button fixation for revision of failed Latarjet. J Shoulder Elbow Surg 2019;28(11):e377–88.

71. Boehm E, Minkus M, Moroder P, et al. Massive graft resorption after iliac crest allograft reconstruction for glenoid bone loss in recurrent anterior shoulder instability. Arch Orthop Trauma Surg 2020;140(7):895–903.

72. Boehm E, Minkus M, Moroder P, et al. Arthroscopic iliac crest bone grafting in recurrent anterior shoulder instability: minimum 5-year clinical and radiologic follow-up. Knee Surg Sports Traumatol Arthrosc 2021;29(1):266–74.

73. Malik SS, Elashry S, Jordan RW, et al. Is there a difference in outcome of arthroscopic iliac crest autograft and allograft in recurrent anterior shoulder instability? Eur J Orthop Surg Traumatol 2020;30(8):1453–61.

74. Hurley ET, Lim Fat D, Farrington SK, et al. Open versus arthroscopic latarjet procedure for anterior shoulder instability: a systematic review and meta-analysis. Am J Sports Med 2019;47(5):1248–53.

75. Taverna E, D'Ambrosi R, Perfetti C, et al. Arthroscopic bone graft procedure for anterior inferior glenohumeral instability. Arthrosc Tech 2014;3(6):e653–60.

76. Steffen V, Hertel R. Rim reconstruction with autogenous iliac crest for anterior glenoid deficiency: forty-three instability cases followed for 5-19 years. J Shoulder Elbow Surg 2013;22(4):550–9.

77. Fortun CM, Wong I, Burns JP. Arthroscopic iliac crest bone grafting to the anterior glenoid. Arthrosc Tech 2016;5(4):e907–12.

78. Oldfield M, Burns J, Wong I. Arthroscopic glenoid bone augmentation using iliac crest autograft is safe and effective for anterior shoulder instability with bone loss. Arthrosc Sports Med Rehabil 2021;3(6):e1671–7.

79. Tokish JM, Fitzpatrick K, Cook JB, et al. Arthroscopic distal clavicular autograft for treating shoulder instability with glenoid bone loss. Arthrosc Tech 2014;3(4):e475–81.

80. Dai F, Yang J, Zhang Q, et al. Arthroscopic autologous scapular spine bone graft for recurrent anterior shoulder dislocation with subcritical (10%-15%) glenoid bone loss. Arthrosc Tech 2022;11(11):e1871–8.

81. Power L, Wong I. Arthroscopic anatomic glenoid repair using distal tibial allograft and an inferior-to-superior capsular shift. Arthrosc Tech 2021;10(1):e221–8.

82. Wong I, John R, Ma J, et al. Arthroscopic anatomic glenoid reconstruction using distal tibial allograft for recurrent anterior shoulder instability: clinical and radiographic outcomes. Am J Sports Med 2020;48(13):3316–21.

83. Wong I, Sparavalo S, Ma J, et al. Podium presentation title: arthroscopic anatomic glenoid reconstruction has excellent outcomes at mid-term follow-up. Arthroscopy 2023;39(6):e25–6.

84. Moga I, Konstantinidis G, Wong IH. The safety of a far medial arthroscopic portal for anatomic glenoid reconstruction: a cadaveric study. Orthop J Sports Med 2018;6(9). https://doi.org/10.1177/2325967118795404. 2325967118795404.

85. Gilat R, Wong SE, Lavoie-Gagne O, et al. Outcomes are comparable using free bone block autografts versus allografts for the management of anterior shoulder instability with glenoid bone loss: a systematic review and meta-analysis of "The Non-Latarjet". Knee Surg Sports Traumatol Arthrosc 2021;29(7):2159–74.

86. Provencher MT, Frank RM, Golijanin P, et al. Distal tibia allograft glenoid reconstruction in recurrent anterior shoulder instability: clinical and radiographic outcomes [published correction appears in arthroscopy. 2018 Mar;34(3):1000]. Arthroscopy 2017;33(5):891–7.

87. Di Giacomo G, Costantini A, de Gasperis N, et al. Coracoid graft osteolysis after the Latarjet procedure for anteroinferior shoulder instability: a computed tomography scan study of twenty-six patients. J Shoulder Elbow Surg 2011;20(6):989–95.

88. Montgomery WH Jr, Wahl M, Hettrich C, et al. Anteroinferior bone-grafting can restore stability in osseous glenoid defects. J Bone Joint Surg Am 2005;87(9):1972–7.

89. Sugaya H. Techniques to evaluate glenoid bone loss. Curr Rev Musculoskelet Med 2014;7(1):1–5.

90. Gasbarro G, Giugale JM, Walch G, et al. Predictive surgical reasons for failure after coracoid process transfers. Orthop J Sports Med 2016;4(12). 2325967116676795.

91. Nourissat G, Doursounian L, Delaroche C, et al. Optimization of bone-block positioning in the Bristow-Latarjet procedure: A biomechanical study. Orthop Traumatol Surg Res 2014;100(5):509–13.

92. Tytherleigh-Strong G, Aresti N, Begum R. Revision guided suture-button bone block stabilization of the shoulder in the presence of significant retained glenoid metalwork. JSES Int 2020;4(4):803–13.

93. Alvi HM, Monroe EJ, Muriuki M, et al. Latarjet fixation: a cadaveric biomechanical study evaluating cortical and cannulated screw fixation. Orthop J Sports Med 2016;4(4). https://doi.org/10.1177/2325967116643533. 2325967116643533.

94. An VV, Sivakumar BS, Phan K, et al. A systematic review and meta-analysis of clinical and patient-reported outcomes following two procedures for recurrent traumatic anterior instability of the shoulder: Latarjet procedure vs. Bankart repair. J Shoulder Elbow Surg 2016;25(5):853–63.

95. Provencher MT, Aman ZS, LaPrade CM, et al. Biomechanical comparison of screw fixation versus a cortical button and self-tensioning suture for the latarjet procedure. Orthop J Sports Med 2018;6(6). https://doi.org/10.1177/2325967118777842. 2325967118777842.

96. Sparavalo S, Jonah L, Ma J, et al. Podium presentation title: screw fixation has better outcomes than button fixation for glenoid reconstruction: matched analysis. Arthroscopy 2023;39(6):e2.

Management of Shoulder Instability in the Overhead Athletes

Mark A. Glover, BS[a],*, Anthony P. Fiegen, MD[b],
Garrett S. Bullock, DPT, DPhil[b], Kristen F. Nicholson, PhD[b],
Nicholas A. Trasolini, MD[b], Brian R. Waterman, MD[b]

KEYWORDS

- Shoulder instability • Overhead athlete • Baseball • Shoulder

KEY POINTS

- Glenohumeral instability in overhead athletes can be debilitating with variable presentation, making it difficult to manage.
- Posterior shoulder instability (ie, "batter's shoulder") is often difficult to differentiate from pain or the sequelae of internal impingement, while anterior and multidirectional instability are usually clinically identifiable.
- Generally, treatment begins with conservative management that focuses on reinforcing proper mechanics with rehabilitation that targets strengthening shoulder stability.
- When this fails or there is an acute or severe injury, operative management is often indicated.
- Further multicenter randomized control trials analyzing surgical techniques, rehabilitation monitoring, and biomechanical analysis are needed to progress the management of shoulder instability in the overhead athlete to a proactive process.

INTRODUCTION

Shoulder instability covers a wide spectrum of glenohumeral joint pathology, ranging from subluxation to dislocation in the anterior, posterior, or multidirectional planes. Instability can be acute, most often in contact-sport athletes, whereas more chronic cases present secondary to repetitive microtrauma, such as seen in the overhead athlete. Overhead athletes participating in sports such as baseball, tennis, volleyball, and swimming perform repetitive, often forceful overhead movements that place significant stress on the static and dynamic stabilizers of the glenohumeral joint, which

[a] Wake Forest University School of Medicine, Winston Salem, NC, USA; [b] Department of Orthopaedic Surgery and Rehabilitation, Wake Forest University School of Medicine, Winston-Salem, NC, USA
* Corresponding author. 1 Medical Center Boulevard, Winston-Salem, NC 27157.
E-mail address: glovermarkalan@gmail.com

Clin Sports Med 43 (2024) 683–703
https://doi.org/10.1016/j.csm.2024.03.024
0278-5919/24/© 2024 Elsevier Inc. All rights reserved.

can ultimately result in injury and instability. Presentation in these athletes can be subtle and nonspecific, especially in the absence of acute trauma or obvious dislocation. Therefore, careful evaluation and a high suspicion are necessary for diagnosis. Once the diagnosis is made, nonoperative as well as surgical management may be indicated based upon the clinical and radiographic findings, which impacts the athlete's return to sport. The purpose of this review is to provide a comprehensive description of shoulder instability in the overhead athlete focusing on management.

ROLE OF SUPPORTIVE STRUCTURES

A key to understanding the pathology of shoulder instability in the overhead athlete is first appreciating the function of anatomic structures essential to stability during the throwing (or overhead athletic) shoulder motion. The stabilizing structures of the glenohumeral joint include joint congruity between the humerus and glenoid, the joint capsule (and resulting negative intracapsular pressure), glenohumeral ligaments, and the glenoid labrum. The dynamic stabilizing structures primarily include the rotator cuff muscles, which aid in stability through concavity compression. To a lesser extent, the long head of the biceps tendon, periscapular muscles, and scapulothoracic position also contribute to stabilization of the glenohumeral joint.[1,2] It is also key to consider physiologic changes that occur in the shoulder of the overhead athletes. The repetitively high forces at extremes of range of motion (ROM) may slowly lead to changes in the stabilizing anatomy. Over time, these changes may progress to dysfunction, injury, and possible instability.

Labrum

The fibrocartilaginous labrum is formed by the glenoid shape and extends the glenoid through its concavity in both width and depth to play an imperative role in articular congruity and shoulder stability. The labrum increases the glenoid concavity and resists against translational forces, withstanding up to 380 N of force during the throwing motion.[3,4] The labrum is also subjected to traction force from the long head of the biceps tendon in addition to overall joint distraction during overhead motion in athletes.[5] Given the high amount of stress, pathology of the labrum is often involved in shoulder stability.

Coracohumeral and Glenohumeral Ligaments

The coracohumeral and glenohumeral ligaments are thickenings of the joint capsule, helping to stabilize the joint via resistance to multiplanar translation in overhead athletes.[6] These structures include the coracohumeral ligament (CHL), the middle glenohumeral ligament (MGHL), superior glenohumeral ligament (SGHL), and the inferior glenohumeral ligament (IGHL), which is further divided into anterior and posterior bands.

The CHL extends from the coracoid process to the rotator cable of the rotator cuff. The CHL functions to resist external rotation and translation during inferiorly directed forces of the adducted arm.[7,8] This can be seen during the deceleration and follow through phases of the throwing motion or during a volleyball spike. Laxity or injury to the CHL may result in increased inferior translation and external rotation of the humeral head.[9,10]

The anterior band of the IGHL (AIGHL) provides stability against anterior and inferior translation forces of the humeral head when the shoulder is in 90° of abduction and external rotation.[11,12] It produces a stable envelope that prevents the humeral head from overrotation and translation during the late cocking phase of throwing, which is associated with peak throwing motion forces.[4,13,14] As a primary restraint during these phases of throwing associated with significant amount of force, the AIGHL is among the most important of the glenohumeral ligaments. The posterior band of the IGHL (PIGHL) limits posterior and inferior translation of the humeral head with the arm in an abducted and internally rotated position. Pathology related to the PIGHL in the overhead athlete may manifest as capsular tightness as seen in glenohumeral internal rotational deficit. This can result in humeral decentering and increase the risk of superior labral injuries or internal impingement. The PIGHL also serves a role in the setting of posterior instability in the overhead athlete.[13,14]

The SGHL and MGHL appear to play a lesser role than the other glenohumeral ligaments in the overhead athlete. With the shoulder in adduction and 90° of abduction with external rotation, the SGHL is taut, suggesting that it plays a role with the CHL to prevent inferior translation of the humeral head.[15] The MGHL, however, is at maximal tension in midrange abduction and provides stability against anterior translation, though there is a great variability in size.[16]

Rotator Cuff

The rotator cuff muscles provide dynamic support of the humeral head during the overhead motion by providing a compressive force to maintain a concentric glenohumeral articulation. The primary role of the rotator cuff is to compress the humeral head against the glenoid. Tears in the rotator cuff are fairly common in overhead athletes.[17] The rotator cuff plays an essential role during the deceleration phase of throwing, maintaining a compressive stabilizing force. Similar to the static stabilizers of the glenohumeral joint, the rotator cuff is subjected to repetitive forces at often the extremes of ROM, resulting in an increased risk of developing injury with possible subsequent instability.[17]

The static and dynamic stabilizing structures of the glenohumeral joint do not function independently, rather, they rely on each other for optimal function. For example, a tight posterior capsule, as often seen in patients with glenohumeral internal rotation deficit, may shift the humeral head anteriorly, subsequently exaggerating stress placed on the subscapularis muscle. Similarly, acute anterior instability, often resulting in anterior inferior labral tears with capsular injury, leaves the subscapularis to provide much of the dynamic support during glenohumeral motion.[17–19] Overhead athletes tend to rely greatly on the subscapularis during the cocking motion of the throw, serve, or stroke, which makes it one of the more common rotator cuff pathologies.[20–22] Repetitive use may also subject the rotator cuff muscles to increased laxity over time with a less dramatic clinical presentation.[23,24]

EPIDEMIOLOGY AND PATHOPHYSIOLOGY

Anterior shoulder instability (ASI) is the most common clinical instability, with an incidence of approximately 0.08 per 1000 person-years.[25,26] Posterior shoulder instability (PSI) is less common with an overall incidence of approximately 0.011 per 1000 person-years. The overall incidence of multidirectional instability (MDI) remains largely unknown due to variation in symptomatology and diagnosis, though accounting for approximately 7% of shoulder surgeries.[27,28] Patients who present with painful anterior instability have often experienced primary or recurrent dislocation.[29] In contrast, pain associated with posterior instability is less often a result of a dislocation event and more likely related to overuse rather than an identifiable injury. MDI is commonly found in sports such as swimming, where an associated increase in physiologic ROM can provide a competitive advantage. However, the overall increase in ROM can result in later pain and dysfunction.[28] Regardless of direction, shoulder instability can be difficult for the athlete and medical professional, and an understanding of the pathophysiology in each respective instability pattern helps guide clinical management.

Anterior Instability

ASI is defined by anterior dislocation or subluxation of the glenohumeral joint with associated pain. ASI commonly affects younger contact-sport athletes, more active populations, as in the case of the overhead athlete.[30] Anterior instability can occur secondary to a single acute event, often an anterior glenohumeral dislocation or secondary to repetitive microtrauma. The repetitive motions performed by overhead athletes over a long period lead to significant and recurrent overhead torque, especially at the limits of ROM.[14] The pathophysiology of anterior instability is associated with damage to or involvement of the anterior labrum, most often the anteroinferior labrum, also known as a Bankart tear. Acute or more chronic anterior instability can also manifest as superior labrum anterior posterior (SLAP) lesions caused by a peel back mechanism, anterior labroligamentous periosteal sleeve avulsion (ALPSA) lesions, and other forms of isolated labrum tears, as well as injuries to the subscapularis, and/or AIGHL (**Figs. 1** and **2**).[31] Both the subscapularis and AIGHL resist anterior translation, and chronic laxity during the overhead motion contributes to instability over time. Compressive forces, along with joint laxity and large anteriorly directed forces during the arm cocking phase of throwing motion, can all lead to anterior labral tears.[32] These structures provide the most important resistance to anterior translation and as a result of chronic or acute changes allow for an increased anterior laxity that can lead to instability.

An important consideration is the degree of osseous involvement, which occurs due to damage to the humeral head in the setting of a Hill–Sachs lesion, or on the glenoid, in the setting of a Bony Bankart lesion (**Fig. 3**). These osseous pathologies can present in 2 ways: either as an acute fracture secondary to a single shoulder dislocation event or as a chronic erosion of the glenoid or humeral head from recurrent instability.[33] Both mechanisms result in bone loss of the glenoid rim or humeral head, which further contribute to glenohumeral instability. Soft tissue stabilizers are unable to compensate for a lack of bony infrastructure as seen with glenoid bone loss. The stability of the

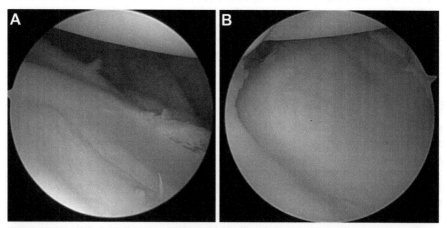

Fig. 1. Arthroscopic images of a 21 year old softball athlete with recurrent ASI secondary to a labral disruption extending anteriorly and posteriorly (*A*) in the left shoulder. Final repair (*B*) showing knotless suture anchor fixation of both anterior and posterior aspects of the labrum.

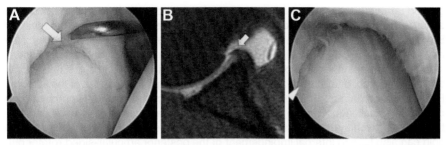

Fig. 2. SLAP lesion in a 17 year old high school baseball player shown arthroscopically (*A*) and under T2-weighted MR imaging (*B*). The peel back mechanism demonstrated arthroscopically, where the labrum rotates medially over the corner of the glenoid during abduction and external rotation of the arm (*C*). *Arrow* in (*A*) is a SLAP lesion, *Arrow* in (*B*) is the SLAP lesion under MR imaging, *Arrow head* in (*C*) is where the labrum rotates medially over the corner of the glenoid.

shoulder is significantly reduced when there is more than 20% bone loss of the glenoid, and this instability can lead to pain, weakness, reduced ROM, and long-term recurrent instability.[34]

Posterior Instability

PSI is less common in overhead athletes, but may present in more subtle manner.[27] In contrast to anterior instability, which is most likely to result in recurrent frank instability events, posterior instability may only be associated with pain and an absence of clinically noticeable instability. However, when present, PSI is especially debilitating for athletes who rely on the overhead motion for performance. Similar to anterior instability, the development of PSI can occur as an acute or more chronic entity, though it is more often multifactorial.[35]

PSI often presents in throwing or overhead athletes with increased pain or reduced velocity of overhead motion.[36,37] Risk factors include osseous abnormalities, mainly

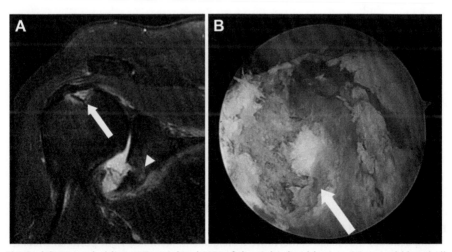

Fig. 3. (*A*) Coronal oblique T2-weighted MRI of the right shoulder in a 27 year old baseball player showing a Hill–Sachs lesion (*arrow*) and concomitant bony Bankart lesion (*arrowhead*). (*B*) Associated arthroscopic imaging showing the Hill–Sachs lesion (*arrow*).

glenoid retroversion, anterior humeral head defects, and glenoid erosion that increase athlete susceptibility to acute on chronic PSI.[38–40] Osseous findings include reverse-Bankart lesions, Kim lesions, and reverse Hill–Sachs lesions. Athletes may also develop PSI after diving onto an outstretched arm or the "batter's shoulder," describing the posterior subluxation of the lead shoulder following a swing on a low and outside pitch, or after missing the ball on a full swing.[39] Regardless of the etiology, PSI is often chronic and multifactorial with less distinct pathologic findings, making diagnosis a challenge.[35] In the setting of PSI, the biomechanics of the overhead motion change, such that the translational mechanics of the humeral head within the glenoid can also lead to internal impingement of the posterior articular-sided rotator cuff with concomitant posterior labral injury (**Figs. 4** and **5**).[37]

Multidirectional Instability

MDI is defined as symptomatic instability or apprehension in greater than one plane and is a common cause of symptomatic shoulder instability in the overhead athlete, especially in swimmers. The improved shoulder motion in patients with MDI may provide a competitive advantage prior to development of pain and dysfunction.[41] MDI can be a debilitating pathology for overhead athletes who rely on a stable shoulder for athletic performance. Although less studied than ASI, MDI is most often a result

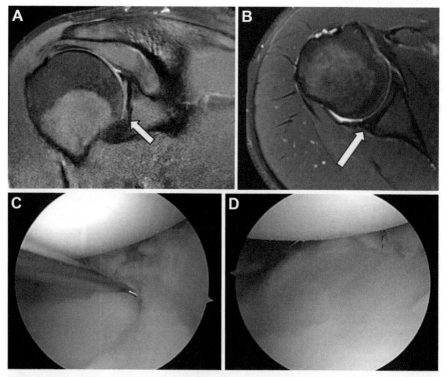

Fig. 4. A 19 year old Division I baseball player with persistent posterior glenohumeral pain during activities that failed conservative management. Identified right posterior shoulder labrum tear on T2-weighted MRI (A, B) and during diagnostic arthroscopy (C). The labral tear was repaired with knotless fixation (D). Arrow in (A) is a posterior labrum tear on sagital view, Arrow is (B) is porterior labrum tear on axial view.

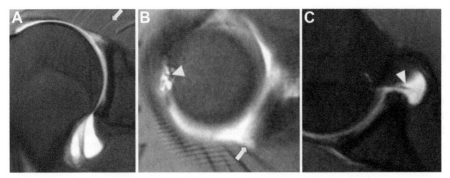

Fig. 5. Coronal (*A*), axial (*B*), and abduction-external rotation (*C*) T1 fat suppressed MR images show increased signal and fraying of the posterosuperior labrum (*arrows*) and fraying of undersurface infraspinatus fibers (*arrowheads*) in a 19 year old male baseball pitcher.

of a wide variety of factors, primarily soft tissue laxity, making it a more chronic pathology.[27,41,42] Chronic etiologies include generalized soft tissue laxity, recurrent microtrauma, redundant capsular elements, proprioceptive imbalances in the glenohumeral supportive structures, as well as congenital and anatomic abnormalities of the glenoid and humeral head. Over time, the suspected summation of these effects allows for laxity in the shoulder and eventual multiplanar subluxation or dislocation.[41]

THROWING MECHANICS
Mechanics in Brief

Overhead athletes subject their arm to a motion sequence that is akin to that of a baseball player delivering a pitch. As such, the baseball pitch is a good representation of most overhead athletes. The throwing motion includes a wind-up, stride, arm cocking, arm acceleration, arm deceleration, and follow through, with the ultimate result of efficient energy transfer from the pitcher to the ball to maximize pitch effectiveness (**Fig. 6**).[5] For this reason, understanding the overhead motion is imperative to conservative and operative management. In a throwing athlete, ball delivery involves distinct phases of motion that subject different anatomy to stress. During the stride, the rear (drive) leg remains connected with the ground and pitching rubber, while the front (stride) leg moves toward the plate. The pitcher uses the force generated by the drive leg and core musculature to hip-hinge and rotate the pelvis during the windup.[42] Once the hip-hinge is completed, the athlete will effectively shift the energy toward the plate during the stride. The arm cocking phase begins around the stride leg foot striking to the ground. Following front foot strike, the pelvis will stop rotating, transferring the

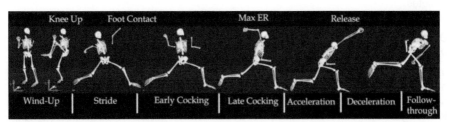

Fig. 6. Phases of pitching in video motion analysis as adapted from Trasolini and colleagues[3] (ER, external rotation).

energy through the torso to the upper extremity, accelerating the throwing arm toward the target. During arm movement toward the target, the torso rotates and tilts forward until stopping just before ball release, resulting in a kinematic transfer of energy through the shoulder as it transitions from external rotation to internal rotation, resulting in elbow extension until final ball release. The arm deceleration phase continues until maximal internal rotation and the torso rotates, tilts forward while the shoulder, arm, upper back, and chest work to decelerate the arm.[5] The follow through is highly dependent upon the athlete's throwing mechanics, but effectively ends with the thrower's upper and low extremities completing arm, torso, and lower extremity deceleration. In the shoulder, the rotator cuff serves an essential role in maintaining shoulder stability during the deceleration phase.

Throwing Analysis

Analysis of the throwing motion via pitching laboratory technology is a current and coming trend for high level athletes and can be applied beyond baseball for other overhead athletes.[5,42] It has been found helpful for evaluating and characterizing the pathobiomechanics in shoulder instability.[4,42–46] Other identifiable mechanics that may play a role in shoulder instability include increased elbow valgus torque and early trunk rotation, which have been presented as independent risk factors for many types of injury including those in the shoulder.[5,47,48] Future study will likely focus on novel attempts at biomechanical analysis. These include double calibration acromion marker cluster approaches focusing on measuring dynamic scapular orientation able to distinguish between glenohumeral and scapulothoracic contributions to shoulder biomechanics, shoulder distraction forces, ground reaction forces, drive leg components such as impulse and slope and their relation to kinematics such as rotational and angular velocities.[5] These aspects of the throwing motion may help identify the specific etiologies of instability in the overhead athletes as well as guide management, especially physical therapy and throwing progression, following conservative or operative management.

Other Sports

In swimmers, the lower extremities are not as involved in the rotation of the shoulder movement with strokes such as the backstroke, breaststroke, and butterfly. However, these techniques involve overhead extension and rotation in order to propel the swimmer forward.[49,50] Despite the relatively decreased energy needed for each stroke, the repetitive nature of swimming remains similar to the principles of throwing.[51] Like swimming, the overhead spike in volleyball and serve in tennis both rely on a similar sequence of upper extremity mechanics, with explosive overhead motion at the bounds of shoulder ROM in an abducted and externally rotated shoulder.[50] As a result, the overall overhead motion of throwers translate well to the discussion of all overhead athletes.

DISCUSSION
In-season Management

In-season management of shoulder instability is challenging for physicians and the athletic training staff. Health care professionals and coaches must prioritize athletes' safety and a safe return to play (RTP). However, in a recent survey on athlete priorities following an injury, athletes cared most about their RTP times.[51] As such, the key to in-season management is setting proper expectation based upon well-established management of overhead athlete shoulder instability. In-season management may involve conservative measures such as functional bracing, physical therapy, or time away from play, as well as more definitive measures such as surgical stabilization.

Functional bracing in overhead athletes can help to temporize an athlete's injury without a complete disruption in their participation in sports.[52] However, in-depth analysis of the effectiveness of bracing is scarce and tends to align more with clinical preference rather than quality studies. The long-term benefits, effects on RTP, or recurrence of instability in those managed with functional bracing remains unclear.

Various criteria have been established to help guide when athletes are able to RTP. One such proposal is that the athlete is to meet 4 criteria: restoration of (1) full ROM and (2) strength as well as the absence of (3) pain and (4) apprehension.[41] This may take between 1 and 3 weeks depending on athlete, demand of sport, position, and severity of instability.[41,53] The timeline to return may also be impacted by hand dominance; however, a current lack of data to suggest a clinically meaningful difference in RTP based on handedness limits this practice.[54–56] Given the fairly quick RTP time of a few weeks, a recent study on overhead athletes that returned within 10 days of injury showed that over half of them underwent off-season surgical management.[53] Overhead athletes that experience a delay in RTP beyond 1 to 3 weeks suggests that the cause is continued insufficient shoulder function or instability, even despite aggressive rehabilitation.[57] The variability in RTP times make early discussion of athlete expectations essential.

Nonoperative Management

Anterior

Nonoperative management of ASI may be successful, especially in the context of lower severity, less structural pathology, athlete and physician preference, and adherence to rehabilitation protocols.[58] Without significant lasting damage of the glenohumeral joint, including fractures, bone loss, osteochondral lesions, or damage to supportive structures, rehabilitation focuses on improving the 4 characteristics described earlier: restoration of full ROM and strength as well as testing for the absence of pain and apprehension.[41] To do this, physical therapy focusing on ROM, strength, scapular stability, as well as observation and improvement of biomechanical factors during exercises and the overhead motion should be implemented.[59,60] For example, 40% of professional baseball players SLAP tears are able to return to preinjury levels of competition via rehabilitation alone.[61,62] However, due to the heterogeneity of nonoperative treatment regimens, analysis of various protocols is limited. In a previous study of long-term outcomes with a mean follow-up of 12 years, a matched cohort between overhead athletes and nonoverhead athletes with ASI suggest that overhead athletes are more likely to experience a greater number of instability events.[63] When characterizing these instability events, they may occur during the rehabilitation process, afterward, or even both, with overhead athletes tending to subluxate more than dislocate, despite having no difference in patient-reported and other clinical outcomes.[63] Overhead athletes experienced an RTP rate of 71% in this study compared to 81% for the nonoverhead athletes. Despite successful conservative management for overhead athletes, there is a lack of a standardized protocol for athletes, making it difficult to definitively suggest a specific rehabilitation protocol.[41] In general, rehabilitation focusing on strength, ROM, scapular stability, and mechanics throughout a sport-specific motion appears to be the best approach.[41]

Posterior

PSI, though relatively uncommon in overhead athletes and thus not well studied, can be managed with multiple protocols. One such protocol suggests a staged approach trial prior to operative management, with progression from pain-free ROM to strengthening and scapulothoracic stabilization, followed by sports specific rehabilitation such as throwing programs.[38,64] Long-term outcomes after nonoperative management of PSI in both overhead athletes and nonoverhead athletes reported a rate of recurrence of 8%, with 54% of patients having continued pain.[37] This suggests that there is a role beyond simply delaying surgery for patients with PSI. An additional study that included both nonoverhead athletes and overhead athletes with PSI showed that patient-reported outcomes were improved following rehabilitation programs, such as the staged approach described above, with all athletes able to RTP.[65] However, these studies do not analyze overhead athletes individually or in subgroup analysis, suggesting further need for more focused studies on this athlete population.

Multidirectional instability

MDI is often multifactorial in nature, making the treatment of these athletes challenging. MDI is associated with increased laxity at baseline. As such, there is a wide array of presentations, making MDI dependent upon a more individualized approach. This individualized approach should consider the demands of the athlete's sport, duration and implications of seasons, and the goals of the respective athletes.[41,66] Therefore, initial treatment of symptomatic MDI should focus on rehabilitation of the specific presented directional instability. Given the likely laxity of the shoulder capsule, labrum, and other ligamentous supports, targeting the muscular support of the shoulder is advisable, specifically the rotator cuff and deltoid to facilitate greater active control of the glenohumeral joint.[67,68]

Surgical Management

A wide variety of operative techniques may be used successfully, with over 14 viable treatments of instability described in the literature.[69] The surgical technique used is often based upon patient or surgeon preference rather than high-quality research.[70–72] While this variability in treatment can be beneficial, allowing for an individualized approach, guidance and trends on surgical technique are necessary to improve expected and repeatable results for athletes. Further considerations of surgical management include larger labral tears in continuity, such as extensive SLAP tears (ie, Type V, VIII, and IX) and/or involvement of the biceps labral insertion with "peel back" phenomenon.[62]

Anterior

There are a number of surgical options for athletes with ASI, including arthroscopic and open techniques, such as capsulolabral or Bankart repair, capsular plication, osseous augmentation, and open labral repair.[73–75] Recurrence rates following arthroscopic capsulolabral repair in overhead athletes range from 0% to 4% with RTP at preinjury level reported from 45% to 82%.[59,76,77] A study evaluating outcomes in baseball players showed an average RTP time of 8.4 months, with only 63% of athletes returning to their preinjury level of play, while interpretation may be limited by the heterogeneity of indications and techniques used in this cohort.[78] Despite research that demonstrates an increased likelihood of overhead athletes to undergo surgical management, their RTP, recurrent instability, and revision rates are not significantly different from nonoverhead athletes.[41,63] Even in the context of heterogenous results, labral repair remains steadfast as the treatment of choice for persistent anterior glenohumeral instability.

In the case of SLAP tears, with and without biceps involvement, treatment algorithms have been proposed for overhead athletes.[62] When surgery is indicated, arthroscopic repair via knotted or increasingly knotless fixation of the torn labrum and/or biceps tenodesis are generally pursued depending on the type of tear, age, provocative physical examination findings, and level or position of the athlete.[62,79,80] Risks and benefits of SLAP tear stabilization, including the possibility of ROM loss and/or residual anterior shoulder pain, must be carefully considered in the overhead throwing athlete that often function at the extremes of shoulder motion.

In the setting of a concomitant Hill–Sachs lesion, capsulolabral repair may be accompanied by the remplissage procedure.[81–83] A significant concern associated with remplissage in overhead athletes is resulting stiffness, which is thought to be related to an increased capsular restraint and reduced secondary shoulder ROM, particularly external rotation in an adducted position.[41] For example, overhead athletes showed poor outcomes with regards to RTP at their preinjury levels when undergoing remplissage.[82] As such, without more extensive analysis on remplissage in overhead athletes, further adoption is currently not recommended and only selectively indicated in overhead athletes.[41,59]

Another consideration in overhead athletes with ASI is bony involvement and specifically, attritional bone loss. While the thresholds are still debated, athletes with glenoid bone loss in excess of approximately 13.5% to 20% may be preferentially considered for reconstructive procedures such as a Latarjet or anterior glenoid bone block reconstruction with allograft or autograft (**Figs. 7** and **8**).[34,84] However, a trial of soft tissue only repair, even in the setting of subcritical bone loss, may be an early option in an attempt to preserve motion and optimize RTP by avoiding the constraints associated with the Latarjet procedure. Importantly, overhead athletes who undergo arthroscopic Latarjet procedures are less likely to successfully RTP than those that do not.[59] The decreased RTP potential is also consistent with open Latarjet procedures, with an RTP rate to preinjury level of approximately 75%.[85] Much like the case of remplissage, this is likely due to reduction in ROM limiting the shoulder's ability to remain stable or even reach preinjury level of biomechanics.

A final consideration in ASI in overhead athletes is rotator cuff involvement. Previous literature suggests that operative fixation of the rotator cuff will more than likely conclude overhead athletes' careers.[86,87] Therefore, current management focuses on debridement for amenable tears, including the involvement of up to 70% of medial-lateral tendon width, rather than repair for athletes who wish to RTP.

In summary, there is a wide variety of techniques available for the surgical management of ASI, which focus on surgeon and athlete preference, with the exception of rotator cuff involvement, remplissage, and Latarjet, as outcomes following these procedures tend to impact the ability to RTP among noncollision, overhead athletes.

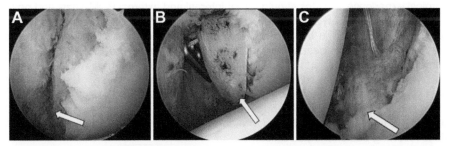

Fig. 7. Anteroinferior bony Bankart lesion (*A*) with repair using iliac crest autograft (*B, C*) in an overhead athlete with acute ASI. *Arrow* in (*A*) is pointing to an anteroinferior bony bankart lesion, *Arrow* in (*B*) is pointing to an illiac crest autograft, and *arrow* in (*C*) is pointing to the illiac crest autograft during fixation within the shoulder.

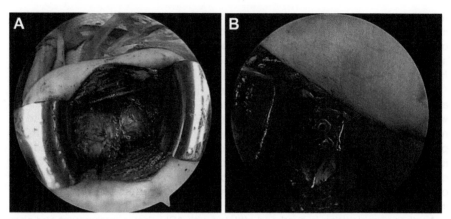

Fig. 8. A 15 year old overhead athlete with recurrent instability following ALPSA lesion repair with continued significant ASI and subsequent bony loss in the form of an irreparable bony Bankart lesion in the right shoulder (*A*). The irreparable bony Bankart lesion was treated with an open Latarjet coracoid transfer using 2 cannulated screws with a rim plate (*B*).

Proper patient selection or surgical technique requires consideration of the condition of stabilizing structures, surgeon preference, and an athlete's expectations.

Posterior

As with ASI, overhead athletes with PSI who are unable to progress following conservative management may be treated with posterior capsulolabral repair with anchor fixation.[88] Well established in the case of PSI is the concern of overtensioning and plication of the posterior shoulder labrum and capsule, as the overhead athletes relies specifically on the extremes of overhead ROM.[89,90] This is due to the possibility that excessive capsular reduction or tension may decrease the necessary ROM for proper throwing mechanics.[38,91] As such, isolated posterior labral repair is recommended with minimal capsulorrhaphy (if necessary) to retention plastic deformation of the IGHL complex. If present, an associated so-called Bennett lesion, or throwers exostosis at the attachment PIGHL, may be decompressed to facilitate better interface for healing. Early immobilization in the "gunslinger" neutral position is beneficial, and scapular and rotator cuff activation occurs early through isometric exercises. Although balancing the impact of posterior stabilization with ROM goals comes with surgical experience, athletes should target internal and external ROM goals and posterior shoulder flexibility during staged rehabilitation.[92–94] A return to throwing program may be initiated in the fourth month of rehabilitation after appropriate criteria for advancement have been achieved.[92] Similarly, a return to batting progression is introduced during the sports-specific phase of rehabilitation, starting with dry swings and hitting from a tee to soft toss and ultimately, simulated hitting.[95] Despite these best practices, athletes vary widely in their return preinjury level of activity following arthroscopic posterior capsulolabral repair (37%–83%), with a revision rate around 9%.[91,96–98] Further characterization of these injuries is important to solidify expectations following posterior stabilization.

Multidirectional instability

MDI follows the same principles, surgical techniques, and surgical selection as PSI and ASI; failed extensive rehabilitation is often treated surgically. Patients diagnosed with MDI should undergo 6 to 12 months of dedicated physical therapy prior to being considered for surgical management, particularly in the absence of trauma and/or labral tears. Historically, surgical options favored open techniques focusing on labral repair with capsular shift,[99,100] although arthroscopic options have shown increasingly equivalent outcomes. This technique is the standard for MDI management as it has a fairly low instability recurrence rate of approximately 4% to 8% at final follow-up.[28,41] Open labral repair with capsular shift may provide stabilization of the shoulder at the cost of performance, as the technique is prone to overtensioning with the resultant loss of abduction and external rotation necessary for overhead athletes. Conversely, arthroscopic pan-capsular plication with a circumferential anchor-based fixation can result in improved capsulolabral bumper and reduction of overall capsular volume with a "pinch tuck" technique. Furthermore, adjunctive lateral rotator interval closure may be considered for individuals with significant multidirectional laxity. However, long-term outcomes have been limited, with a similar concern for overtensioning with subsequently reduced ROM at the expense of increased stability.[101]

Further Recommendations

The treatment of shoulder instability, in most instances, should begin with a trial of nonoperative management. A focus on shoulder ROM, strength, and biomechanics is essential to optimize dynamic shoulder stability throughout overhead motion. When conservative management fails, critical or combined subcritical bone loss is present, or acute, first-time shoulder dislocation occurs, surgical repair may be preferentially considered. Given the risk of impairing native ROM essential to the overhead athlete, the minimal operative technique to restore stability is advisable, with avoidance of reducing capsular volume when feasible. This is in stark contrast to the non-overhead athlete, where capsular volume reduction is often included in a comprehensive surgical approach to reduce the recurrence of instability.

PHYSICAL THERAPY AND RETURN TO THROWING PROGRAM
Physical Therapy

Physical therapy following shoulder instability is integral and may take a variety of forms dependent on the type of instability present. Given the biomechanical changes seen in these overhead athletes overtime, attention to the specific needs of the sport are necessary during initial, more standardized rehabilitation. In a recent systematic review, postoperative sling use was recommended, along with elbow, wrist, and hand ROM exercises.[102] Further, full passive foreword flexion was achieved around 3 weeks, with active ROM by around 5 weeks, and normal motion by 10 weeks postoperatively. Various protocols provided recommendations on a return to sport-specific exercises around 17 weeks following surgery, though there remains variability between Latarjet and Bankart repair protocols with regard to exercise and motion goal recommendations.[102,103] As the general timeline of rehabilitation following surgery continues to solidify, research comparing types of surgery and accompanying rehabilitation is essential to optimize athlete outcomes.

Throwing and Rehabilitation Programs

Effective rehabilitation and throwing programs, such as USA Pitch Smart, are essential in the RTP process.[104] These programs are not limited to focus on the upper extremity, as core control and leg strength are foundational to the throwing motion, and ensuring proper mechanics during the return to throwing is imperative to a successful return to

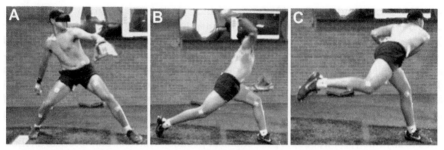

Fig. 9. Visual motion technology with attached video-motion sensors showing a pitcher in the stride (*A*), late cocking phase (*B*), and follow through (*C*) phases.

sport.[105] In the context of the volume of throwing in baseball, additional considerations include pitch or throwing counts, appropriate rest, and proper conditioning to decrease injury risk associated with shoulder instability and overall health.[5,54]

To optimize performance recovery, early interval throwing programs have thus far relied on throwing distance and velocity to estimate training load and to guide progression of sporting activities.[106,107] New technology, including pitching laboratories and field-accessible throwing analysis make estimating strain on the athlete increasingly accurate (**Fig. 9**).[107-109] With the development of accurate monitoring of throwing mechanics and stress, a more individualized and flexible throwing programs may be used. Future developments in this technology may even be predictive, such that current objective and subjective mechanics can advise adaptation to avoid or correct pathomechanics prior to injury. Examples include research on variables derived from ground reaction force curves that may predict variation in pitching mechanics before the athlete can identify these changes (see **Fig. 6**; **Fig. 10**). Adapting to these improvements in rehabilitation is key to continue the shift from a reactive to a more proactive approach for the management of shoulder instability in the overhead athlete.

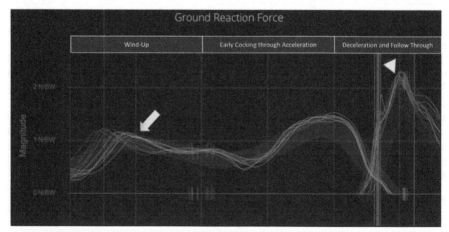

Fig. 10. Demonstrative ground reaction force curve of the drive leg (*arrow*) and stride leg (*arrowhead*) during the pitching motion. Forces measured in Newton per body weight overtime. Labeled phases of the pitching motion correlate with those noted in **Fig. 6**.

SUMMARY

Shoulder instability in overhead athletes can be debilitating with variable presentation, making it difficult to manage. In general, treatment begins with conservative management with a focus on reinforcing proper mechanics with rehabilitation that targets strengthening shoulder stability. When this fails or there is an acute or severe injury, operative management may be indicated. During labral repair and capsulorrhaphy, it is important to understand that some level of laxity relates to performance in an overhead athlete, such that overstabilization may impede ability and affect performance. The incorporation of video-motion analysis of overhead athletes may serve as a way to proactively detect pathomechanics and either improve postoperative rehabilitation or avoid injury before onset. Further multicenter randomized control trials focusing on surgical techniques, improvements in rehabilitation monitoring, and biomechanical analysis are needed to progress the management of shoulder instability in the overhead athlete from reactive to proactive.

CLINICS CARE POINTS

- In-season management is variable and should consider bracing, physical therapy, time away from sport, and surgical fixation based on the presentation and athlete preference.
- Despite heterogenous long-term outcomes, labral repair remains standard in the treatment of shoulder instability for overhead athletes.
- During labral repair and capsulorrhaphy, some level of laxity relates to performance in an overhead athlete. Overstabilization may impede ability and affect performance.
- Operative fixation of the rotator cuff will more than likely conclude overhead athletes' careers.
- Physical therapy is variable by sport and type of instability. Protocols should be based upon expected progression in the context of the athlete's sport.

DISCLOSURE

The authors have no relevant disclosures.

REFERENCES

1. Goetti P, Denard PJ, Collin P, et al. Shoulder biomechanics in normal and selected pathological conditions. EFORT Open Rev 2020;5(8):508–18.
2. Duman N, Özer M. Radiological and clinical evaluation of long head of biceps tendon function in the glenohumeral joint. Jt Dis Relat Surg 2023;34(1):98–107.
3. Yeh ML, Lintner D, Luo ZP. Stress distribution in the superior labrum during throwing motion. Am J Sports Med 2005;33(3):395–401.
4. Wardell M, Creighton D, Kovalcik C. Glenohumeral instability and arm pain in overhead throwing athletes: a correlational study. Int J Sports Phys Ther 2022; 17(7):1351–7.
5. Trasolini NA, Nicholson KF, Mylott J, et al. Biomechanical Analysis of the Throwing Athlete and Its Impact on Return to Sport. Arthrosc Sports Med Rehabil 2022;4(1):e83–91.
6. Veeger HE, van der Helm FC. Shoulder function: the perfect compromise between mobility and stability. J Biomech 2007;40(10):2119–29.

7. Kuhn JE, Bey MJ, Huston LJ, et al. Ligamentous restraints to external rotation of the humerus in the late-cocking phase of throwing. A cadaveric biomechanical investigation. Am J Sports Med 2000;28(2):200–5.

8. Huffman GR, Tibone JE, McGarry MH, et al. Path of glenohumeral articulation throughout the rotational range of motion in a thrower's shoulder model. Am J Sports Med 2006;34(10):1662–9.

9. Borsa PA, Laudner KG, Sauers EL. Mobility and stability adaptations in the shoulder of the overhead athlete: a theoretical and evidence-based perspective. Sports Med 2008;38(1):17–36.

10. Gelber JD, Soloff L, Schickendantz MS. The thrower's shoulder. J Am Acad Orthop Surg 2018;26(6):204–13.

11. Massimini DF, Boyer PJ, Papannagari R, et al. In-vivo glenohumeral translation and ligament elongation during abduction and abduction with internal and external rotation. J Orthop Surg Res 2012;7:29.

12. Yi M, Yang F, An J, et al. Effect of glenohumeral ligaments on posterior shoulder stabilization: a biomechanical study. Am J Transl Res 2023;15(3):1953–63.

13. Thompson SF, Guess TM, Plackis AC, et al. Youth baseball pitching mechanics: a systematic review. Sports Health 2018;10(2):133–40.

14. Chalmers PN, Wimmer MA, Verma NN, et al. The relationship between pitching mechanics and injury: a review of current concepts. Sports Health 2017;9(3):216–21.

15. Sahara W, Yamazaki T, Inui T, et al. The glenohumeral micromotion and influence of the glenohumeral ligaments during axial rotation in varying abduction angle. J Orthop Sci 2020;25(6):980–5.

16. Funakoshi T, Takahashi T, Shimokobe H, et al. Arthroscopic findings of the glenohumeral joint in symptomatic anterior instabilities: comparison between overhead throwing disorders and traumatic shoulder dislocation. J Shoulder Elbow Surg 2023;32(4):776–85.

17. Economopoulos KJ, Brockmeier SF. Rotator cuff tears in overhead athletes. Clin Sports Med 2012;31(4):675–92.

18. Lin DJ, Wong TT, Kazam JK. Shoulder injuries in the overhead-throwing athlete: epidemiology, mechanisms of injury, and imaging findings. Radiology 2018;286(2):370–87.

19. Tooth C, Gofflot A, Schwartz C, et al. Risk factors of overuse shoulder injuries in overhead athletes: a systematic review. Sports Health 2020;12(5):478–87.

20. Escamilla RF, Andrews JR. Shoulder muscle recruitment patterns and related biomechanics during upper extremity sports. Sports Med 2009;39(7):569–90.

21. Medina G, Bartolozzi AR 3rd, Spencer JA, et al. The thrower's shoulder. JBJS Rev 2022;10(3).

22. Moradi M, Hadadnezhad M, Letafatkar A, et al. Efficacy of throwing exercise with TheraBand in male volleyball players with shoulder internal rotation deficit: a randomized controlled trial. BMC Muscoskel Disord 2020;21(1):376.

23. Thomas SJ, Blubello A, Peterson A, et al. Master swimmers with shoulder pain and disability have altered functional and structural measures. J Athl Train 2021;56(12):1313–20.

24. Hibberd EE, Oyama S, Spang JT, et al. Effect of a 6-week strengthening program on shoulder and scapular-stabilizer strength and scapular kinematics in division I collegiate swimmers. J Sport Rehabil 2012;21(3):253–65.

25. Owens BD, Dawson L, Burks R, et al. Incidence of shoulder dislocation in the United States military: demographic considerations from a high-risk population. J Bone Joint Surg Am 2009;91(4):791–6.

26. Galvin JW, Ernat JJ, Waterman BR, et al. The epidemiology and natural history of anterior shoulder instability. Curr Rev Musculoskelet Med 2017;10(4):411–24.

27. Brelin A, Dickens JF. Posterior shoulder instability. Sports Med Arthrosc Rev 2017;25(3):136–43.

28. Longo UG, Rizzello G, Loppini M, et al. Multidirectional instability of the shoulder: a systematic review. Arthroscopy 2015;31(12):2431–43.

29. Boileau P, Zumstein M, Balg F, et al. The unstable painful shoulder (UPS) as a cause of pain from unrecognized anteroinferior instability in the young athlete. J Shoulder Elbow Surg 2011;20(1):98–106.

30. Arner JW, Peebles LA, Bradley JP, et al. Anterior shoulder instability management: indications, techniques, and outcomes. Arthroscopy 2020;36(11):2791–3.

31. Burkhart SS, Morgan CD, Kibler WB. The disabled throwing shoulder: spectrum of pathology Part I: pathoanatomy and biomechanics. Arthroscopy 2003;19(4):404–20.

32. Kibler WB, Thomas SJ. Pathomechanics of the throwing shoulder. Sports Med Arthrosc Rev 2012;20(1):22–9.

33. Parvaresh KC, Vargas-Vila M, Bomar JD, et al. Anterior glenohumeral instability in the adolescent athlete. JBJS Rev 2020;8(2):e0080.

34. Yamamoto N, Itoi E, Abe H, et al. Effect of an anterior glenoid defect on anterior shoulder stability: a cadaveric study. Am J Sports Med 2009;37(5):949–54.

35. Robinson CM, Aderinto J. Recurrent posterior shoulder instability. J Bone Joint Surg Am 2005;87(4):883–92.

36. Bäcker HC, Galle SE, Maniglio M, et al. Biomechanics of posterior shoulder instability - current knowledge and literature review. World J Orthoped 2018;9(11):245–54.

37. Lee J, Woodmass JM, Bernard CD, et al. Nonoperative management of posterior shoulder instability: what are the long-term clinical outcomes? Clin J Sport Med 2022;32(2):e116–20.

38. Sheean AJ, Kibler WB, Conway J, et al. Posterior labral injury and glenohumeral instability in overhead athletes: current concepts for diagnosis and management. J Am Acad Orthop Surg 2020;28(15):628–37.

39. Millett PJ, Clavert P, Hatch GF 3rd, et al. Recurrent posterior shoulder instability. J Am Acad Orthop Surg 2006;14(8):464–76.

40. Chang ES, Greco NJ, McClincy MP, et al. Posterior shoulder instability in overhead athletes. Orthop Clin N Am 2016;47(1):179–87.

41. Arguello AM, Till SE, Reinholz AK, et al. Camp CL. Managing shoulder instability in the overhead athlete. Curr Rev Musculoskelet Med 2022;15(6):552–60.

42. Weber AE, Kontaxis A, O'Brien SJ, et al. The biomechanics of throwing: simplified and cogent. Sports Med Arthrosc Rev 2014;22(2):72–9.

43. Illyés A, Kiss RM. Electromyographic analysis in patients with multidirectional shoulder instability during pull, forward punch, elevation and overhead throw. Knee Surg Sports Traumatol Arthrosc 2007;15(5):624–31.

44. Kibler WB, Wilkes T, Sciascia A. Mechanics and pathomechanics in the overhead athlete. Clin Sports Med 2013;32(4):637–51.

45. Jobe FW, Moynes DR, Tibone JE, et al. An EMG analysis of the shoulder in pitching. A second report. Am J Sports Med 1984;12(3):218–20.

46. Dillman CJ, Fleisig GS, Andrews JR. Biomechanics of pitching with emphasis upon shoulder kinematics. J Orthop Sports Phys Ther 1993;18(2):402–8.

47. Hurd WJ, Kaufman KR. Glenohumeral rotational motion and strength and baseball pitching biomechanics. J Athl Train 2012;47(3):247–56.

48. Stokes H, Eaton K, Zheng NN. Shoulder external rotational properties during physical examination are associated with injury that requires surgery and shoulder joint loading during baseball pitching. Am J Sports Med 2021;49(13): 3647–55.

49. Perry J. Anatomy and biomechanics of the shoulder in throwing, swimming, gymnastics, and tennis. Clin Sports Med 1983;2(2):247–70.

50. Pozzi F, Plummer HA, Shanley E, et al. Preseason shoulder range of motion screening and in-season risk of shoulder and elbow injuries in overhead athletes: systematic review and meta-analysis. Br J Sports Med 2020;54(17): 1019–27.

51. Bien DP, Dubuque TJ. Considerations for late stage acl rehabilitation and return to sport to limit re-injury risk and maximize athletic performance. Int J Sports Phys Ther 2015;10(2):256–71.

52. Baker HP, Krishnan P, Meghani O, et al. Protective sport bracing for athletes with mid-season shoulder instability. Sports Health 2023;15(1):105–10.

53. Buss DD, Lynch GP, Meyer CP, et al. Nonoperative management for in-season athletes with anterior shoulder instability. Am J Sports Med 2004;32(6):1430–3.

54. Otley T, Myers H, Lau BC, et al. Return to sport after shoulder stabilization procedures: a criteria-based testing continuum to guide rehabilitation and inform return-to-play decision making. Arthrosc Sports Med Rehabil 2022;4(1): e237–46.

55. Falsone SA, Gross MT, Guskiewicz KM, et al. One-arm hop test: reliability and effects of arm dominance. J Orthop Sports Phys Ther 2002;32(3):98–103.

56. Rangavajjula A, Hyatt A, Raneses E, et al. Return to play after treatment of shoulder labral tears in professional hockey players. Phys Sportsmed 2016;44(2): 119–25.

57. Dickens JF, Owens BD, Cameron KL, et al. Return to play and recurrent instability after in-season anterior shoulder instability: a prospective multicenter study. Am J Sports Med 2014;42(12):2842–50.

58. Hurley ET, Matache BA, Wong I, et al. Anterior shoulder instability international consensus group. anterior shoulder instability part i-diagnosis, nonoperative management, and bankart repair-an international consensus statement. Arthroscopy 2022;38(2):214–23.e7.

59. Trinh TQ, Naimark MB, Bedi A, et al. Clinical outcomes after anterior shoulder stabilization in overhead athletes: an analysis of the moon shoulder instability consortium. Am J Sports Med 2019;47(6):1404–10.

60. Clesham K, Shannon FJ. Arthroscopic anterior shoulder stabilisation in overhead sport athletes: 5-year follow-up. Ir J Med Sci 2019;188(4):1233–7.

61. Frantz TL, Shacklett AG, Martin AS, et al. Biceps tenodesis for superior labrum anterior-posterior tear in the overhead athlete: a systematic review. Am J Sports Med 2021;49(2):522–8.

62. Fortier LM, Menendez ME, Kerzner B, et al. SLAP tears: treatment algorithm. Arthroscopy 2022;38(12):3103–5.

63. Wilbur RR, Shirley MB, Nauert RF, et al. Anterior shoulder instability in throwers and overhead athletes: long-term outcomes in a geographic cohort. Am J Sports Med 2022;50(1):182–8.

64. Gouveia K, Kay J, Memon M, et al. Return to Sport after surgical management of posterior shoulder instability: a systematic review and meta-analysis. Am J Sports Med 2022;50(3):845–57.

65. Blacknall J, Mackie A, Wallace WA. Patient-reported outcomes following a physiotherapy rehabilitation programme for atraumatic posterior shoulder subluxation. Shoulder Elbow 2014;6(2):137–41.
66. Warby SA, Pizzari T, Ford JJ, et al. The effect of exercise-based management for multidirectional instability of the glenohumeral joint: a systematic review. J Shoulder Elbow Surg 2014;23(1):128–42.
67. Warby SA, Ford JJ, Hahne AJ, et al. Comparison of 2 exercise rehabilitation programs for multidirectional instability of the glenohumeral joint: a randomized controlled trial. Am J Sports Med 2018;46(1):87–97.
68. Watson L, Warby S, Balster S, et al. The treatment of multidirectional instability of the shoulder with a rehabilitation programme: Part 2. Shoulder Elbow 2017;9(1): 46–53.
69. Griffith R, Fretes N, Bolia IK, et al. Return-to-sport criteria after upper extremity surgery in athletes-a scoping review, part 1: rotator cuff and shoulder stabilization procedures. Orthop J Sports Med 2021;9(8). 23259671211021827.
70. Friedman LGM, Lafosse L, Garrigues GE. Global perspectives on management of shoulder instability: decision making and treatment. Orthop Clin N Am 2020; 51(2):241–58.
71. Cole BJ, Warner JJ. Arthroscopic versus open Bankart repair for traumatic anterior shoulder instability. Clin Sports Med 2000;19(1):19–48.
72. Ernstbrunner L, De Nard B, Olthof M, et al. Long-term results of the arthroscopic bankart repair for recurrent anterior shoulder instability in patients older than 40 years: a comparison with the open latarjet procedure. Am J Sports Med 2020; 48(9):2090–6.
73. Hurley ET, Manjunath AK, Bloom DA, et al. Arthroscopic bankart repair versus conservative management for first-time traumatic anterior shoulder instability: a systematic review and meta-analysis. Arthroscopy 2020;36(9):2526–32.
74. Coyner KJ, Arciero RA. Shoulder instability: anterior, posterior, multidirectional, arthroscopic versus open, bone block procedures. Sports Med Arthrosc Rev 2018;26(4):168–70.
75. Jones KJ, Kahlenberg CA, Dodson CC, et al. Arthroscopic capsular plication for microtraumatic anterior shoulder instability in overhead athletes. Am J Sports Med 2012;40(9):2009–14.
76. Harada Y, Yokoya S, Sumimoto Y, et al. Prevalence of rotator cuff tears among older tennis players and its impact on clinical findings and shoulder function. J Sport Rehabil 2022;31(7):849–55.
77. Lau BC, Pineda LB, Johnston TR, et al. Return to play after revision anterior shoulder stabilization: a systematic review. Orthop J Sports Med 2021;9(3). 2325967120982059.
78. Park JY, Lee JH, Oh KS, et al. Return to play after arthroscopic treatment for shoulder instability in elite and professional baseball players. J Shoulder Elbow Surg 2019;28(1):77–81.
79. Wilk KE, Macrina LC, Cain EL, et al. The recognition and treatment of superior labral (slap) lesions in the overhead athlete. Int J Sports Phys Ther 2013;8(5): 579–600.
80. Waterman BR, Newgren J, Richardson C, et al. High rate of return to sporting activity among overhead athletes with subpectoral biceps tenodesis for Type II SLAP Tear. Arthroscopy 2023;39(1):11–6.
81. Gouveia K, Harbour E, Athwal GS, et al. Return to sport after arthroscopic bankart repair with remplissage: a systematic review. Arthroscopy 2023;39(4): 1046–59.e3.

82. Garcia GH, Wu HH, Liu JN, et al. Outcomes of the remplissage procedure and its effects on return to sports: average 5-year follow-up. Am J Sports Med 2016; 44(5):1124–30.

83. Horinek JL, Menendez ME, Narbona P, et al. Remplissage yields similar 2-year outcomes, fewer complications, and low recurrence compared to latarjet across a wide range of preoperative glenoid bone loss. Arthroscopy 2022;38(10): 2798–805.

84. Yamamoto N, Itoi E. Osseous defects seen in patients with anterior shoulder instability. Clin Orthop Surg 2015;7(4):425–9.

85. Abdul-Rassoul H, Galvin JW, Curry EJ, et al. Return to sport after surgical treatment for anterior shoulder instability: a systematic review. Am J Sports Med 2019;47(6):1507–15.

86. Alrabaa RG, Lobao MH, Levine WN. Rotator cuff injuries in tennis players. Curr Rev Musculoskelet Med 2020;13(6):734–47.

87. Liu JN, Garcia GH, Gowd AK, et al. Treatment of partial thickness rotator cuff tears in overhead athletes. Curr Rev Musculoskelet Med 2018;11(1):55–62.

88. Leivadiotou D, Ahrens P. Arthroscopic treatment of posterior shoulder instability: a systematic review. Arthroscopy 2015;31(3):555–60.

89. McClincy MP, Arner JW, Bradley JP. Posterior shoulder instability in throwing athletes: a case-matched comparison of throwers and non-throwers. Arthroscopy 2015;31(6):1041–51.

90. Radkowski CA, Chhabra A, Baker CL 3rd, et al. Arthroscopic capsulolabral repair for posterior shoulder instability in throwing athletes compared with non-throwing athletes. Am J Sports Med 2008;36(4):693–9.

91. Vaswani R, Arner J, Freiman H, et al. Risk factors for revision posterior shoulder stabilization in throwing athletes. Orthop J Sports Med 2020;8(12). 2325967120967652.

92. Goldenberg BT, Goldsten P, Lacheta L, et al. Rehabilitation following posterior shoulder stabilization. Int J Sports Phys Ther 2021;16(3):930–40.

93. Gharisia O, Lohman E, Daher N, et al. Effect of a novel stretching technique on shoulder range of motion in overhead athletes with glenohumeral internal rotation deficits: a randomized controlled trial. BMC Muscoskel Disord 2021; 22(1):402.

94. Tahran Ö, Yeşilyaprak SS. Effects of modified posterior shoulder stretching exercises on shoulder mobility, pain, and dysfunction in patients with subacromial impingement syndrome. Sports Health 2020/Apr;12(2):139–48.

95. Monti R. Return to hitting: an interval hitting progression and overview of hitting mechanics following injury. Int J Sports Phys Ther 2015;10(7):1059–73.

96. Kercher JS, Runner RP, McCarthy TP, et al. Posterior labral repairs of the shoulder among baseball players: results and outcomes with minimum 2-year follow-up. Am J Sports Med 2019;47(7):1687–93.

97. McClincy MP, Arner JW, Thurber L, et al. Arthroscopic capsulolabral reconstruction for posterior shoulder instability is successful in adolescent athletes. J Pediatr Orthop 2020;40(3):135–41.

98. Chan S, O'Brien LK, Waterman BR, et al. Low risk of recurrence after posterior labral repair of the shoulder in a high-risk united states military population. Arthrosc Sports Med Rehabil 2020;2(1):e47–52.

99. Voigt C, Schulz AP, Lill H. Arthroscopic treatment of multidirectional glenohumeral instability in young overhead athletes. Open Orthop J 2009;3:107–14.

100. Ren H, Bicknell RT. From the unstable painful shoulder to multidirectional instability in the young athlete. Clin Sports Med 2013;32(4):815–23.

101. Carlson Strother CR, McLaughlin RJ, Krych AJ, et al. Open shoulder stabilization for instability: anterior labral repair with capsular shift. Arthrosc Tech 2019;8(7):e749–54.

102. DeFroda SF, Mehta N, Owens BD. Physical therapy protocols for arthroscopic bankart repair. Sports Health 2018/Jun;10(3):250–8.

103. Fleisig GS, Barrentine SW, Escamilla RF, et al. Biomechanics of overhand throwing with implications for injuries. Sports Med 1996;21(6):421–37.

104. Axe M, Hurd W, Snyder-Mackler L. Data-based interval throwing programs for baseball players. Sports Health 2009;1(2):145–53.

105. Cisco S, Miller Semon M, Moraski P, et al. Distance-based throwing programs for baseball players from little league to high school. Pediatr Phys Ther 2019; 31(3):297–300.

106. Hermanns CA, Coda RG, Cheema S, et al. Variability in rehabilitation protocols after superior labrum anterior posterior surgical repair. Kans J Med 2021;14: 243–8.

107. Boddy KJ, Marsh JA, Caravan A, et al. Exploring wearable sensors as an alternative to marker-based motion capture in the pitching delivery. PeerJ 2019;7: e6365.

108. Nicholson KF, Mylott JA, Waterman BR, et al. Pitching biomechanics normative values and kinetic differences by competition level. J Surg Orthop Adv 2022; 31(3):177–80.

109. Seroyer ST, Nho SJ, Bach BR, et al. The kinetic chain in overhand pitching: its potential role for performance enhancement and injury prevention. Sports Health 2010;2(2):135–46.

Rehabilitation and Return to Sport following Operative and Nonoperative Treatment of Anterior Shoulder Instability

Zachary J. Herman, MD, Rajiv P. Reddy, BS, Alex Fails, DPT,
Albert Lin, MD*, Adam Popchak, PT, PhD

KEYWORDS

• Anterior shoulder instability • Postoperative rehabilitation • Return to sport criteria

KEY POINTS

• Regardless of the treatment intervention employed, rehabilitation following anterior shoulder instability should focus on the preservation of motion and strengthening.
• Rehabilitation interventions differ slightly based on the operative intervention that was performed.
• A well-informed, shared return to sport (RTS) decision after anterior shoulder instability should involve an assessment of an athlete's pain levels and tolerance, psychological readiness for RTS, shoulder range of motion, strength, sport-specific power and endurance, and functional assessments that incorporate necessary components of the kinetic chain.

INTRODUCTION

Anterior glenohumeral instability is common among young athletes and typically presents following a traumatic injury.[1,2] Although anterior shoulder instability can be treated nonoperatively, current literature suggests operative management may result in lower recurrent rates compared to nonoperative treatment.[3] Operative treatment options include open or arthroscopic Bankart repair, remplissage, Latarjet, and other bone block augmentation procedures.[4] As no consensus on how to optimize outcomes following surgery and rehabilitation has been established, there has been growing interest in the rehabilitation process and timing of returning an athlete to sport following these management options for anterior shoulder instability. The purpose of

Department of Orthopaedic Surgery, UPMC Freddie Fu Sports Medicine Center, University of Pittsburgh, 3200 South Water Street, Pittsburgh, PA, USA
* Corresponding author. UPMC Freddie Fu Sports Medicine Center, University of Pittsburgh, 3200 South Water Street, Pittsburgh, PA 15203.
E-mail address: lina2@upmc.edu

Clin Sports Med 43 (2024) 705–722
https://doi.org/10.1016/j.csm.2024.03.025

this article is to review the current rehabilitation and return to sport (RTS) protocols for various nonoperative and operative management strategies following anterior shoulder instability events.

NONOPERATIVE MANAGEMENT

The best course of management for patients following primary traumatic anterior shoulder dislocation is up for debate. A Cochrane systematic review[5] suggests that surgical management should be the first choice for younger male individuals participating in activities that place high demands on the shoulder complex, while another showed moderate-quality evidence that nearly half of patients were able to avoid recurrence with nonoperative management after anterior glenohumeral joint dislocation.[6]

Regardless, if a shared decision-making process results in the choice of nonoperative management, immobilization in a standard sling should be limited to 1 week and weaning should be encouraged as the patient becomes more comfortable.[7] Short-term immobilization can limit decreases in strength and motor control related to disuse. Sling positioning in external rotation (ER) and increased duration of sling use have not been shown to decrease recurrence rates.[8,9] To date, no evidence suggests a role for corticosteroids or orthobiologics in the management of primary anterior glenohumeral dislocation.

During the first 10 to 14 days of conservative management following primary traumatic anterior shoulder dislocation, rehabilitation should emphasize the restoration of range of motion (ROM), early activation of the rotator cuff and scapular muscles through submaximal contractions, and activities to address proprioception and motor control.[10] Isometric contractions may be emphasized in this phase. Psychological risk factors and kinesiophobia should also be addressed with patient education encouraging active movement and use of the injured shoulder for daily activities as symptoms and comfort allow. Referrals for mental health care should be made when deemed appropriate to help avoid protracted recovery times. Social support from rehabilitation professionals has been identified as an important contributor to increased patient satisfaction and decreased depression postinjury.[11]

As pain and inflammation subside after the initial postinjury phase, a progressive neuromuscular strengthening program incorporating the kinetic chain and plyometric activity as appropriate should be initiated. Interventions should be matched to the patient's irritability level and activity demands. A staged approach for rehabilitation classification based on irritability levels has been previously described and can be useful to guide progression for these patients.[12] Strengthening and controlled active ROM should be gradually progressed in position from at the side, to mid-ROM, and eventually into provocative end-range positions under progressively increased loads that are specific to the demands of a patient's desired activities. In general, rehabilitation programs incorporating neuromuscular control and the kinetic chain have demonstrated superior patient outcomes when compared to strengthening alone for those recovering from shoulder instability.[10,13,14] A description of general phased rehabilitation approach with general timelines and overarching objectives is provided in **Table 1**. A corresponding detailed rehabilitation progression is provided in Appendix 1. It should be emphasized that these phases are not mutually exclusive and patients will often progress in a nonlinear manner and at differing rates. For example, a patient may be progressing through midrange strengthening activities and have periods of higher tissue irritability levels and require more controlled ROM activities along with submaximal isometrics to allow symptoms to subside.

Table 1
Phased approach to rehabilitation for shoulder instability

	Weeks 0–6	Weeks 6–8	Weeks 8–10	Weeks 10–12	Weeks >12
		Staged Recovery of ROM (II)			
	Tissue Protection (I)		Period of Strengthening (III)		Functional Optimization (IV)
Symptom modulation	✔				
Motor control		✔	✔	✔	
Activation		✔	✔	✔	
Acquisition			✔	✔	
Assimilation				✔	
Functional optimization					✔

Return to Sport and the Rehabilitation Setting

There is no current consensus on timing or criteria for RTS decision-making after an anterior shoulder instability event. Specific rehabilitation endpoints may vary greatly by sport, and many functional tests, though widely used, have not been fully explored in the literature. A 2022 evidence-based Consensus statement on shoulder injury provides an overview of 6 domains that should be considered when making RTS decisions.[15] These domains include (1) pain, (2) active shoulder ROM, (3) strength, power, and endurance, (4) the kinetic chain, (5) psychological readiness, and (6) sport-specific activities. Pain levels can be assessed via self-report with measures such as the numeric pain rating scale (ie, 0–10 rating indicating no pain to extreme pain).[16] There is some debate regarding whether an athlete should be pain free prior to a return to previous performance levels, as there is likely to be situations in which this will be unavoidable. An assessment of risk and risk tolerance can be utilized if some pain persists with sport participation,[17] and pain that impacts performance should be seriously considered prior to allowing an athlete to return to play. ROM criteria for RTS will vary with sport-specific demands, and in some cases, a loss of ROM may persist but have no impact on an athlete's performance (football linebacker), while for others, return to full ROM is essential (baseball pitcher). In the case of nonoperative management of anterior shoulder instability, there should be a reasonable expectation for the athlete to achieve full, preinjury ROM of the involved shoulder due to the lack of expected postoperative changes. Strength, power, and endurance testing needs may differ by sport. Broadly, minimum strength recommendations are to aim for 10% increased rotator cuff strength on the dominant arm compared to the nondominant and an external/internal rotation strength ratio of at least 65% (measured isokinetically), but up to 100% (if measured isometrically).[18] A comprehensive RTS decision-making process should also include functional testing that can encompass the above domains of strength, power, and endurance, as well as the kinetic chain and sport-specific activities. Some of the most commonly studied and used functional tests are the closed kinetic chain upper extremity stability test (CKCUEST),[19–21] the single-arm seated shot-put test,[22,23] the athletic shoulder test (ASH),[24–27] and the upper quarter Y-balance test[21,28,29] (**Fig. 1**).

As noted previously, no specific set of criteria for RTS decision-making has been established. Some literature has described potential specific testing batteries to aid RTS decision-making with promising initial results demonstrating validity and

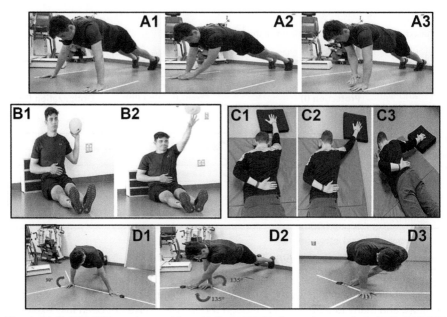

Fig. 1. (*A.1*) CKCUEST starting position; (*A.2*) CKCUEST alternating touch 1; (*A.3*) CKCUEST alternating touch 2; (*B.1*) Single-arm seated shot-put test starting position; (*B.2*) Single-arm seated shot-put test ending position; (*C.1*) ASH test I-position; (*C.2*) ASH test Y-position; (*C.3*) ASH test T-position; (*D.1*) Upper quarter Y-balance test medial reach; (*D.2*) Upper quarter Y-balance test superolateral reach; (*D.3*) Upper quarter Y-balance test inferolateral reach.

decrease recurrence rates,[30,31] while others have provided expert opinion and clinical commentaries on potential testing avenues.[32,33] At a minimum, a well-informed, shared RTS decision after anterior shoulder instability should involve an assessment of an athlete's pain levels and tolerance, psychological readiness for RTS, shoulder ROM, strength, sport-specific power and endurance, and functional assessments that incorporate necessary components of the kinetic chain.

Evidence for RTS outcomes with nonoperative management of anterior shoulder instability suggests a high rate of return to activity, but also a high rate of recurrence and continued symptoms. Buss and colleagues,[34] Tokish and colleagues,[35] and Dickens and colleagues[36] have all illustrated this. Additionally, a recent systematic review demonstrated a high level of RTS (76.5%) across the literature, but with a low-rate (51.5%) of RTS at (or above) the same level as prior to injury.[37] In that review, the overall recurrence rate was 54.7% for the included studies and was higher (78.7%) for collision athletes specifically.[37] Though not exclusively in athletes, a long-term outcomes (median follow-up time = 17 years) study in 2022 found similar results.[38] In this relatively young cohort (median age = 19 years), the recurrence of instability was 37.5% and 58.4% of patients had recurrent pain at some point during clinical follow-up. Further, it is well known that individuals who fail nonoperative management and suffer recurrent instability have higher risk of biomechanical alterations and further injury, including labral tear progression as well as glenoid and humeral bone loss with known risk of increased failures rates following subsequent, standard Bankart repair.[39–41] Lastly, it is imperative to remember that outcomes of successful RTS and recurrent instability are not synonymous, and the decision to RTS should be weighed against the significant risk factors.

ARTHROSCOPIC BANKART REPAIR

Most often, arthroscopic Bankart repair is indicated in cases of capsulolabral injury without significant bone loss following anterior shoulder instability events.[42] Recently, attention has been given to rehabilitation protocols with accelerated, early ROM as multiple studies have supported its use in functional recovery, reduced postoperative pain, and earlier return to activity with no increase in recurrence.[43] A level 1 randomized study by Kim and colleagues[44] reported on the outcomes of 62 patients with shoulder instability, randomizing them into 2 groups: early accelerated rehabilitation versus conventional rehabilitation. The authors concluded that early accelerated rehabilitation does not increase recurrence, with final patient-reported outcomes comparable to conventional rehabilitation.[44]

Rehabilitation following surgical stabilization has been dependent on time frames, with 4 phases making up the rehabilitation protocol.[45] Phase I is dependent on tissue healing and begins immediately after surgery to the first 4 weeks postoperatively. The primary goal is the protection of the surgical repair and ROM. The first 2 weeks should incorporate minimal stress to allow for healing and scar formation.[46] After the first 2 weeks, moderate stresses can be applied to promote tissue remodeling and maturation via a defined, protected ROM protocol. Pendulum exercises, rope/pulley exercises, and wand exercises can be used to obtain reasonable passive range of motion (PROM) and active-assisted range of motion (AAROM) goals of forward flexion (FF) to 90°, ER to 30°, and internal rotation (IR) to 45°.[45] Submaximal isometric strengthening within protected ROM is also incorporated.[45,46]

Phase II begins 4 to 6 weeks postoperatively and involves a gradual increase in ROM, submaximal tissue loading, and dynamic stabilization while continuing to protect the surgical repair and control pain and inflammation. PROM and AAROM with increases in FF, ER, and IR are performed, and active range of motion (AROM) in FF, ER, and IR begins in this phase with the goal of full AROM FF by completion of this phase. Isometric strengthening continues and isotonic strengthening exercises are introduced.[43,45]

The goals of phase III include the preservation of the surgical repair and continued increase in strength, endurance, and neuromuscular proprioception. The athlete should still avoid overhead and contact sports at this time, but activities such as jogging and cycling are allowed.[43] Rehabilitation in this phase focuses on terminal ROM stretching and strengthening exercises with goals of painless shoulder AROM with strength comparable to the uninjured side by phase completion.[43]

The RTS/function phase (phase IV) begins next and requires an athlete to establish and maintain full AROM/PROM while continuing to improve strength, power, and endurance. Throwers should begin a return to throwing program during this phase, and contact athletes should continue to develop strength and neuromuscular proprioception.[43,47] This phase usually continues until 4 to 6 months postoperatively, as these time-based restrictions have been used most commonly to protect before full returning to play.[48,49] However, the effectiveness of time-based clearance methods following surgical stabilization of the shoulder has been questioned, as recurrent instability in athletes after surgical stabilization has been reported as high as 23%,[50] and rates of return to preinjury level have ranged from 50% to 80%.[51,52] While standardized RTS testing has been popularized following anterior cruciate ligament reconstruction, with objective measurements of strength, endurance, and functional testing driving the decision-making process of returning to sport,[53,54] similar methods of assessing appropriate strength and restoration of functional ability for RTS following shoulder stabilization surgery are underdeveloped. In 2020, Wilson and colleagues[55] sought to construct objective criteria for returning to sport following shoulder stabilization surgery. Using a battery of strength and functional testing, the authors found that despite athletes being 6 months from operative intervention, a substantial number did not meet expected objective recovery goals.[55] They concluded that strength and functional testing, rather than arbitrary passage of time, may be better to assess return to play following shoulder stabilization.[55] These objective criteria-based return-to-sport (CBRTS) testing protocols continue to be developed and validated,[56] and most recently, Drummond Junior and colleagues[30] has shown that athletes undergoing CBRTS testing following arthroscopic Bankart repair are less likely to experience recurrent instability than those who are cleared to RTS based on time from surgery alone. These promising results are likely to shape further research on the RTS decision-making paradigm following shoulder stabilization surgery as current evidence suggests that objective CBRTS testing proves superior over time-based clearance in terms of outcomes following RTS after shoulder stabilization.[30] An example of a CBRTS protocol is provided in **Table 2**.

REMPLISSAGE AND OPEN BANKART REPAIR

Rehabilitation following remplissage in accordance with arthroscopic Bankart repair follows a very similar protocol to that described above and RTS results following this combination of procedures has been promising. However, consideration of stress across the healing infraspinatus is recommended. Therefore, rehabilitation following remplissage generally incorporates an approximately 6 week period of limitation with aggressive stretching/tensioning of the infraspinatus and no greater than submaximal activation of the external rotators of the glenohumeral joint. Davis and colleagues[57] found in their 2023 systematic review and meta-analysis that odds of RTS at any level were significantly higher after Bankart repair plus remplissage compared to Latarjet or Bankart repair alone. In addition, open Bankart repair continues to provide surgeons with an option for operatively managing shoulder instability in athletes. In a 2021 systematic review, AlSomali and colleagues[58] found an overall recurrent instability rate of 8.5% and a high RTS rate of 87%. However, special consideration should be given to the open nature of this procedure in the rehabilitation process if a subscapular peel or tenotomy approach is utilized. Caution with passive and active-assisted ER and active IR in the first 4 to 6 weeks postoperatively is suggested due to the healing subscapularis.[43]

LATARJET AND OTHER BONE BLOCK PROCEDURES

The Latarjet and other bone block procedures have been shown to be reliable treatments for patients with recurrent instability, particularly in young athletes with glenoid bone loss.[59–61]

While there is a growing body of studies supporting the efficacy of Latarjet and other bone block procedures, there is no clear consensus on postoperative rehabilitation protocols, with substantial heterogeneity from one provider to another. Many of the existing rehabilitation protocols after bone block procedures have been derived from level IV and V evidence. Beletsky and colleagues[62] reviewed 31 publicly available protocols from both academic orthopedic programs as well as private sports medicine practices and found significant variability between rehabilitation exercise protocols and motion goal recommendations.

In general, rehabilitation after bone block procedures classically consists of 5 phases[63]: (1) protection, (2) active ROM, (3) strengthening, (4) progression to functional training, and (5) sports-specific activities.

Table 2
Criteria-based return to sport testing protocol example

Assessment	Involved	Uninvolved	Pass/Fail Criteria	Results
ROM				
ER @ 90°			Fail if:	
IR @ 90°			1) Total ROM difference of >5°	
Total arc			2) IR deficit >15° in involved	
Strength				
Isometric ER @ 0°			Goal: ≥90% of uninvolved with dynamometer	
Isometric IR @ 0°			Goal: ≥90% of uninvolved with dynamometer	
Isometric ER @ 90°			Goal: ≥90% of uninvolved with dynamometer	
Isometric IR @ 90°			Goal: ≥90% of uninvolved with dynamometer	
Isokinetic ER @ 60°/s *if available			Goal: ≥90% of uninvolved with dynamometer	
Isokinetic IR @ 60°/s *if available			Goal: ≥90% of uninvolved with dynamometer	
Isokinetic ER @ 180°/s *if available			Goal: ≥90% of uninvolved with dynamometer	
Isokinetic ER @ 180°/s *if available			Goal: ≥90% of uninvolved with dynamometer	
Functional				
CKCUEST			Goal: ≥21 touches; no apprehension	
Unilateral seated shot-put test			Goal: Involved dominant: 95%–100% of uninvolved Goal: Involved nondominant: 80% of uninvolved	
Upper quarter Y-balance test			Goal: Normalized reach ≥90% of contralateral limb in all directions	
ASH test			Goal: ≥90% net peak force of contralateral limb	
Overall recommendation:			Rationale	

The goals of the protection phase include protecting the bony augmentation and subscapularis repair while optimizing tissue healing, controlling for swelling, and preventing stiffness. The arm is immobilized in a sling for 4 weeks with ER limited to less than 30°. Early PROM exercises are initiated during this time. Scapulothoracic exercises and active ROM of uninvolved joints including the elbow, wrist, and neck are encouraged.

The goals of the AROM phase are to improve active shoulder motion and increase muscular endurance of the shoulder complex. The sling is discontinued at this time, and the patient should have adequate PROM. AAROM exercises are initiated followed by AROM exercises. AROM can be started in supine, side-lying, or prone positions to reduce the effects of gravity, progressing to standing as endurance improves. Isotonic exercises should focus on high-volume training with 15 to 25 repetitions for 2 to 3 sets.

Oftentimes, FF will progress faster than ER, and ER deficits have been shown to persist after Latarjet.[64,65] Given the higher probability of restricted ER, rehabilitation should closely monitor ER ROM progression and address any deficits more aggressively starting at 10 weeks.

The goals of the strengthening phase are to improve muscular strength while challenging neuromuscular control. This begins at around the 10 week postoperative period. Progressive strengthening of the subscapularis, biceps brachii, and pectoralis major and minor muscles is initiated while taking care not to stress the capsule with aggressive overhead activity. Loads that correspond to a repetition range of an 8 to 12 for 3 to 6 sets should be used. Rehabilitation exercises that include kinetic activation in single leg squat, split squat, and half and tall kneeling positions while adding distal resistance should be utilized at the end of this phase.

The goals of the functional training phase are to progress to preinjury levels of function while maximizing power development. This phase begins around the 16 week postoperative period. At this stage, patients can initiate overhead strengthening activities. Plyometric exercises can be used to enhance fast twitch muscle fibers and improve neuromuscular control.

After completion of the prior 4 phases, the athlete has demonstrated enough ROM, neuromuscular control, strength, and power to start a return to play progression. This phase will be dependent on the sport the patient is returning to and consists of sport-specific drills.

However, despite generalized rehabilitation protocols, RTS timing and criteria remain controversial. In a systematic review of 2134 patients spanning 36 studies, Hurley and colleagues[66] reported a wide discrepancy in return to play criteria, with time-based clearance most often utilized (66.7% of studies), followed by computed tomographic imaging (25% of studies), and physical examination (11.1% of studies). Among the studies utilizing time-based clearance for return to play, 3 months was the most commonly used time-point for clearance (35.4% of studies), and average return to play occurred at an average of 5.8 months postoperatively.[66] However, recent studies have called into question the reliability and validity of utilizing time-based clearance or physical examination to determine the readiness for RTS.[30] Similar to the recent trend seen in arthroscopic Bankart repair, surgeons have increasingly used CBRTS testing protocols after bone block augmentation procedures to allow for more critical evaluation of multiple components of functionality, including strength and endurance. Compared to manual muscle testing, isokinetic and isometric dynamometry often used in CBRTS testing have been shown to better assess rotation strength while controlling for positioning, translational stresses, speed, and rotational forces.[67] Furthermore, endurance testing allows for the evaluation of shoulder girdle fatigue, which is often overlooked during physical examination.[56]

Despite the clearance method, multiple systematic reviews have demonstrated good-to-excellent clinical outcomes after bone block procedures, with high rates of RTS ranging from 72% to 96.8% and low recurrent instability rates around 7%.[37,66] More specifically, a systematic review by Hurley and colleagues[66] of 2134 patients found an RTS rate after open Latarjet of 88.2% overall and 90.3% in overhead athletes. Studies have also demonstrated similar RTS outcomes between open and arthroscopic Latarjet.[61] Other bone block procedures including distal tibial allograft and iliac crest autografts were studied in a pooled meta-analysis of 623 patients by Gilat and colleagues,[68] who found an overall RTS rate of 88%. Hurley and colleagues[69] found that common reasons for failure to RTS after Latarjet included persistent pain and apprehension, feeling like it was a natural end to their sports career, and thoughts of having to undergo repeat surgery and rehabilitation.

Assessing Psychological Readiness

Regardless of the management strategy utilized following an anterior shoulder instability event, psychological readiness to RTS should be evaluated prior to clearance. The Shoulder Instability-Return to Sport Index (SIRSI) provides a framework for this evaluation.[70] The SIRSI was adapted from the Anterior Cruciate Ligament-Return to Sport after Injury scale and has been validated as a reproducible scale that identifies patients who are not ready to RTS after an episode of shoulder instability, whether they undergo operative or nonoperative management.[70,71] It is comprised of 12 items, and athletes are asked to answer questions based on a 0 to 10 scale, 0 being "not confident at all," and 10 being "full confident."[70]

Implementing tools such as the SIRSI score have proven beneficial as a psychological assessment of a patient's readiness to RTS following shoulder instability events.[70,72]

Rossi and colleagues[71,73] and Kelley and colleagues[74] found that following arthroscopic Bankart repair, patients who RTS and those who returned to their preinjury sports level were significantly more psychologically ready than those who did not return. Additionally, Hurley and colleagues[69] found that poor psychological readiness was a key factor preventing patients from returning to play after Latarjet. Using the SIRSI scale, these authors found that thoughts of having to repeat surgery and rehabilitation again were significantly associated with decreased RTS.[69] Thus, assessing psychological readiness is a critical piece of the RTS decision-making process following management of anterior shoulder instability and should be addressed during the rehabilitation period.

SUMMARY

As anterior shoulder instability continues to plague athletes, it is imperative to define appropriate rehabilitation protocols that lead to the most successful functional outcomes and RTS. Regardless of the treatment intervention employed, rehabilitation should focus on the preservation of motion and strengthening. When appropriate in the rehabilitation protocol, RTS testing should be criteria based, rather than time based, with a special focus given to psychological readiness in order to promote successful return to athletics and prevention of recurrent instability episodes in the future.

CLINICS CARE POINTS

- Rehabilitation following anterior shoulder instability should focus on recovery of strength and range of motion.
- Rehabilitation should be tailored to the specific surgical intervention performed.
- A well-informed, shared return to sport (RTS) decision should involve assessment of an athlete's pain, psychological readiness to return, shoulder range of motion, sport-specific power/endurance, and functional assessments that incorporate necessary components of the kinetic chain.

DISCLOSURE

A. Lin: Stryker/Tornier: Paid Consultant/IP, Arthrex: Paid Consultant/IP, American Shoulder and Elbow Surgeon: Committee or board member, American Orthopedic Society for Sports Medicine: Committee or board member, ISAKOS: Committee or board member, Rotator Cuff Study Group: Committee or board member, Knee Surgery, Sports Traumatology, Arthroscopy: Editorial or governing board, JBJS Case Connector: Associate Editor, Arthroscopy: Editorial or governing board, JISAKOS: Editorial or governing board, American Journal of Sports Medicine: Reviewer, Journal of American Academy of Orthopedic Surgeons: Reviewer, Knee Surgery, Sports Traumatology, Arthroscopy: Reviewer, Journal of Shoulder and Elbow Surgery: Reviewer, Journal of Bone and Joint Surgery: Reviewer. No other authors have anything to disclose.

REFERENCES

1. Dumont GD, Russell RD, Robertson WJ. Anterior shoulder instability: a review of pathoanatomy, diagnosis and treatment. Curr Rev Musculoskelet Med 2011;4(4):200–7.
2. Varacallo M, Musto MA, Mair SD. Anterior Shoulder Instability. St. Petersburg, FL: StatPearls Publishing; 2022. p. 1–7.
3. Van Spanning SH, Verweij LPE, Priester-Vink S, et al. Operative Versus Nonoperative Treatment Following First-Time Anterior Shoulder Dislocation: A Systematic Review and Meta-Analysis. JBJS Reviews 2021;9(9). https://doi.org/10.2106/JBJS.RVW.20.00232.
4. Glazebrook H, Miller B, Wong I. Anterior Shoulder Instability: A Systematic Review of the Quality and Quantity of the Current Literature for Surgical Treatment. Orthop J Sports Med 2018;6(11). 2325967118805983.
5. Handoll HH, Almaiyah MA, Rangan A. Surgical versus non-surgical treatment for acute anterior shoulder dislocation. Cochrane Database Syst Rev 2004;2004(1):CD004325.
6. Kavaja L, Lahdeoja T, Malmivaara A, et al. Treatment after traumatic shoulder dislocation: a systematic review with a network meta-analysis. Br J Sports Med 2018;52(23):1498–506.
7. Smith BI, Bliven KC, Morway GR, et al. Management of primary anterior shoulder dislocations using immobilization. J Athl Train 2015;50(5):550–2.
8. Whelan DB, Kletke SN, Schemitsch G, et al. Immobilization in External Rotation Versus Internal Rotation After Primary Anterior Shoulder Dislocation: A Meta-analysis of Randomized Controlled Trials. Am J Sports Med 2016;44(2):521–32.
9. Paterson WH, Throckmorton TW, Koester M, et al. Position and duration of immobilization after primary anterior shoulder dislocation: a systematic review and meta-analysis of the literature. J Bone Joint Surg Am 2010;92(18):2924–33.
10. Eshoj HR, Rasmussen S, Frich LH, et al. Neuromuscular Exercises Improve Shoulder Function More Than Standard Care Exercises in Patients With a Traumatic Anterior Shoulder Dislocation: A Randomized Controlled Trial. Orthop J Sports Med 2020;8(1):2325967119896102.
11. Yang J, Schaefer JT, Zhang N, et al. Social support from the athletic trainer and symptoms of depression and anxiety at return to play. J Athl Train 2014;49(6):773–9.
12. McClure PW, Michener LA. Staged Approach for Rehabilitation Classification: Shoulder Disorders (STAR–Shoulder). Phys Ther 2015;95(5):791–800.
13. Burkhead Jr W, Rockwood Jr C. Treatment of instability of the shoulder with an exercise program. JBJS 1992;74(6):890–6.
14. Bateman M, Osborne SE, Smith BE. Physiotherapy treatment for atraumatic recurrent shoulder instability: updated results of the Derby Shoulder Instability Rehabilitation Programme. J Arthrosc Jt Surg 2019;6(1):35–41.

15. Schwank A, Blazey P, Asker M, et al. 2022 Bern Consensus Statement on Shoulder Injury Prevention, Rehabilitation, and Return to Sport for Athletes at All Participation Levels. J Orthop Sports Phys Ther 2022;52(1):11–28.

16. Mintken PE, Glynn P, Cleland JA. Psychometric properties of the shortened disabilities of the Arm, Shoulder, and Hand Questionnaire (QuickDASH) and Numeric Pain Rating Scale in patients with shoulder pain. J Shoulder Elbow Surg 2009;18(6):920–6.

17. Shrier I. Strategic Assessment of Risk and Risk Tolerance (StARRT) framework for return-to-play decision-making. Br J Sports Med 2015;49(20):1311–5.

18. Cools AM, Vanderstukken F, Vereecken F, et al. Eccentric and isometric shoulder rotator cuff strength testing using a hand-held dynamometer: reference values for overhead athletes. Knee Surg Sports Traumatol Arthrosc 2016;24(12):3838–47.

19. Pontillo M, Spinelli BA, Sennett BJ. Prediction of in-season shoulder injury from preseason testing in division I collegiate football players. Sports Health 2014; 6(6):497–503.

20. Roush JR, Kitamura J, Waits MC. Reference Values for the Closed Kinetic Chain Upper Extremity Stability Test (CKCUEST) for Collegiate Baseball Players. N Am J Sports Phys Ther 2007;2(3):159–63.

21. Taylor JB, Wright AA, Smoliga JM, et al. Upper-Extremity Physical-Performance Tests in College Athletes. J Sport Rehabil 2016;25(2):146–54.

22. Chmielewski TL, Martin C, Lentz TA, et al. Normalization considerations for using the unilateral seated shot put test in rehabilitation. J Orthop Sports Phys Ther 2014;44(7):518–24.

23. Negrete RJ, Hanney WJ, Kolber MJ, et al. Reliability, minimal detectable change, and normative values for tests of upper extremity function and power. J Strength Cond Res 2010;24(12):3318–25.

24. Ashworth B, Hogben P, Singh N, et al. The Athletic Shoulder (ASH) test: reliability of a novel upper body isometric strength test in elite rugby players. BMJ Open Sport Exerc Med 2018;4(1):e000365.

25. Trunt A, Fisher BT, MacFadden LN. Athletic shoulder test differences exist bilaterally in healthy pitchers. Int J Sports Phys Ther 2022;17(4):715.

26. Tooth C, Forthomme B, Croisier J-L, et al. The Modified-Athletic Shoulder Test: Reliability and validity of a new on-field assessment tool. Phys Ther Sport 2022; 58:8–15.

27. Królikowska A, Mika A, Plaskota B, et al. Reliability and validity of the athletic shoulder (ASH) test performed using portable isometric-based strength training device. Biology 2022;11(4):577.

28. Gorman PP, Butler RJ, Plisky PJ, et al. Upper Quarter Y Balance Test: reliability and performance comparison between genders in active adults. J Strength Cond Res 2012;26(11):3043–8.

29. Westrick RB, Miller JM, Carow SD, et al. Exploration of the y-balance test for assessment of upper quarter closed kinetic chain performance. Int J Sports Phys Ther 2012;7(2):139–47.

30. Drummond Junior M, Popchak A, Wilson K, et al. Criteria-based return-to-sport testing is associated with lower recurrence rates following arthroscopic Bankart repair. J Shoulder Elbow Surg 2021;30(7s):S14–20.

31. Jure D, Blache Y, Degot M, et al. The S-STARTS Test: Validation of a Composite Test for the Assessment of Readiness to Return to Sport After Shoulder Stabilization Surgery. Sports Health 2022;14(2):254–61.

32. Otley T, Myers H, Lau BC, et al. Return to Sport After Shoulder Stabilization Procedures: A Criteria-Based Testing Continuum to Guide Rehabilitation and Inform

Return-to-Play Decision Making. Arthrosc Sports Med Rehabil 2022;4(1): e237–46.

33. Wilk KE, Bagwell MS, Davies GJ, et al. Return to Sport Participation Criteria Following Shoulder Injury: A Clinical Commentary. Int J Sports Phys Ther 2020; 15(4):624–42.

34. Buss DD, Lynch GP, Meyer CP, et al. Nonoperative Management for In-Season Athletes with Anterior Shoulder Instability. Am J Sports Med 2004;32(6):1430–3.

35. Dickens JF, Rue JP, Cameron KL, et al. Successful Return to Sport After Arthroscopic Shoulder Stabilization Versus Nonoperative Management in Contact Athletes With Anterior Shoulder Instability: A Prospective Multicenter Study. Am J Sports Med 2017;45(11):2540–6.

36. Tokish JM, Thigpen CA, Kissenberth MJ, et al. The Nonoperative Instability Severity Index Score (NISIS): A Simple Tool to Guide Operative Versus Nonoperative Treatment of the Unstable Shoulder. Sports Health 2020;12(6):598–602.

37. Hurley ET, Colasanti CA, Haskel JD, et al. Return to play after non-operative management of primary anterior shoulder instability a systematic review. Bull Hosp Jt Dis 2023;81(2):118–24.

38. Novakofski KD, Melugin HP, Leland DP, et al. Nonoperative management of anterior shoulder instability can result in high rates of recurrent instability and pain at long-term follow-up. J Shoulder Elbow Surg 2022;31(2):352–8.

39. Vaswani R, Gasbarro G, Como C, et al. Labral Morphology and Number of Preoperative Dislocations Are Associated With Recurrent Instability After Arthroscopic Bankart Repair. Arthroscopy 2020;36(4):993–9.

40. Fox MA, Drain NP, Rai A, et al. Increased Failure Rates After Arthroscopic Bankart Repair After Second Dislocation Compared to Primary Dislocation With Comparable Clinical Outcomes. Arthroscopy 2023;39(3):682–8.

41. Yoshida M, Takenaga T, Chan CK, et al. Altered shoulder kinematics using a new model for multiple dislocations-induced Bankart lesions. Clin Biomech 2019;70: 131–6.

42. White AE, Patel NK, Hadley CJ, et al. An Algorithmic Approach to the Management of Shoulder Instability. J Am Acad Orthop Surg Glob Res Rev 2019;3(12): e19.00168.

43. Lloyd G, Day J, Lu J, et al. Postoperative Rehabilitation of Anterior Glenohumeral Joint Instability Surgery: A Systematic Review. Sports Med Arthrosc Rev 2021; 29(2):54–62.

44. Kim SH, Ha KI, Cho YB, et al. Arthroscopic anterior stabilization of the shoulder: two to six-year follow-up. J Bone Joint Surg Am 2003;85(8):1511–8.

45. Popchak A, Patterson-Lynch B, Christain H, et al. Rehabilitation and return to sports after anterior shoulder stabilization. Ann Joint 2017;2(10).

46. Gaunt BW, Shaffer MA, Sauers EL, et al. The American Society of Shoulder and Elbow Therapists' consensus rehabilitation guideline for arthroscopic anterior capsulolabral repair of the shoulder. J Orthop Sports Phys Ther 2010;40(3): 155–68.

47. Gibson J, Kerss J, Morgan C, et al. Accelerated rehabilitation after arthroscopic Bankart repair in professional footballers. Shoulder Elbow 2016;8(4):279–86.

48. Memon M, Kay J, Cadet ER, et al. Return to sport following arthroscopic Bankart repair: a systematic review. J Shoulder Elbow Surg 2018;27(7):1342–7.

49. Ciccotti MC, Syed U, Hoffman R, et al. Return to Play Criteria Following Surgical Stabilization for Traumatic Anterior Shoulder Instability: A Systematic Review. Arthroscopy 2018;34(3):903–13.

50. Donohue MA, Owens BD, Dickens JF. Return to Play Following Anterior Shoulder Dislocation and Stabilization Surgery. Clin Sports Med 2016;35(4):545–61.

51. Ide J, Maeda S, Takagi K. Arthroscopic Bankart repair using suture anchors in athletes: patient selection and postoperative sports activity. Am J Sports Med 2004;32(8):1899–905.

52. Garofalo R, Mocci A, Moretti B, et al. Arthroscopic treatment of anterior shoulder instability using knotless suture anchors. Arthroscopy 2005;21(11):1283–9.

53. Joreitz R, Lynch A, Popchak A, et al. Criterion-based rehabilitation program with return to sport testing following ACL reconstruction: a case series. Int J Sports Phys Ther 2020;15(6):1151–73.

54. Gokeler A, Dingenen B, Hewett TE. Rehabilitation and return to sport testing after anterior cruciate ligament reconstruction: where are we in 2022? Arthrosc Sports Med Rehabil 2022;4(1):e77–82.

55. Wilson KW, Popchak A, Li RT, et al. Return to sport testing at 6 months after arthroscopic shoulder stabilization reveals residual strength and functional deficits. J Shoulder Elbow Surg 2020;29(7s):S107–14.

56. Popchak A, Poploski K, Patterson-Lynch B, et al. Reliability and validity of a return to sports testing battery for the shoulder. Phys Ther Sport 2021;48:1–11.

57. Davis WH, DiPasquale JA, Patel RK, et al. Arthroscopic remplissage combined with bankart repair results in a higher rate of return to sport in athletes compared with Bankart repair alone or the Latarjet procedure: a systematic review and meta-analysis. Am J Sports Med 2023;51(12):3304–12.

58. AlSomali K, Kholinne E, Van Nguyen T, et al. Outcomes and Return to Sport and Work After Open Bankart Repair for Recurrent Shoulder Instability: A Systematic Review. Orthop J Sports Med 2021;9(10):23259671211026907.

59. Baverel L, Colle PE, Saffarini M, et al. Open Latarjet Procedures Produce Better Outcomes in Competitive Athletes Compared With Recreational Athletes: A Clinical Comparative Study of 106 Athletes Aged Under 30 Years. Am J Sports Med 2018;46(6):1408–15.

60. Ernat JJ, Rakowski DR, Hanson JA, et al. High rate of return to sport and excellent patient-reported outcomes after an open Latarjet procedure. J Shoulder Elbow Surg 2022;31(8):1704–12.

61. Hurley ET, Ben Ari E, Lorentz NA, et al. Both Open and Arthroscopic Latarjet Result in Excellent Outcomes and Low Recurrence Rates for Anterior Shoulder Instability. Arthrosc Sports Med Rehabil 2021;3(6):e1955–60.

62. Beletsky A, Naami E, Lu Y, et al. The Minimally Clinically Important Difference and Substantial Clinical Benefit in Anterior Cruciate Ligament Reconstruction: A Time-to-Achievement Analysis. Orthopedics 2021;44(5):299–305.

63. Bradley H, Lacheta L, Goldenberg BT, et al. Latarjet Procedure for the Treatment of Anterior Glenohumeral Instability in the Athlete - Key Considerations for Rehabilitation. Int J Sports Phys Ther 2021;16(1):259–69.

64. Griesser MJ, Harris JD, McCoy BW, et al. Complications and re-operations after Bristow-Latarjet shoulder stabilization: a systematic review. J Shoulder Elbow Surg 2013;22(2):286–92.

65. Sinha S, Kar S, Naik AK, et al. Decreased motion with normal strength after Latarjet procedure has minimal impact on return to activity. Knee Surg Sports Traumatol Arthrosc 2021;29(8):2579–86.

66. Hurley ET, Montgomery C, Jamal MS, et al. Return to Play After the Latarjet Procedure for Anterior Shoulder Instability: A Systematic Review. Am J Sports Med 2019;47(12):3002–8.

67. Ellenbecker TS. Muscular strength relationship between normal grade manual muscle testing and isokinetic measurement of the shoulder internal and external rotators. Isokinet Exerc Sci 1996;6:51–6.

68. Gilat R, Wong SE, Lavoie-Gagne O, et al. Outcomes are comparable using free bone block autografts versus allografts for the management of anterior shoulder instability with glenoid bone loss: a systematic review and meta-analysis of "The Non-Latarjet". Knee Surg Sports Traumatol Arthrosc 2021;29(7):2159–74.

69. Hurley ET, Davey MS, Montgomery C, et al. Analysis of Athletes Who Did Not Return to Play After Open Latarjet. Orthop J Sports Med 2022;10(2):23259671211071082.

70. Gerometta A, Klouche S, Herman S, et al. The Shoulder Instability-Return to Sport after Injury (SIRSI): a valid and reproducible scale to quantify psychological readiness to return to sport after traumatic shoulder instability. Knee Surg Sports Traumatol Arthrosc 2018;26(1):203–11.

71. Rossi LA, Pasqualini I, Brandariz R, et al. Relationship of the SIRSI Score to Return to Sports After Surgical Stabilization of Glenohumeral Instability. Am J Sports Med 2022;50(12):3318–25.

72. Pasqualini I, Rossi LA, Brandariz R, et al. The Short, 5-Item Shoulder Instability-Return to Sport After Injury Score Performs as Well as the Longer Version in Predicting Psychological Readiness to Return to Sport. Arthroscopy 2023;39(5):1131–8.e1.

73. Rossi LA, Pasqualini I, Tanoira I, et al. Factors That Influence the Return to Sport After Arthroscopic Bankart Repair for Glenohumeral Instability. Open Access J Sports Med 2022;13:35–40.

74. Kelley TD, Clegg S, Rodenhouse P, et al. Functional Rehabilitation and Return to Play After Arthroscopic Surgical Stabilization for Anterior Shoulder Instability. Sports Health 2022;14(5):733–9.

APPENDIX 1: DETAILED REHABILITATION PROGRESSION

Activity	0–3 wk	3–6 wk	6–9 wk	9–12 wk	12–16 wk	16+ wk
Tissue protection	Sling immobilization for all activities other than physical therapy (PT) exercises Strict protection of • Infraspinatus (arthroscopic Bankart) • Subscapularis (open Bankart and Latarjet)	Only PROM through the beginning of sling discharge Strict protection of • Infraspinatus (arthroscopic Bankart) • Subscapularis (open Bankart and Latarjet)	End of strict tissue protection Stepwise increase in loading of all structures in shoulder	No overpressure to the anterior capsule in the abducted-externally rotated position All mobilizations to occur only with surgeon orders*	NA	NA
ROM	120° maximum PROM flexion 30° maximum PROM ER at ≤20° shoulder abduction	135° (to tolerance) PROM flexion 45° maximum PROM ER at ≤20° shoulder abduction	155° PROM flexion 65° PROM ER at ≤45° shoulder abduction in the scapular plane At 8-wk postop: 45° maximum PROM ER at 90° shoulder abduction in the scapular plane	PROM ER to frontal plane after achieving 90° shoulder abduction in the scapular plane 90° (or available end-range) ER at 90° shoulder abduction frontal plane Goal: ROM within 5° of the contralateral side	Achievement of all ROM goals	NA

(continued on next page)

(*continued*)

Activity	0–3 wk	3–6 wk	6–9 wk	9–12 wk	12–16 wk	16+ wk
Joint mobilizations/overpressure	Contraindicated	Contraindicated	*At 8 wk postop:* *Only with surgeon orders* If significant deviations from ROM goals and pathologic stiffness present, initiate glenohumeral (GH) mobilizations in 45° of scapular abduction (*distraction, posterior, and inferior glides only*) *Contraindicated in absence of surgeon orders*	*Only with surgeon orders* If significant deviations from ROM goals and pathologic stiffness present, initiate GH mobilizations in 45° of scapular abduction (*distraction, posterior, and inferior glides only*) *Contraindicated in absence of surgeon orders*	*At 12 wk postop:* If significant deviations from ROM goals and pathologic stiffness present, GH mobilizations, beginning in midrange, progressing to end-range/restricted position (*begin anterior glides*)	As required, no restrictions
Proprioception	Contraindicated	*1–2 wk prior to sling discharge:* (approximately wk 5) Finger-tip pressure rhythmic stabilization; joint positioning; scapular muscle activation *At sling discharge:* Scapular rhythmic stabilization/	Rhythmic stabilization with increasing load during resistance activities	Progress from isolated patterns and progress to complex, multiplanar patterns	*Complex, multiplanar patterns:* Slow reversal-hold relax Protected plyometrics	Unprotected plyometrics

Summary of Rehabilitation Progression (continued)

Strengthening	Contraindicated	AAROM at the beginning of sling discharge AROM at complete sling discharge Finger-tip pressure only No external resistance	AROM progressing to Maximal Isometrics Use of "place and holds" for elevation Rhythmic stabilization with increasing load *Week-8:* start progressive resistance exercises (PREs) pending criteria are achieved (allow free weights) External and internal rotations strengthening before loading in scapular plane abduction *Week-8+:* Weight-bearing exercises	Progress to elastic resistance	Specific, targeted strengthening based on interim strength testing results Progressive strengthening for the rotator cuff, scapular stabilizers, and shoulder girdle muscles	Progressive strengthening activities for the rotator cuff, scapular stabilizers, and shoulder girdle muscles

Summary of Rehabilitation Progression (continued)

Functional training	Contraindicated	Contraindicated	Contraindicated	Contraindicated	Dynamic exercises and power development Closed-kinetic chain over open-kinetic chain exercises	Progression of functional-based and activity-specific exercises

(continued on next page)

(continued)

Activity	0–3 wk	3–6 wk	6–9 wk	9–12 wk	12–16 wk	16+ wk
Plyometrics	Contraindicated	Contraindicated	Contraindicated	Contraindicated	Protected plyometrics: Limit and protect ROM ROM increasing progression and lessening support of anterior capsule Progress from general movements to specific movements	Initiate unprotected plyometrics

Posterior Instability

Posterior instability

Biomechanics and Pathoanatomy of Posterior Shoulder Instability

Edward J. Testa, MD, Michael J. Kutschke, MD, Elaine He, BA,
Brett D. Owens, MD*

KEYWORDS

- Posterior shoulder instability • Glenohumeral instability • Biomechanics
- Posterior subluxation • Posterior dislocation

KEY POINTS

- Posterior glenohumeral instability encompasses a spectrum of pathology related to various anatomic features, including capsuloligamentous anatomy and bony constraints.
- The posterior capsulolabral complex, including the posterior band of the inferior glenohumeral ligament, as well as the posterior labrum, are both essential static soft tissue elements providing posterior glenohumeral stability, and are a common therapeutic target.
- Critical posterior glenoid bone loss, severe retroversion, and engaging humeral lesions must be addressed to adequately restore shoulder stability.
- Emerging concepts such as posterior acromial morphology may play an additional pathoanatomic role in posterior shoulder instability, but further research is needed to characterize its relevance.

INTRODUCTION

Posterior glenohumeral instability is an underrecognized shoulder pathology that accounts for approximately 2% to 10% of all glenohumeral instability cases.[1,2] Estimates of posterior instability incidence have ranged from 4.64 to 23.9 per 100,000 person-years in the general population[2,3] to upwards of 184 per 100,000 person-years in young, active populations such as military personnel and participants in over-head or contact sports.[2,4–6] Recurrent posterior instability is commonly the result of repetitive microtrauma but can also develop following a posterior shoulder dislocation or in the context of hyperlaxity.[7] Posterior shoulder instability represents a diagnostic challenge and is missed in up to 79% of patients.[8–10] Unlike anterior instability, patients with posterior shoulder instability often present with a primary complaint of pain and

Department of Orthopedics, The Warren Alpert Medical School of Brown University, Providence, RI, USA
* Corresponding author. 1 Kettle Point Avenue, East Providence, RI 029014.
E-mail address: owensbrett@gmail.com

Clin Sports Med 43 (2024) 723–735
https://doi.org/10.1016/j.csm.2024.03.026
0278-5919/24/© 2024 Elsevier Inc. All rights reserved.

may not necessarily report any perceived instability or recall an identifiable mechanism of injury.[11,12]

While many initially considered posterior shoulder instability to simply be the counterpart of anterior instability, surgeons now recognize posterior shoulder instability as a distinct clinical and pathoanatomic entity. Posterior shoulder stability depends upon a complex interplay between soft tissue and osseous restraints that are distinct from anterior instability. For example, the glenoid version has been shown to play a substantial role in posterior shoulder instability, and can be targeted as a therapeutic modality to enhance shoulder stability.[13,14] In recent years, there has been improved awareness and understanding of posterior instability, with a concomitant growing body of biomechanical and clinical work in this field. Therefore, in the current article, we seek to review the pathoanatomy and biomechanics of posterior shoulder instability. This review will focus on evaluating the morphologic features, such as glenoid and humeral bone loss and capsuloligamentous pathology, in addition to reviewing the biomechanical literature which defines our current understanding of the pathoanatomy of posterior shoulder instability.

DISCUSSION
Pathoanatomy

Capsuloligamentous anatomy
There are several key soft tissue and bony constraints to the glenohumeral joint that confer stability, and, when injured, deficient, or otherwise incompetent, can lead to posterior shoulder instability. Beginning with capsuloligamentous anatomy, the role of the inferior glenohumeral ligament complex (IGHLC) has long been and remains an active area of investigation.[15–19] Grossly, the posterior capsule is thinner, yet more capacious than its anterior counterpart.[18] Histologically, the IGHLC is comprised of anterior and posterior bands of collagen representing the anterior IGHL and posterior IGHL (PIGHL), respectively, which are joined by a thickened area of the inferior capsule termed the axillary pouch.[18] Of specific relevance to this topic is the PIGHL, which originates from the glenoid surface and/or adjacent bone and labrum ranging from the 7 to 9 o'clock position on the glenoid face.[18,20] The entirety of the IGHLC inserts along the proximal humerus in either a "collar-like" or "v-shaped" fashion, with the PIGHL attaching directly adjacent to the articular margin of the humeral head in either scenario.[18] Due to its material properties and anatomic orientation, the PIGHL is critical to posterior shoulder stability when the glenohumeral joint is abducted 90° and forward flexed 30° (with respect to the plane of the scapula).[19,21] When incompetent, this structure can be a cause of recurrent posterior instability (**Fig. 1**).

Glenoid labrum
The glenoid labrum is well known to be a robust static stabilizer to the glenohumeral joint and affords deeper concavity and conformity to the glenohumeral articulation, increases the suction cup effect of the joint, and serves as a soft tissue boundary to humeral head translation.[22–24] Although substantial variation exists among individuals in labral width and thickness, the posterior labrum is typically larger than the anterior labrum.[25,26] In cross-section, the shape of the posterior labrum may also differ from the anterior labrum. Most commonly, the labrum has a triangular shape in roughly 50% of individuals; however, this shape may be rounded in up to 33% of posterior labrums, compared with only 17% in anterior labrums.[27] Additionally, the posterior capsular tissue inserting onto the labrum is not as robust as its anterior counterpart, with the posterior band of the IGHL thinner than the anterior band in 75% of individuals.[25] Disruption to the posterior labrum can lead to increased propensity for

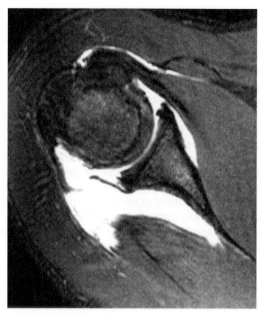

Fig. 1. An axial magnetic resonance arthrogram image of a patient with recurrent posterior instability and an avulsion of the posterior band of the inferior glenohumeral ligament from the humeral head.

posterior shoulder subluxation or dislocation (**Fig. 2**A and B). When this is the case, arthroscopic surgical repair of the posterior capusulolabral tissue with or without augmentation is the recommended management of this injury as it provides improved glenohumeral biomechanics, enhances posterior stability, and contributes to excellent patient-reported outcomes.[28–33]

Glenoid bony anatomy
As mentioned, the congruence of the glenohumeral articulation is an essential component of shoulder stability. However, multiple posterior shoulder instability events can

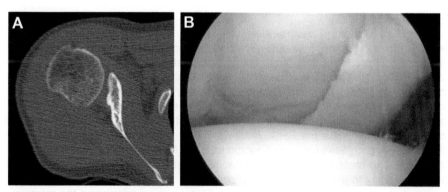

Fig. 2. (*A*) A computed tomography axial slice of a patient with severe glenoid dysplasia and posterior shoulder instability. (*B*) An arthroscopic view of the same shoulder, demonstrating a hypertrophic and torn posterior labrum, as viewed from a high posterolateral viewing portal. Note the hypertrophic labral tear on the right side of the image.

lead to posterior glenoid bone loss and subsequent glenoid retroversion, both of which further potentiate the problem. Although originally designed to assess anterior glenoid lesions, one accepted technique in quantifying posterior glenoid bone loss is the best-fit circle method.[34] This approach uses the area of missing bone within a circle best-fit to the radius of curvature of the inferior aspect of the glenoid face to quantify the amount of glenoid bone loss. While this has been a widely applied technique, the contralateral comparison method compares the width of the affected glenoid to the unaffected contralateral glenoid to determine the percentage of bone loss, though bone deficiency can be bilateral in dysplasia cases. Recent work by Kuberakani and colleagues[35] demonstrated superior intra- and interobserver reliability with the contralateral comparison technique versus the best-fit circle method (0.98 vs 0.91 and 0.88 and 0.77, respectively). The percentage of posterior glenoid bone that must be deficient to be considered critical posterior glenoid bone loss remains of active area of investigation. One recent case-control study of 75 patients demonstrated a 10 times higher failure rate of arthroscopic posterior capsulolabral repair in the setting of 11% posterior glenoid bone loss and 25 times higher with 15% bone loss suggesting a point at which soft tissue repair alone may not be sufficient for managing this subset of patients.[36]

Glenoid retroversion
Closely related to posterior glenoid bone loss, and one of the most important pathoanatomic differences between anterior and posterior shoulder instability, is glenoid retroversion.[14,37] Normally, the glenoid is positioned in between 5 and 6° of retroversion.[38] However, it is conceivable and has been demonstrated clinically that those with increased retroversion experience posterior shoulder instability more frequently than those with normal retroversion contributing to preferential posterior wear of the glenoid and eventual glenoid bone loss.[13] Owens and colleagues[39] demonstrated that pathologic glenoid retroversion is closely connected with glenoid bone loss, as glenoid retroversion greater than 10° is associated with increased posterior glenoid bone loss. This recurrent process in conjunction with the deterioration of the posterior soft tissue constraints can make treating patients with recurrent posterior shoulder instability in the setting of increased retroversion and critical bone loss considerably difficult, and may require glenoid vault reconstruction with or without a scapular neck osteotomy.

Humeral head
Humeral sided lesions (ie, reverse Hill-Sachs lesions (RHSL)) must also be considered when addressing posterior shoulder instability. More commonly occurring following frank dislocations rather than more subtle presentations of posterior shoulder instability, RHSLs can vary in size, position, and clinical significance.[40,41] Computed tomography (CT) or magnetic resonance imaging (MRI) should be obtained to evaluate for the specific anatomic nature of a humeral sided bony lesion.[42] Lesions are commonly classified via their size relative to the articular surface: lesions are considered small when the RHSL involves 0% to 20% to 25%, medium between 20% to 25%, and 45% to 50% and greater as large. Moroder and colleagues reported a technique to measure RSHLs, with specific attention to assessing for lesions that would be likely to engage in the posterior glenoid, similar to the on-track, off-track concept of anterior shoulder instability.[43–45] These authors introduced the measurement of an angle which may be prone to re-engagement (ie, the gamma angle). This angle is measured from the bicipital groove to the most posterior aspect of the RHSL, with a measurement of greater than 90° thought to be susceptible to

re-engagement (**Fig. 3**).[46] They performed a subsequent analysis evaluating bipolar bony lesions in posterior shoulder instability, finding that, similar to its anterior counterpart, glenoid bone loss can make even noncritical size lesions engage and thus prone to redislocation.[44]

Acromion

Historically, surgeons have considered the osseus restraint of the posterior glenoid on the humeral head as the primary bony constraint of the glenoid. In recent years however, the acromion has become increasingly implicated as a risk factor for shoulder instability.[47–52] The first mentions of any potential connection between the acromion and posterior instability was in the form of posterior acromial augmentation to treat unidirectional posterior shoulder instability.[52] Per his report, Scapinelli and his colleagues demonstrated good results with performing a scapular spine autograft to the posterolateral acromion to provide a mechanical buttress to the humeral head in the management of posterior instability.[52] While his work did not directly suggest the acromion to be a pathoanatomic structure in these patients, he indirectly proposed the importance of acromial morphology in posterior instability by using the acromion as a therapeutic target.

Subsequently, Meyer and colleagues[51] found that a tall and flat acromion was highly associated with posterior instability when compared with anterior instability or a group of control patients. These authors posed the concept that a lower, more tilted acromion may serve a mechanical advantage when it comes to posterior instability by providing a buttress to the humeral head and thus decreasing its propensity for instability episodes. Another group sought to examine the relationship between acromial morphology and posterior glenoid bone loss in posterior instability patients.[50] These researchers determined that the same risk factors identified by Meyer and colleagues for posterior instability—a high, flat acromion—were also associated with increased posterior glenoid bone loss. Again, this expands the literature suggesting the potential pathoanatomic connection between posterior acromial morphology and posterior shoulder instability.[50]

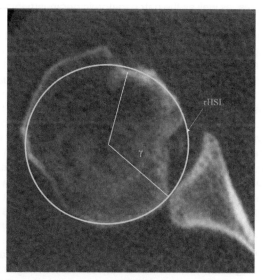

Fig. 3. An axial CT slice of a large reverse Hill-Sachs lesion, with a gamma angle of greater than 90°.

Biomechanics

The complex balance between active and passively stabilizing soft tissue and osseous restraints affords the shoulder the greatest range of motion of all joints in the human body.[53,54] Unfortunately, this wide range of motion also comes at the price of the greatest risk of instability. Initially thought to be the biomechanical converse to anterior shoulder instability, researchers have assessed the biomechanics of posterior instability and characterize this unique phenomenon as a distinct pathoanatomical process. In the following section, we will review the relevant literature and highlight the biomechanical features of the structures associated with posterior shoulder stability.

Position of instability

Posterior shoulder dislocations are well-described to occur in the setting of three primary, concurrent humeral positions: flexion to 90°, internal rotation, and adduction.[55–58] Patients who present with posterior shoulder instability as the result of microtrauma and subluxation episodes often experience symptoms during activities such as bench press, pushups, or blocking in football as the forces imparted on the shoulder in this position reproduces pain from posterorinferior labral tears.[14] However, several biomechanical studies have also tested posterior shoulder stability using less forward humeral flexion and varying degrees of humeral abduction with the shoulder in neutral rotation, simulating the posterior load-and-shift testing position.[21,59,60] For example, 30° of humeral flexion with an abducted shoulder is the position in which the posterior band of the inferior glenohumeral ligament becomes the primary antero-posterior stabilizer of the glenohumeral joint, describing an important pathoanatomic connection to this scapulohumeral position.[21]

Capsulolabral complex biomechanics

The PIGHL and the posterior labrum are essential soft tissue structures implicated in posterior shoulder instability, and are therapeutic targets for repair when nonoperative management of posterior labral tear fails.[61] The anatomic and biomechanical properties of these structures, as well as the pathoanatomic derangements when injured, are of particular importance in this clinical context.

The PIGHL biomechanically differs appreciably from the anterior band of the IGHL. Bigliani and colleagues[16] demonstrated that the tensile properties of the PIGHL are inferior to that of the anterior pouch and superior band, as the posterior band is thinner and exhibits a lower strain to failure. Ticker and colleagues also evaluated the geometric and strain-rate dependent properties of the IGHL, once again finding that the posterior band was thinner, demonstrated inferior tensile stress to failure, and lower bone-to-bone and mid-substance strains than the other regions of the ligament.[62] When combined with a posterior labral lesion, a posterior capsular injury results in a significant increase in the posterior and inferior translation of the humeral head, demonstrating the bidirectional (ie, posterior and inferior) importance of this ligament.[63] This group also found increased humeral head translation when adding a rotator interval injury (superior glenohumeral ligament and coracohumeral ligament), suggesting the importance of the superior capsule in posterior shoulder stability. This is in accordance with a biomechanical study performed by Harryman and colleagues[64] in 1992, which identified significant posteroinferior instability when sectioning the rotator interval and improved resistance to posterior and inferior translation when imbricating the rotator interval. On the contrary, Mologne and colleagues[65] found no increase in resistance to posterior translation when adding an arthroscopic rotator interval closure after posterior capsulolabral repair, but did find a significant decrease in external rotation following this procedure. As a result, controversy remains as to the biomechanical relevance of the rotator interval on posterior shoulder instability.

The posterior labrum acts as both a bumper to posterior humeral head translation, but also an essential component of the suction effect maintaining humeral head concentricity within the glenoid. Many cadaveric biomechanical studies have demonstrated increasing humeral head translation or decreased force to translate the humeral head posteriorly and/or inferiorly in the context of a posterior labral tear when studying posterior shoulder instability.[59,60,63,66] In a cadaveric biomechanical study of posteroinferior labral lesions, Wellman and colleagues[63] found an 86% increase in posterior humeral head translation and a 31% increase in inferior translation when simulating a posterior Bankart lesion. Accordingly, Waltz and colleagues[67] reported that a posterior labral repair significantly decreases the posterior–inferior translation of the humeral head up to 2.3 mm when compared with labral tear states when applying 75 N of posteroinferior force to the humeral head using a cadaveric model. These results demonstrate the biomechanical importance of posterior labral repairs in restoring posterior shoulder stability, but as we will highlight in the upcoming section, labral repair alone may be insufficient to restore posterior stability in the context of severe posterior glenoid bony deficiency.

Glenoid bone loss and retroversion

The glenoid is an essential osseous restraint to both anterior and posterior shoulder instability. As previously described, the glenoid is a concave structure, with a central depression and elevation eccentrically throughout its circular arc. On average, the glenoid is retroverted approximately 5 to 6° relative to the plane of the scapula.[38] Several glenoid abnormalities can predispose to posterior shoulder instability including higher degrees of retroversion, loss of glenoid concavity and tilt, or posterior glenoid bone loss from recurrent instability episodes.[13,60,68]

While the pathoanatomic features and surgical treatments for anterior instability have been well-established over the years, only more recently have surgeons emphasized posterior glenoid bone loss in recurrent posterior instability. Nacca and colleagues[60] performed a cadaveric biomechanical study to evaluate the critical amount of posterior glenoid bone loss at which a posterior labral repair alone would be insufficient to restore shoulder stability. This group found that an osseous defect of greater than 20% of the glenoid width could not be effectively stabilized with a reverse Bankart repair alone. Waltz and colleagues attempted another biomechanical study to evaluate the effectiveness of a reverse Bankart repair in the setting of posterior glenoid bone loss, finding that smaller-sized osseous defects could be stabilized with a reverse Bankart repair alone. However, in their larger defect group (>25% of the glenoid width), labral repair alone could not restore stability to the native state.[67]

The biomechanical effect of glenoid retroversion has also been studied regarding both glenohumeral osteoarthritis and posterior shoulder stability. In a study aimed to evaluate the amount of posterior glenoid wear before posterior humeral head subluxation occurred (ie, in the case of a Walch B2 glenoid), Bryce and colleagues[69] found that posterior humeral head translation increased with even 5° of posterior glenoid bone loss (equating to 2.5° of glenoid retroversion) depending on the position of the humerus. When considering posterior shoulder instability, Levins and colleagues[59] found in their cadaveric biomechanical study that each degree of retroversion accounted for a 3.5% decrease in resistance to posterior humeral head translation. Their results also suggested that repairing the posterior labrum does not restore posterior shoulder stability when retroversion exceeds 20 to 25°, implying that bony anatomy may be more relevant at higher degrees of glenoid retroversion. Ernstbrunner and colleagues[70] performed a biomechanical analysis of a posterior glenoid opening-wedge osteotomy using a J-shaped iliac crest graft, finding that reconstructing the glenoid to 0° of retroversion significantly improved shoulder stability in the setting of either a posterior labral lesion or posterior glenoid bone loss (**Fig. 4**). Similarly, Marcaccio and colleagues[66] found a posterior glenoid opening wedge osteotomy to be a useful biomechanical option in the treatment of posterior glenoid bone loss. However, while a posterior glenoid osteotomy appears to be biomechanically beneficial, the clinical results are suboptimal; at long-term follow-up, these patients have unfortunately high rates of glenohumeral arthritis.[71]

Humeral head

The biomechanical data assessing humeral head lesions in posterior shoulder instability are limited.[44,46] To the best of our knowledge, there are no cadaveric biomechanical studies performed in this realm. Moroder and colleagues has however performed the previously mentioned analysis to assess for engagement in bipolar bone defects.

This group used 19 cases of posterior shoulder dislocations with no posterior glenoid bony defects. They performed various measurements using CT scans, created virtual posterior glenoid defects, all with the goal of identifying the size and location of RHSL and amount of posterior glenoid bone loss that could lead to re-engagement. The authors found that each millimeter of posterior glenoid bone loss decreased the range of achievable humeral internal rotation prior to the re-engagement of the RHSL by 2.3° (also known as the delta angle).[44]

Acromion

There is limited biomechanical data assessing the role of acromial morphology in posterior shoulder instability. Testa and colleagues[72] performed a cadaveric biomechanical study evaluating the utility of a posterior acromial bone block in the treatment posterior shoulder instability. Their results found that posterior acromial augmentation

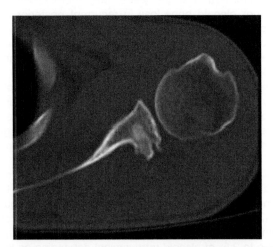

Fig. 4. A CT image in the axial plane of a shoulder after a posterior glenoid opening wedge osteotomy was performed. (Image courtesy of Elselvier Open Access publication; and Citation: Waltenspül, M, Häller, T, Ernstbrunner, L, Wyss, S, Wieser, K, Gerber, C: Long-term results after posterior open glenoid wedge osteotomy for posterior shoulder instability associated with excessive glenoid retroversion. J Shoulder Elbow Surg 2022;31:81–89.[68])

with a scapular spine bone block is biomechanically effective at restoring the force required to translate the humeral head posteriorly, and produces superior resistance force to humeral head translation than a posterior capsulolabral repair alone. Future biomechanical research in this area will be interesting to characterize any biomechanical relationship between posterior acromial morphology and posterior shoulder instability.

SUMMARY

Posterior glenohumeral instability encompasses a spectrum of pathology related to various anatomic features, including capsuloligamentous anatomy and bony constraints. While much attention is paid to the posterior capsulolabral complex, the osseous anatomy is of great importance when considering the biomechanical stability of the shoulder. Critical posterior glenoid bone loss, severe retroversion, and engaging humeral lesions must be addressed to adequately restore shoulder stability. Emerging concepts such as posterior acromial morphology may play an additional pathoanatomic role in posterior shoulder instability, but further research is needed to characterize its relevance.

CLINICS CARE POINTS

- Posterior glenohumeral instability encompasses a spectrum of pathology related to various anatomic features, including capsuloligamentous anatomy and bony constraints.

- The posterior capsulolabral complex, including the posterior band of the inferior glenohumeral ligament, as well as the posterior labrum, are both essential static soft tissue elements providing posterior glenohumeral stability, and are a common therapeutic target

- Critical posterior glenoid bone loss, severe retroversion, and engaging humeral lesions must be addressed to adequately restore shoulder stability.

- Emerging concepts such as posterior acromial morphology may play an additional pathoanatomic role in posterior shoulder instability, but further research is needed to characterize its relevance.

DISCLOSURE

No relevant disclosures.

REFERENCES

1. McLaughlin HL. Posterior dislocation of the shoulder. J Bone Joint Surg Am 1952; 24 A(3):584–90.
2. Woodmass JM, Lee J, Wu IT, et al. Incidence of posterior shoulder instability and trends in surgical reconstruction: a 22-year population-based study. J Shoulder Elbow Surg 2019;28(4):611–6.
3. Zacchilli MA, Owens BD. Epidemiology of shoulder dislocations presenting to emergency departments in the United States. J Bone Joint Surg Am 2010; 92(3):542–9.
4. Bokshan SL, Kotchman HM, Li LT, et al. Incidence of Posterior Shoulder Instability in the United States Military: Demographic Considerations From a High-Risk Population. Am J Sports Med 2021;49(2):340–5.

5. Lanzi JT, Chandler PJ, Cameron KL, et al. Epidemiology of Posterior Glenohumeral Instability in a Young Athletic Population. Am J Sports Med 2017;45(14): 3315–21.

6. Yow BG, Wade SM, Bedrin MD, et al. The Incidence of Posterior and Combined AP Shoulder Instability Treatment with Surgical Stabilization Is Higher in an Active Military Population than in the General Population: Findings from the US Naval Academy. Clin Orthop Relat Res 2021;479(4):704.

7. Robinson CM, Seah M, Akhtar MA. The epidemiology, risk of recurrence, and functional outcome after an acute traumatic posterior dislocation of the shoulder. J Bone Joint Surg Am 2011;93(17):1605–13.

8. Hatzis N, Kaar TK, Wirth MA, et al. The often overlooked posterior dislocation of the shoulder. Tex Med 2001;97(11):62–7.

9. Hawkins RJ, Neer CS, Pianta RM, et al. Locked posterior dislocation of the shoulder. J Bone Joint Surg Am 1987;69(1):9–18.

10. Rowe CR, Zarins B. Chronic unreduced dislocations of the shoulder. J Bone Joint Surg Am 1982;64(4):494–505.

11. Teske LG, Arvesen J, Kissenberth MJ, et al. Athletes diagnosed with anterior and posterior shoulder instability display different chief complaints and disability. J Shoulder Elbow Surg 2021;30(7S):S21–6.

12. Bernhardson AS, Murphy CP, Aman ZS, et al. A Prospective Analysis of Patients With Anterior Versus Posterior Shoulder Instability: A Matched Cohort Examination and Surgical Outcome Analysis of 200 Patients. Am J Sports Med 2019; 47(3):682–7.

13. Brewer BJ, Wubben RC, Carrera GF. Excessive retroversion of the glenoid cavity. A cause of non-traumatic posterior instability of the shoulder. J Bone Joint Surg Am 1986;68(5):724–31.

14. Wolfe JA, Elsenbeck M, Nappo K, et al. Effect of Posterior Glenoid Bone Loss and Retroversion on Arthroscopic Posterior Glenohumeral Stabilization. Am J Sports Med 2020;48(11):2621–7.

15. Bey MJ, Hunter SA, Kilambi N, et al. Structural and mechanical properties of the glenohumeral joint posterior capsule. J Shoulder Elbow Surg 2005;14(2):201–6.

16. Bigliani LU, Pollock RG, Soslowsky LJ, et al. Tensile properties of the inferior glenohumeral ligament. J Orthop Res 1992;10(2):187–97.

17. Diop A, Maurel N, Blancheton A, et al. The biomechanical effect of injury and repair of the inferior glenohumeral ligament on glenohumeral stability: Contribution of the posterior band. Clin BioMech 2022;91:105540. https://doi.org/10.1016/j.clinbiomech.2021.105540.

18. O'Brien SJ, Neves MC, Arnoczky SP, et al. The anatomy and histology of the inferior glenohumeral ligament complex of the shoulder. Am J Sports Med 1990; 18(5):449–56.

19. Warner JJP, Caborn DNM, Berger R, et al. Dynamic capsuloligamentous anatomy of the glenohumeral joint. J Shoulder Elbow Surg 1993;2(3):115–33.

20. Koga A, Itoigawa Y, Wada T, et al. Anatomic Analysis of the Attachment of the Posteroinferior Labrum and Capsule to the Glenoid: A Cadaveric Study. Arthrosc J Arthrosc Relat Surg 2020;36(11):2814–9.

21. O'Brien SJ, Schwartz RS, Warren RF, et al. Capsular restraints to anterior-posterior motion of the abducted shoulder: A biomechanical study. J Shoulder Elbow Surg 1995;4(4):298–308.

22. Howell SM, Galinat BJ. The glenoid-labral socket. A constrained articular surface. Clin Orthop Relat Res 1989;(243):122–5.

23. Ishikawa H, Henninger HB, Kawakami J, et al. A stabilizing role of the glenoid labrum: the suction cup effect. J Shoulder Elbow Surg 2023;32(5):1095–104.

24. Lazarus MD, Sidles JA, Harryman DT, et al. Effect of a Chondral-Labral Defect on Glenoid Concavity and Glenohumeral Stability. A Cadaveric Model. J Bone Joint Surg 1996;78(1):94–102.

25. Chloros G, Haar P, Loughran T, et al. Imaging of Glenoid Labrum Lesions. Clin Sports Med 2013;32:361–90.

26. De Maeseneer M, Van Roy P, Shahabpour M. Normal MR imaging anatomy of the rotator cuff tendons, glenoid fossa, labrum, and ligaments of the shoulder. Radiol Clin 2006;44(4):479–87.

27. Park YH, Lee JY, Moon SH, et al. MR arthrography of the labral capsular ligamentous complex in the shoulder: imaging variations and pitfalls. AJR Am J Roentgenol 2000;175(3):667–72.

28. Antosh IJ, Tokish JM, Owens BD. Posterior Shoulder Instability: Current Surgical Management. Sport Health 2016;8(6):520–6.

29. DeLong JM, Jiang K, Bradley JP. Posterior Instability of the Shoulder: A Systematic Review and Meta-analysis of Clinical Outcomes. Am J Sports Med 2015;43(7):1805–17.

30. Kim S, Ha K, Yoo J, et al. Kim's lesion: An incomplete and concealed avulsion of the posteroinferior labrum in posterior or multidirectional posteroinferior instability of the shoulder. Arthrosc J Arthrosc Relat Surg 2004;20(7):712–20.

31. Kim SH, Ha KI, Park JH, et al. Arthroscopic Posterior Labral Repair and Capsular Shift for Traumatic Unidirectional Recurrent Posterior Subluxation of the Shoulder. The Journal of Bone and Joint Surgery-American 2003;85(8):1479–87.

32. Metcalf MH, Pon JD, Harryman DT, et al. Capsulolabral augmentation increases glenohumeral stability in the cadaver shoulder. J Shoulder Elbow Surg 2001;10(6):532–8.

33. Young BL, Corpus KT, Scarola G, et al. Outcomes of posterior labral repair with or without concomitant high-grade glenohumeral chondral pathology: a retrospective cohort with minimum 2-year follow-up. J Shoulder Elbow Surg 2021;30(12):2720–8.

34. Huijsmans PE, Haen PS, Kidd M, et al. Quantification of a glenoid defect with three-dimensional computed tomography and magnetic resonance imaging: A cadaveric study. J Shoulder Elbow Surg 2007;16(6):803–9.

35. Kuberakani K, Aizawa K, Yamamoto N, et al. Comparison of best-fit circle versus contralateral comparison methods to quantify glenoid bone defect. J Shoulder Elbow Surg 2020;29(3):502–7.

36. Arner JW, Ruzbarsky JJ, Midtgaard K, et al. Defining Critical Glenoid Bone Loss in Posterior Shoulder Capsulolabral Repair. Am J Sports Med 2021;49(8):2013–9.

37. Owens BD, Campbell SE, Cameron KL. Risk Factors for Posterior Shoulder Instability in Young Athletes. Am J Sports Med 2013;41(11):2645–9.

38. Serrano N, Kissling M, Krafft H, et al. CT-based and morphological comparison of glenoid inclination and version angles and mineralisation distribution in human body donors. BMC Muscoskel Disord 2021;22(1):849.

39. Owens B, Slaven S, LeClere L, et al. Glenoid Bone Loss After First-Time Posterior Instability Events: A Prospective Cohort Study. Orthopaedic Journal of Sports Medicine 2021;9(7_suppl4):2325967121S00238. https://doi.org/10.1177/2325967121S00238.

40. Guehring M, Lambert S, Stoeckle U, et al. Posterior shoulder dislocation with associated reverse Hill-Sachs lesion: treatment options and functional outcome after a 5-year follow up. BMC Muscoskel Disord 2017;18(1):442.

41. Testa EJ, Byrne R, Petit L, et al. Open treatment of posterior glenoid bone loss and bipolar bone loss. Annals of Joint 2023;8. https://doi.org/10.21037/aoj-23-25.

42. Bock P, Kluger R, Hintermann B. Anatomical reconstruction for Reverse Hill-Sachs lesions after posterior locked shoulder dislocation fracture: a case series of six patients. Arch Orthop Trauma Surg 2007;127(7):543–8.

43. G G, E I, SS B. Evolving concept of bipolar bone loss and the Hill-Sachs lesion: From "engaging/non-engaging" lesion to "on-track/off-track" lesion. Arthroscopy 2014;30(1):90–8.

44. Moroder P, Plachel F, Tauber M, et al. Risk of Engagement of Bipolar Bone Defects in Posterior Shoulder Instability. Am J Sports Med 2017;45(12):2835–9.

45. Moroder P, Tauber M, Hoffelner T, et al. Reliability of a new standardized measurement technique for reverse Hill-Sachs lesions in posterior shoulder dislocations. Arthroscopy 2013;29(3):478–84.

46. Moroder P, Runer A, Kraemer M, et al. Influence of defect size and localization on the engagement of reverse Hill-Sachs lesions. Am J Sports Med 2015;43(3):542–8.

47. Lopez CD, Ding J, Bixby EC, et al. Association between shoulder coracoacromial arch morphology and anterior instability of the shoulder. JSES Int 2020;4(4):772–9.

48. Beeler S, Hasler A, Götschi T, et al. Different acromial roof morphology in concentric and eccentric osteoarthritis of the shoulder: a multiplane reconstruction analysis of 105 shoulder computed tomography scans. J Shoulder Elbow Surg 2018;27(12):e357–66.

49. Gerber C, Sigrist B, Hochreiter B. Correction of Static Posterior Shoulder Subluxation by Restoring Normal Scapular Anatomy Using Acromion and Glenoid Osteotomies: A Case Report. JBJS Case Connector 2023;13(2):e23.00060.

50. Livesey MG, Bedrin MD, Baird MD, et al. Acromion Morphology is Associated with Glenoid Bone Loss in Posterior Glenohumeral Instability. J Shoulder Elbow Surg 2023;32(9):1850–6.

51. Meyer DC, Ernstbrunner L, Boyce G, et al. Posterior Acromial Morphology Is Significantly Associated with Posterior Shoulder Instability. J Bone Joint Surg Am 2019;101(14):1253–60.

52. Scapinelli R. Posterior addition acromioplasty in the treatment of recurrent posterior instability of the shoulder. J Shoulder Elbow Surg 2006;15(4):424–31.

53. Bäcker HC, Galle SE, Maniglio M, et al. Biomechanics of posterior shoulder instability - current knowledge and literature review. World J Orthoped 2018;9(11):245–54.

54. Blasier RB, Soslowsky LJ, Malicky DM, et al. Posterior glenohumeral subluxation: active and passive stabilization in a biomechanical model. J Bone Joint Surg Am 1997;79(3):433–40.

55. Hawkins RJ, Koppert G, Johnston G. Recurrent posterior instability (subluxation) of the shoulder. J Bone Joint Surg Am 1984;66(2):169–74.

56. Ovesen J, Nielsen S. Anterior and posterior shoulder instability. A cadaver study. Acta Orthop Scand 1986;57(4):324–7.

57. Antosh IJ, Tokish JM, Owens BD. Posterior Shoulder Instability. Sport Health 2016;8(6):520–6.

58. Brelin A, Dickens JF. Posterior Shoulder Instability. Sports Med Arthrosc Rev 2017;25(3):136–43.

59. Levins J, Badida R, Garcia-Lopez E, et al. The Influence of Glenoid Retroversion on Posterior Shoulder Instability: A Cadaveric Study (214). Orthopaedic Journal

of Sports Medicine 2021;9(10_suppl5):2325967121S00322. https://doi.org/10.1177/2325967121S00322.

60. Nacca C, Gil JA, Badida R, et al. Critical Glenoid Bone Loss in Posterior Shoulder Instability. Am J Sports Med 2018;46(5):1058–63.

61. Itoigawa Y, Itoi E. Anatomy of the capsulolabral complex and rotator interval related to glenohumeral instability. Knee Surg Sports Traumatol Arthrosc 2016; 24(2):343–9.

62. Ticker JB, Bigliani LU, Soslowsky LJ, et al. Inferior glenohumeral ligament: geometric and strain-rate dependent properties. J Shoulder Elbow Surg 1996;5(4): 269–79.

63. Wellmann M, Blasig H, Bobrowitsch E, et al. The biomechanical effect of specific labral and capsular lesions on posterior shoulder instability. Arch Orthop Trauma Surg 2011;131(3):421–7.

64. Harryman DT, Sidles JA, Harris SL, et al. The role of the rotator interval capsule in passive motion and stability of the shoulder. J Bone Joint Surg Am 1992;74(1): 53–66.

65. Mologne TS, Zhao K, Hongo M, et al. The addition of rotator interval closure after arthroscopic repair of either anterior or posterior shoulder instability: effect on glenohumeral translation and range of motion. Am J Sports Med 2008;36(6): 1123–31.

66. Marcaccio SE, O'Donnel RM, Schilkowsky R, et al. Posterior Glenoid Osteotomy With Capsulolabral Repair Improves Resistance Forces in a Critical Glenoid Bone Loss Model. Orthopaedic Journal of Sports Medicine 2022;10(3): 23259671221083579. https://doi.org/10.1177/23259671221083579.

67. Waltz RA, Brown J, Brady AW, et al. Biomechanical Evaluation of Posterior Shoulder Instability With a Clinically Relevant Posterior Glenoid Bone Loss Model. Am J Sports Med 2023;51(9):2443–53.

68. Inui H, Sugamoto K, Miyamoto T, et al. Glenoid shape in atraumatic posterior instability of the shoulder. Clin Orthop Relat Res 2002;403:87–92.

69. Bryce CD, Davison AC, Okita N, et al. A biomechanical study of posterior glenoid bone loss and humeral head translation. J Shoulder Elbow Surg 2010;19(7): 994–1002.

70. Ernstbrunner L, Borbas P, Ker AM, et al. Biomechanical Analysis of Posterior Open-Wedge Osteotomy and Glenoid Concavity Reconstruction Using an Implant-Free, J-Shaped Iliac Crest Bone Graft. Am J Sports Med 2022;50(14): 3889–96.

71. Waltenspül M, Häller T, Ernstbrunner L, et al. Long-term results after posterior open glenoid wedge osteotomy for posterior shoulder instability associated with excessive glenoid retroversion. J Shoulder Elbow Surg 2022;31(1):81–9.

72. Testa EJ, Morrissey P, Albright JA, et al. A Posterior Acromial Bone Block Augmentation Is Biomechanically Effective at Restoring the Force Required To Translate the Humeral Head Posteriorly in a Cadaveric, Posterior Glenohumeral Instability Model. Arthroscopy 2024;S0749-8063(24)00058-6.

Arthroscopic Management of Posterior Shoulder Instability

Benjamin B. Rothrauff, MD, PhD[a], Justin W. Arner, MD[b],
James P. Bradley, MD[b],*

KEYWORDS

- Arthroscopic surgery • Capsulolabral repair • Posterior instability • Shoulder

KEY POINTS

- Posterior shoulder instability is a distinct subcategory of shoulder instability with an incidence higher than previously reported.
- Nonoperative interventions including physical therapy and avoidance of provocative activities are the first-line of treatment.
- Patients with generalized ligamentous laxity and posterior shoulder instability should fully exhaust a rehabilitation program before surgical treatment is considered.
- Excellent outcomes and return to play at mid-term follow-up can be expected following arthroscopic posterior capsulolabral repair: (1) durable outcomes have been shown recently with long-term follow-up and (2) decreased glenoid bone width, female gender, concomitant rotator cuff injury, and the use of less than 3 anchors are the risk factors for failure.
- Throwing athletes have a slightly less predictable outcome after surgery while American football players have the most reliable positive results.

INTRODUCTION

Once thought to be relatively uncommon, posterior shoulder instability is increasingly identified, with an incidence of posterior capsulolabral injury equal to or exceeding that of anterior pathology.[1,2] The growing recognition of the prevalence of posterior shoulder instability, coupled with a thorough history and physical examination, has facilitated a prompt and accurate diagnosis. Nevertheless, greater physician knowledge and education is still needed. Surgical treatment has progressed from open suture-only procedures to anatomic patient-specific arthroscopic knotless

[a] Department of Orthopaedic Surgery, University of Pittsburgh Medical Center, Pittsburgh, PA, USA; [b] Burke and Bradley Orthopaedics, Department of Orthopaedic Surgery, University of Pittsburgh Medical Center, Pittsburgh, PA, USA
* Corresponding author. Burke and Bradley Orthopaedics, 200 Delafield Rd., Suite 4010, Pittsburgh, PA 15215.
E-mail address: bradleyjp@upmc.edu

Clin Sports Med 43 (2024) 737–753
https://doi.org/10.1016/j.csm.2024.03.027
0278-5919/24/© 2024 Elsevier Inc. All rights reserved.

sportsmed.theclinics.com

suture anchor repair. Further knowledge regarding risk factors for posterior shoulder instability and failure of its surgical treatment are still necessary, with ongoing research investigating the influence of labral and glenoid morphology, including the effect of posterior glenoid bone loss.

HISTORY

While posterior shoulder injuries can present with traumatic locked posterior shoulder instability, athletes most frequently have pathology secondary to repetitive microtrauma leading to recurrent posterior subluxation (RPS).[3] RPS tends to affect a subset of athletes, including overhead throwers, baseball hitters, golfers, tennis players, butterfly and freestyle swimmers, paddling sport athletes, weightlifters, rugby players, military service members, and football lineman.[4] Repetitive microtrauma inherent in these sporting activities can produce posterior capsular attenuation and posterior labral tears ultimately resulting in symptomatic RPS. Regardless of sport, patients with RPS often have vague and ambiguous complaints of diffuse pain and shoulder fatigue without a distinct complaint of instability, making this diagnosis difficult and in contrast to the more primary complaint of instability accompanying anterior shoulder instability.[3]

Despite a similar presentation of signs and symptoms, throwers have a unique mechanism of posterior shoulder injury which involves an avulsion of the posterior capsulolabral complex (PCLC) or a labral flap tear. RPS in throwers can be caused by several mechanisms with a common pathway involving deceleration and eccentric loading during the throwing cycle, leading to repetitive microtrauma. Throwers commonly have a tight posterior inferior capsule (glenohumeral internal rotation deficient) which leads to repetitive microtrauma after ball release, and thus progressive tearing can occur. Similarly, throwers are prone to develop superior labrum anterior posterior (type IIb SLAP) tears with continued stress on the tension band causing posterior extension along the labrum resulting in RPS. A more dynamic pathology involves an imbalance of a weak or contracted pectoralis major muscle which allows the latissimus to pull the humeral head posteroinferiorly. Mechanical symptoms or pain during follow-through as well as loss of velocity and control (commonly high and outside) are the typical complaint in this population. Like other athletes, instability is not the predominant issue. In those with a dynamic muscle imbalance, pain is typically seen at or just before ball release.[5,6]

Despite being less common, posterior shoulder instability can be caused by traumatic injury, often from a posteriorly directed force to the anterior shoulder with the shoulder in a position of flexion, internal rotation, and adduction. The most common indirect causes are accidental electrocution and convulsive seizures, although these are relatively uncommon in the general population. Recurrent or locked posterior shoulder dislocations from macrotrauma are rare in the athletic population. However, a high clinical index of suspicion should be maintained in the trauma setting as a locked posterior dislocation may be overlooked in up to 80% of situations, often due to a failure to recognize posterior shoulder prominence and mechanical block to external rotation in the emergency department. Concomitant pathologies are common with posterior shoulder instability and include reverse Hill–Sachs lesions, reverse bony Bankart lesions, capsular ligament avulsions, excessive humeral or glenoid retroversion, glenoid hypoplasia, or glenoid bone loss.

SIGNS AND SYMPTOMS

As opposed to a history of a traumatic shoulder subluxation or frank dislocation that frequently accompanies anterior shoulder instability, the more often insidious nature of posterior shoulder instability especially necessitates a thorough history and physical examination while maintaining a high index of suspicion. A minority of patients with RPS will have a history of a posterior dislocation requiring formal reduction. Likewise, a chief complaint of instability is less common than pain with specific activities, particularly in the provocative position (90° of forward flexion, adduction, and internal rotation). Throwing athletes will often complain of requiring increased time to warm-up before games and requiring longer durations to recovery between games. Bernhardson and colleagues[3] matched a cohort of patients with anterior or posterior instability and found that those with posterior shoulder instability typically had no identifiable injury, with pain being the primary complaint.

A specific history of the athlete's sport, position, and training regimen is equally critical in deducing the pathogenesis and specific pathology associated with RPS. Mechanical symptoms, specifically clicking, clunking, or crepitation with motion, should also be noted. Crepitation can often be reproduced during examination and may be caused by discrete pathology of the PCLC.

Physical Examination

- Inspection for skin dimpling, atrophy, and scapular motion (including winging or dyskinesia)
- Palpation for tenderness (especially along the posterior glenohumeral joint)
- Active and passive range of motion in the coronal, sagittal, and axial planes
- Strength testing
- Evaluation for impingement
- Assessment for generalized ligamentous laxity (9 point Beighton scale)
- Shoulder laxity
  - Load and shift test for anterior and posterior translation
  - Sulcus sign (both in neutral and external rotation) for inferior translation
    - Sulcus sign graded as 3+ that remains 2+ in external rotation is pathognomonic for multidirectional instability (MDI)
  - Gagey test for inferior shoulder instability
- Specific tests
  - Jerk test
  - Kim test
  - Circumduction test
  - Active compression or O'Brien's test (**Fig. 1**)
  - osterior instability test / dynamic posterior instability test (**Fig. 2**)
  - Whipple/modified Whipple (**Fig. 3**)

Imaging

- Plain radiographs including an axillary, anteroposterior (AP), AP oblique (Grashey), and scapular Y view
  - Reverse Hill–Sachs lesions of the humeral head
    - Lesser tuberosity fracture
  - Glenoid pathology (retroversion, rim fractures, and hypoplasia)
    - Additional West Point axillary view can be useful
  - Bony humeral avulsion of the glenohumeral ligaments (HAGLs)
- MRI
  - Labrum
    - Kim classification can specifically describe posterior labral tear morphology
      - Type I, incomplete detachment
      - Type II (the "Kim lesion"), a concealed complete detachment

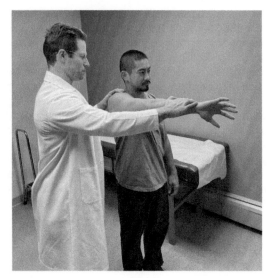

Fig. 1. Active compression (O'Brien's) test. With the shoulder in a position of 90° forward elevation and 10° adduction from the sagittal plan, the arm is internally rotated. Resistance of downward pressure will illicit pain. A positive test is confirmed with improvement in pain when downward force is applied to the now externally rotated arm (palm up).

- Type III, chondrolabral erosion
- Type IV, flap tear of the posteroinferior labrum
○ Concomitant injuries are common and must be evaluated and treated appropriately
    ■ Capsular rents or tears

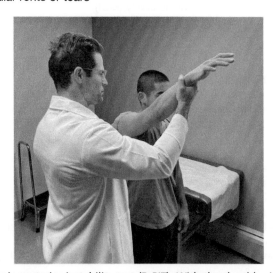

Fig. 2. The dynamic posterior instability test (D-PIT). With the shoulder in 135° of forward flexion and the elbow fully extended, the patient applied a downward force in a throwing motion as the examiner provides resistance. Posterior shoulder pain indicates a positive test. The modified D-PIT involves the examiner stabilizing the posterior humeral head by applying pressure, often improving the patient's pain.

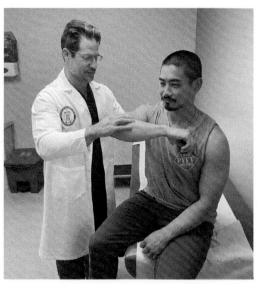

Fig. 3. The Whipple test. With the shoulder of interest forward flexed to 90° and the hand placed on the contralateral shoulder, the patient provides an upward force resisted by the examiner, producing posterior shoulder pain. The modified Whipple test involves the examiner stabilizing the posterior humeral head by pushing on it with his or her thumb. Improvement in pain is expected.

- ■ HAGL lesion
- ■ Reverse HAGL lesion
- ■ SLAP (including posterior extension, SLAP VIII–X)
- ■ Cartilage lesions
- ■ Rotator cuff tears
- ■ Biceps tendon
- ■ Subscapularis integrity
- ○ Posterior labrum periosteal sleeve avulsion
- ○ Evaluate boney parameters
  - ■ Glenoid version: risk factor for posterior instability
  - ■ Glenoid width: risk factor for failure of arthroscopic posterior capsulolabral repair
- • Dynamic MRI
  - ○ Demonstrate labral peel-back in the abduction and external rotation position, consistent with posterosuperior labral tear (or type VIII SLAP tear)
- • Magnetic resonance arthrogram
  - ○ Findings of glenoid dysplasia, posterior humeral head subluxation, and increased posterior capsular volume are independent risk factors in patients with posterior labral tears who develop posterior instability
- • Computed tomography
  - ○ Evaluate bone loss and glenoid version
  - ○ Locked posterior dislocation

Indications and Contraindications

Many patients with RPS can be managed successfully without surgery, depending on their activities and goals. While there remains no consensus on what constitutes failure of conservative treatment, a period of 6 months of physical therapy before consideration of surgical treatment has been proposed by some.[7] Effective rehabilitation includes avoidance of aggravating activities, restoration of a full range of motion, and shoulder strengthening with particular emphasis on the rotator cuff, posterior deltoid, and periscapular musculature. While rehabilitation can often diminish the functional disability and pain associated with RPS, recurrent subluxation seen in this pathology may persist.

Surgical consideration is given to patients failing extensive physical therapy protocols. Indications for arthroscopic posterior stabilization include active patients and athletes with continued disabling isolated RPS typically with a posterior labral tear or patients with antecedent microtrauma leading to a posterior labral tear. Patients with MDI with a primary posterior component and voluntary positional posterior instability have less reliable surgical outcomes and nonoperative treatments should be the mainstay. Surgical consideration for an in-season athlete is made on a case-by-case basis and depends on the severity of symptoms, current level of (compromised) performance, sport (eg, contact vs noncontact), position (eg, thrower vs nonthrower), competitive level (eg, recreational vs professional), timing of season (eg, preseason vs championships), and so forth. Generally, an athlete is permitted to complete the competitive season if there was no singular acute injury event, normal strength is maintained, and the athlete has passed a milestone-based, progressive return to sport rehabilitation protocol.

Contraindications of arthroscopic repair include patients who have not completed an appropriate rehabilitation program, a large engaging reverse Hill–Sachs lesion requiring subscapularis transfer or an osteochondral allograft, and a large reverse bony Bankart lesion, patients with muscular voluntary instability and underlying psychogenic disorders, and patients unable or unwilling to comply with postoperative limitations. In those with extensive glenoid bone loss or extensive poor soft tissue quality, a posterior bone block augmentation, typically with iliac crest autograft or distal tibia allograft, can be considered. Ongoing research seeks to elucidate what constitutes critical bone loss that necessitates posterior bone block augmentation.[8] Glenoid osteotomy has been described as a treatment of posterior shoulder instability secondary to excessive glenoid retroversion, but a high rate of posterior instability and arthritis may result.[9] A recent study on long-term outcomes following glenoid osteotomy for excessive glenoid retroversion found nearly universal recurrence of posterior shoulder instability (86%); therefore, the study investigators recommended against this procedure.[10] In agreement, we do not believe glenoid osteotomies for the correction of abnormal version are a reliable treatment option and have found the above-mentioned treatment options to result in successful surgical outcomes.

Arthroscopic Surgical Technique

Anesthesia and positioning

Arthroscopic posterior shoulder capsulolabral repair can be performed with general endotracheal anesthesia with or without use of a preoperative interscalene block for pain control. The authors prefer to perform instability surgery in the lateral decubitus position, although a recent systematic review found equivalent outcomes in comparing the beach chair versus lateral decubitus positioning.[11] An inflatable beanbag with an axillary roll and foam cushions are used to protect bony prominences such as the peroneal nerve at the neck of the fibula. The full upper extremity is sterility prepared to the level of the sternum anteriorly and the medial border of the scapula posteriorly. The operative shoulder is positioned in 45° of abduction and 20° of forward flexion with 10 pounds of traction.

Landmarks, incisions, and portals

After sterile draping, the bony landmarks, including the coracoid process, distal clavicle, and acromion, are highlighted with a marking pen. The glenohumeral joint is insufflated with 50 mL of sterile saline using an 18 gauge spinal needle. A posterior portal is then established 1 cm distal and 1 cm lateral to a standard posterior portal, facilitating anchor placement in the glenoid rim. A switching stick placed through the posterior portal is then used in an inside-to-outside technique to establish an anterior portal high in the rotator interval. An accessory 7 o'clock portal can be made percutaneously for inferior anchor placement.

Examination

Examination under anesthesia. Before positioning the patient in the lateral decubitus position, an examination under anesthesia is performed on the supine patient. A load-and-shift maneuver is performed with the arm in 90° of abduction and neutral rotation where a posteriorly directed force is applied in an attempt to translate the humeral head over the posterior glenoid. In order to assess inferior instability, axial traction is applied to the adducted arm in the neutral position to elicit a potential sulcus sign. A 3+ sulcus sign that remains 2+ or greater in external rotation is considered pathognomonic for MDI. The contralateral unaffected shoulder is examined in the same manner, with examination findings on both shoulders appropriately documented.

Diagnostic arthroscopy. Systematic evaluation of labrum, capsule, biceps tendon, subscapularis, rotator interval, rotator cuff, and articular surfaces is performed by diagnostic arthroscopy of the glenohumeral joint. Notably, lesions commonly seen in the setting of posterior shoulder instability include a posterior labral tear, patulous posterior capsule, labral fraying and splitting, capsular tears, and undersurface partial thickness rotator cuff tears. Following establishment of the anterior portal, an anterior cannula is placed (Partially Threaded 5.75 × 7 mm, Arthrex, Naples, FL). After the glenohumeral joint has been viewed from the posterior portal, the arthroscope is switched to the anterior portal to allow for visualization of the posterior capsule and labrum. A switching stick can be used to place a posterior 8.25 or 9 mm distally threaded clear cannula (Arthrex, Naples, FL), allowing passage of an arthroscopic probe and other instruments to probe the posterior labrum for evidence of tears. Smaller cannulas are avoided as they will not accommodate a 45° suture hook. The labrum is initially prepared while viewing from the posterior portal using a 70° arthroscope, with instruments being used across the glenoid from the anterior portal as this permits a superior angle of attack.

Specific Steps

Preparation for repair

- The labrum is visualized from both the anterior and posterior portals to determine tear size and morphology (**Fig. 4**).
- Viewing from the posterior portal, the torn labrum is mobilized from the glenoid using an arthroscopic chisel and rasp (**Fig. 5**).
- The glenoid rim is decorticated using a motorized synovial shaver to achieve a bleeding edge (**Fig. 6**).
- If capsular plication is needed, a meniscal rasp is used to abrade the capsule adjacent to the labral tear.

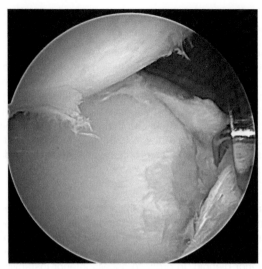

Fig. 4. Posterior labral tear. Diagnostic arthroscopy revealing a posterior and inferior labral tear, with separation of the labrum from the glenoid exaggerated by the retracting probe.

Labral repair and placement of suture anchors

- Suture anchors are placed at the articular margin of the glenoid rim; Knotless anchors are recommended to avoid complications of knot abrasion, knot migration, repair strength, and surgical efficiency.
- A posterior labral tear involving the 6 to 9 o'clock position (clockface position in reference to a right shoulder) is typically repaired with suture anchors at the 6:30, 7:30, 8:30, and 9:30 positions, constituting a slightly superior-directed vector of suture tension.

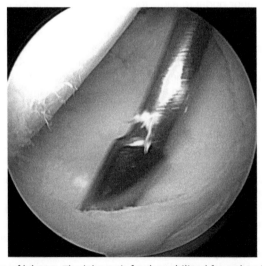

Fig. 5. Mobilization of labrum. The labrum is freely mobilized from the glenoid rim using an arthroscopic chisel.

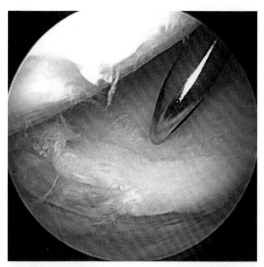

Fig. 6. Glenoid preparation. The glenoid rim is decorticated using a motorized synovial shaver to achieve a bleeding edge.

- We prefer anchors close to the 6 o'clock position be placed percutaneously using a 7 o'clock portal using a 1.8 mm knotless FiberTak or 3.0 mm BioComposite Knotless SutureTak (Arthrex Naples, FL) to minimize capsular injury and obtain the ideal angle.
- To initiate the capsulolabral repair, a suture passer device is inserted through the posterior portal. The tip of the suture passer is pierced through the capsule and delivered on the articular side of the torn labrum (**Fig. 7**). The passer can be advanced superiorly, re-entering the joint at the edge of the glenoid articular cartilage in order to shift the capsule superiorly. The direction of the curve of the passer is opposite of the side of the operative shoulder (eg, left curve on suture passer needle for right operative shoulder)
- When utilizing a 1.8 mm knotless FiberTak or 3.0 mm BioComposite Knotless SutureTak (Arthrex Naples, FL), the anchor is first placed and then the polydioxanone suture (PDS) is passed. The self-tensioning loop apparatus is then utilized.
- As noted, the capsulolabral repair suture is advanced in a slightly superior direction: the 7 o' clock position is advanced to the 7:30 suture anchor, and the 8 o'' clock labral tear position is advanced to the 8:30 suture anchor.
- The posterior band of the inferior glenohumeral ligament must be appropriately tensioned to re-establish posterior stability.
- When capsular laxity is appreciated in addition to a labral tear, the suture passer is advanced through the posterior capsule approximately 1 cm lateral to the edge of the labral tear and then is advanced underneath the labral tear to the edge of the articular cartilage.
- The size of the "bite" depends in part on the degree of capsular laxity and the sport to which the athlete will return (eg, contact vs throwing)
- Throwers should not undergo large capsular plications, but contact athletes (ie, American football lineman) with capsular laxity benefit from capsular advancement.

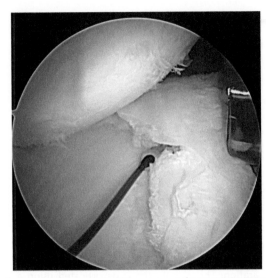

Fig. 7. Initiation of capsulolabral repair. Using a curved suture passer pierced through the peripheral capsule and advanced under the labrum, emerging between the glenolabral junction, a PDS suture is advanced into the joint.

- Acute injuries, which often lack the capsular stretching associated with chronic repetitive microtrauma, often do not require the same degree of capsular advancement.
- For suture passage, the PDS is fed into the glenohumeral joint and the suture passer is withdrawn through the posterior cannula.
- The PDS is then retrieved using an arthroscopic suture. The suture tape is then pulled through a loop formed in the end of the PDS suture.
- In pulling the most lateral PDS suture, which has not been tied to the tape suture, through the posterior portal, the suture tape is then shuttled around the labrum and capsule.
- A drill guide is placed on the edge of the articular margin. The authors prefer a ShaverDrill (Arthrex Naples, FL) for anchor drilling as it is disposable and therefore always sharp while eliminating the need for a reusable drill and batteries.
- With exception to the 6 o'clock percutaneously placed anchor, we prefer 2.4 mm or 2.9 mm BioComposite PushLock suture anchors (depending on the size of the glenoid) with SutureTape (Arthrex Naples, FL) in more superior locations because of the ease of use and their knotless manor. Suture tape provides a larger surface area for distribution of force through tissue, increasing the pull-through strength.
- After drilling, the suture tape is passed through the anchor islet on the surgical field. The anchor is advanced into drill hole on the glenoid rim (**Fig. 8**) and the suture is tensioned appropriately under direct visualization to assure appropriate tissue tension (**Fig. 9**).
- With the final knotless construct in place, the posterior bumper has been restored to its anatomic position (**Fig. 10**).
- If following the above-mentioned capsulolabral repair, the capsule requires further tension, suture capsulorrhaphies can be added in the intervals between the suture anchors directly to the newly secured labrum; it is our experience that this is rarely needed.

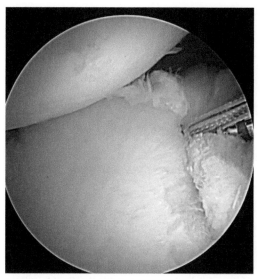

Fig. 8. Suture anchor placement. After drilling a bone tunnel at the glenoid rim, a 2.4 or 2.9 mm BioComposite PushLock suture anchor is advanced into the bone tunnel.

- If capsular laxity is the main pathology without a labral tear, suture anchors should still be used for capsular plication.
- If knot tying is performed by the operating surgeon, we prefer the sliding, locking Weston knot because of its low profile.
- The rotator interval is no longer closed in typical posterior capsulolabral repair.

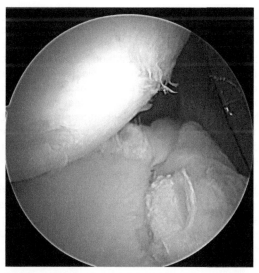

Fig. 9. Tensioning of suture to restore capsulolabral tension. The suture tape on the knotless suture anchor can be progressively tensioned until the labrum is secured against the glenoid rim and the physiologic capsular tension is restored.

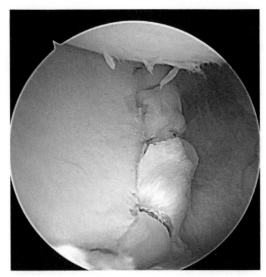

Fig. 10. Restoration of capsulolabral anatomy. With the final knotless construct in placed, the posterior bumper has been restored to its anatomic position.

Capsular closure

- A PDS suture is passed through the posterior capsular portal rent using the suture passer, with retrieval of the suture with an arthroscopic penetrator.
- The PDS is then tied blindly in the cannula, closing the posterior capsular rent to avoid a stress riser (**Fig. 11**).

Technical Alternatives and Pitfalls

There is ongoing debate regarding the superiority of lateral decubitus or beach chair position when treating posterior shoulder instability, with a recent systematic review suggesting largely equivalent clinical outcomes.[12] We prefer the lateral position, feeling it provides better access to both the anterior and posterior labrum. With regard to posterior instability surgery, the combined application of 10 pounds of traction in the position of 45° of abduction and 20° of forward flexion effectively displaces the humeral head anteriorly and inferiorly, providing excellent visualization of the posterior labrum. Additionally, we prefer to inject the glenohumeral joint with 40 to 50 mL of sterile saline before introduction of the arthroscope through the posterior portal. The inflated joint promotes safer insertion of the camera, limiting risk to the articular cartilage. While a 30° arthroscope is most commonly used, a 70° may be utilized to aid in visualization.

Localization of the posterior portal in a position that is too superior or medial can make difficult the placement of suture anchors. We, therefore, place the posterior portal approximately 1 cm inferior and 1 cm lateral to standard posterior portals. Insufflation of the joint before placement of the portal is helpful to distend the capsule and allow an improved trajectory for anchor placement in the glenoid. A spinal needle can be used in positioning an auxiliary portal at the 7 o'clock position approximately 1 cm lateral to the glenoid rim when coming through the posterior capsule. We recommend a percutaneous kit in this location to minimize capsular damage.

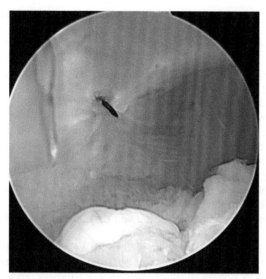

Fig. 11. Posterior capsule closure. The posterior portal is closed to prevent rent propagation and loss of posterior capsular tension.

Postoperative considerations

Rehabilitation and return-to-play recommendations. While there is a lack of consensus on how to rehabilitate after posterior shoulder stabilization most effectively,[13] all described rehabilitation programs entail a graded progression back to increasingly strenuous activities, such as sports. Our preferred rehabilitation program is as follows:

- Initially the posterior capsule must be protected by avoidance of extremes of internal rotation. Immobilization in an UltraSling (DonJoy, Carlsbad, CA) is performed for 6 weeks, with approximately 30° of shoulder abduction.
- Gentle passive pain-free range-of-motion exercises are begun almost immediately. For the first 4 weeks, we allow 90° of forward flexion and external rotation to 0°
- At 6 weeks, the sling is discontinued. Active-assisted range-of-motion exercises and gentle passive range of motion exercises are progressed, and pain-free gentle internal rotation is implemented.
- At 2 to 3 months postsurgery, mobilization is further progressed to achieve full passive and active motion. Stretching exercises for the anterior and posterior capsule are instituted.
- By 4 months, a painless shoulder is expected. Eccentric strength training, with emphasis on the rotator cuff and periscapular musculature, is advanced.
- At 5 months, isotonic and isokinetic exercises are progressed.
- At 4 to 6 months, throwing athletes undergo isokinetic testing. Achieving at least 80% strength and endurance compared with the uninvolved side permits the start of an integrated throwing protocol and/or sport-specific rehabilitation protocol.
- The throwing protocol begins with an easy-tossing program at a distance of 20 feet without a windup. Stretching and the application of heat to increase circulation before throwing sessions are essential.

- By 7 months, light throwing with an easy windup to 30 feet is allowed 2 or 3 days per week for 10 minutes per session.
- By 9 months, long, easy throws from the mid-outfield (150–200 feet) are permitted.
- By 10 months, stronger throws from the outfield are allowed, reaching home plate on only 1 or 2 bounces.
- At 11 months, pitchers are allowed to throw at half to three-quarter speed from the mound, with emphasis on technique and accuracy.
- By 12 months, throwers are allowed to throw at three-quarter to full speed. When able to perform full-speed throwing for 2 consecutive weeks, return to full competition is permitted.
- Nonthrowing athletes and nonathletes are managed by different criteria than throwing athletes, which permits early return to sporting activities. Notably, when patients are able to achieve at least 80% strength and endurance at the 6 month isokinetic testing compared with the uninvolved side, a sport-specific program can begin.
- Power athletes and contact athletes, such as weightlifters and football players, can generally return to full competition by 6 to 9 months postsurgery. Noncontact athletes such as golfers, basketball players, swimmers, and cheerleaders can generally return to full competition by 6 to 8 months.

Complications. Surgical complications after arthroscopic posterior shoulder capsulo-labral repair are rare, with recurrent instability being the most common adverse outcome. Given that posterior shoulder instability most commonly presents with insidious pain in the absence of a traumatic injury, it can be difficult to identify recurrent instability, as compared to frank dislocation or subluxation commonly seen in anterior instability surgical failure. Recurrent and persistent pain with an inability to return to activities may indicate surgical failure. MRI can be helpful in identifying recurrent posterior capsulolabral tearing, but regardless of imaging findings, physical therapy should be the first line of treatment. In addition to recurrent posterior capsulolabral tearing, cartilage deficiencies or anchor arthropathy caused by prominent anchors or knots should also be considered.[14,15] Axillary nerve injury may also occur with aberrant 7 o'clock portal placement or when grabbing too large of a capsular bite inferiorly on the glenoid. The rotator cuff should also be closely evaluated.

A 2015 systematic review of 19 studies investigating arthroscopic posterior shoulder stabilization reported a combined revision rate of 7.6%.[16] Recent literature by our group found revision to be necessary in 6.4% of primary surgeries at average 8.9 year follow-up. This was a nonthrowing cohort of 297 shoulders which previously underwent capsulolabral repair with suture anchors. Risk factors for failure were dominant shoulder, female gender, concomitant rotator cuff injury, and the use of 3 or fewer anchors, and smaller glenoid bone width. Although patients improved from their preoperative status, revision surgery resulted in poorer outcomes and return to sport when compared to primary cases.[17] A similar trend was confirmed in a more recent study of 53 patients with an average follow-up of 15.4 years.[18] Glenoid version was not a risk factor for surgical failure but has been reported to be a risk factor for initially developing posterior instability.[17,19] Another study by our group evaluating revision in contact athletes found a lower incidence of 5.4% at minimum 4 year and average 13 year follow-up. Again, smaller glenoid bone width and higher preoperative instability were risk factors for failure with return to play also being inferior to patients who did not undergo revision.[20] In thrower data from our group, revision rate was higher (8.9%) with female gender being a risk factor for surgical failure with poorer return to sport rates. Revision posterior shoulder capsulolabral repair can be considered after failure of conservative treatments including physical therapy and possibly injections, with leukocyte-poor platelet-rich plasma being preferred by the authors. Revision surgery following failed posterior shoulder stabilization is the topic of another chapter included in this book.

DISCUSSION

In defining success through clinical outcome scores, patient satisfaction, and return to sport, arthroscopic stabilization of posterior shoulder instability is successful in 80% to 90% of cases at mid-term follow-up,[16,21] with durable benefit seen at long-term follow-up of 15.4 years.[18] Return to sports rates are high in athletes from all sports; however, throwers tend to have slightly less predictable outcomes. Contact athletes, and American football players in particular, fair the best postoperatively.[6,22] Arthroscopic methods have become the gold standard as they afford the ability to perform simultaneous anterior, superior, and posterior repair if necessary and avoid splitting the deltoid and rotator cuff, which is required in open repairs. Patients with partial thickness rotator cuff tears who underwent debridement have been shown by our group not to have inferior outcomes.[23] We prefer knotless capsulolabral fixation as it is more efficient, stronger, and avoids the possibility of knot damage to the cartilage or soft tissue.[24] A directed physical therapy program postsurgery is vital to a successful outcome.

SUMMARY

Posterior shoulder instability is a distinct subcategory of shoulder instability with an incidence higher than previously reported. Pain is typically the primary complaint, with pathology due to repetitive microtrauma being more common than a specific traumatic event. If nonoperative treatment fails, arthroscopic posterior capsulolabral repair has been shown to result in excellent outcomes and return to sport, with American football players having the best outcomes and throwers being slightly less predictable. Risk factors for surgical failure include decreased glenoid bone width, rotator cuff injury, female gender, and the use of less than 3 anchors. Ongoing research efforts seek to further identify risk factors for surgical failure, including the role of posterior bone glenoid bone loss and its implication for possible posterior bone block augmentation.

CLINICS CARE POINTS

Pearls

- The authors prefer the lateral decubitus position during arthroscopy to allow better access to both the anterior and the posterior labrum.

- Placing the shoulder in 10 pounds of traction in the position of 45° of abduction and 20° of forward flexion displaces the humeral head anteriorly and inferiorly, bringing the posterior labrum into view.

- The authors recommend the posterior portal be placed 1 cm lower and 1 cm more lateral than a typical viewing portal to allow for the ideal angle for anchor placement.
  Insufflation of the joint before placement of the portal is helpful to distend the capsule and allow an improved trajectory for anchor placement in the glenoid.

- Patient-specific capsular plication should be done with the labral repair based on tissue quality and activity with suture anchors.

- Knotless anchors should be utilized when possible as they are faster, have greater pull-through strength, allow more anatomic repair, and minimize the risk of cartilage abrasion associated with knotted suture anchors.
- A 7 o'clock portal can be helpful for placement of anchors near the 6 o'clock position.
- A small percutaneous posterior portal should be considered when using a 7 o'clock portal to minimize injury to the native capsule.
- Closure of the posterior capsular rent created by the surgical cannulas is recommended.

Pitfalls

- Suture anchors should be used for capsulolabral repair.
- Difficulty in the placement of suture anchors can be encountered if the posterior portal is located too far superior or medial in the posterior capsule. If this occurs, one can pull back the cannula, and close the capsular rent, and replace the posterior cannula in the proper trajectory.
- In those with large shoulders, a longer cannula (7–9 cm) may be necessary.
- A spinal needle can be used to help determine the appropriate location of the 7 o'clock portal with the ideal capsular entry being 1 cm lateral to the glenoid rim and at a 45° angle.
- If the posterior capsule is not closed, widening of portal holes can occur and lead to capsular insufficiency.

DISCLOSURE

B.B. Rothrauff discloses educational support from Mid-Atlantic Surgical Systems. J.W. Arner discloses educational and travel support from Arthrex, United States, grant support from DJO, hospitality payments from Mid-Atlantic Surgical Systems and Smith + Nephew, and is an AOSSM committee member. J.P. Bradley discloses royalties from Arthrex, consulting fees from Arthrex and DJO, and is an AOSSM board member.

REFERENCES

1. Alexeev M, Kercher JS, Levina Y, et al. Variability of glenoid labral tear patterns: a study of 280 sequential surgical cases. J shoulder Elb Surg 2021;30(12):2762–6.
2. Kibler W Ben, Grantham WJ, Pike JSM, et al. Glenoid Labral Injuries Are More Common Posteriorly Than Superiorly and Are Combined Across Multiple Areas of the Glenoid. Arthrosc Sport Med Rehabil 2021;4(2):e535–44.
3. Bernhardson AS, Murphy CP, Aman ZS, et al. A Prospective Analysis of Patients With Anterior Versus Posterior Shoulder Instability: A Matched Cohort Examination and Surgical Outcome Analysis of 200 Patients. Am J Sports Med 2019; 47(3):682–7.
4. Bradley JP, McClincy MP, Arner JW, et al. Arthroscopic capsulolabral reconstruction for posterior instability of the shoulder: a prospective study of 200 shoulders. Am J Sports Med 2013;41(9):2005–14.
5. Chang ES, Greco NJ, McClincy MP, et al. Posterior Shoulder Instability in Overhead Athletes. Orthop Clin North Am 2016;47(1):179–87.
6. McClincy MP, Arner JW, Bradley JP. Posterior Shoulder Instability in Throwing Athletes: A Case-Matched Comparison of Throwers and Non-Throwers. Arthroscopy 2015;31(6):1041–51.
7. Goldenberg BT, Goldsten P, Lacheta L, et al. Rehabilitation Following Posterior Shoulder Stabilization. Int J Sports Phys Ther 2021;16(3):930–40.

8. Dickens JF, Hoyt BW, Kilcoyne KG, et al. Posterior Glenoid Bone Loss and Instability: An Evidence-based Approach to Diagnosis and Management. J Am Acad Orthop Surg 2023;31(9):429–39.

9. Sardar H, Lee S, Horner NS, et al. Indications and outcomes of glenoid osteotomy for posterior shoulder instability: a systematic review. Shoulder Elb 2023;15(2): 117–31.

10. Waltenspül M, Häller T, Ernstbrunner L, et al. Long-term results after posterior open glenoid wedge osteotomy for posterior shoulder instability associated with excessive glenoid retroversion. J shoulder Elb Surg 2022;31(1):81–9.

11. Moeller EA, Houck DA, McCarty EC, et al. Outcomes of Arthroscopic Posterior Shoulder Stabilization in the Beach-Chair Versus Lateral Decubitus Position: A Systematic Review. Orthop J Sport Med 2019;7(1):2325967118822452.

12. de SA D, Sheean AJ, Morales-Restrepo A, et al. Patient Positioning in Arthroscopic Management of Posterior-Inferior Shoulder Instability: A Systematic Review Comparing Beach Chair and Lateral Decubitus Approaches. Arthroscopy 2019;35(1):214–24.e3.

13. Dacey S, Meghani O, Dove JH, et al. Lack of Consensus in Rehabilitation Protocols After Posterior Shoulder Stabilization. Orthop J Sport Med 2023;11(5): 23259671231161589.

14. Waltz RA, Wong J, Peebles AM, et al. Postoperative Stiffness and Pain After Arthroscopic Labral Stabilization: Consider Anchor Arthropathy. Arthroscopy 2021;37(11):3266–74.

15. Ruzbarsky JJ, Waltz RA, Peebles AM, et al. Anchor Arthropathy of the Shoulder Joint After Instability Repair: Outcomes Improve With Revision Surgery. Arthroscopy 2021;37(12):3414–20.

16. Delong JM, Jiang K, Bradley JP. Posterior Instability of the Shoulder: A Systematic Review and Meta-analysis of Clinical Outcomes. Am J Sports Med 2015; 43(7):1805–17.

17. Bradley JP, Arner JW, Jayakumar S, et al. Risk Factors and Outcomes of Revision Arthroscopic Posterior Shoulder Capsulolabral Repair. Am J Sports Med 2018; 46(10):2457–65.

18. Rothrauff BB, Arner JW, Talentino SE, et al. Minimum 10-Year Clinical Outcomes After Arthroscopic Capsulolabral Repair for Isolated Posterior Shoulder Instability. Am J Sports Med 2023;51(6):1571–80.

19. Owens BD, Campbell SE, Cameron KL. Risk factors for posterior shoulder instability in young athletes. Am J Sports Med 2013;41(11):2645–9.

20. Bradley JP, Arner JW, Jayakumar S, et al. Revision Arthroscopic Posterior Shoulder Capsulolabral Repair in Contact Athletes: Risk Factors and Outcomes. Arthroscopy 2020;36(3):660–5.

21. Gouveia K, Kay J, Memon M, et al. Return to Sport After Surgical Management of Posterior Shoulder Instability: A Systematic Review and Meta-analysis. Am J Sports Med 2022;50(3):845–57.

22. Arner JW, McClincy MP, Bradley JP. Arthroscopic Stabilization of Posterior Shoulder Instability Is Successful in American Football Players. Arthroscopy 2015; 31(8):1466–71.

23. Arner JW, McClincy MP, Bradley JP. In Throwers With Posterior Instability, Rotator Cuff Tears Are Common but Do Not Affect Surgical Outcomes. Am J Orthop 2018; 47(1). https://doi.org/10.12788/ajo.2018.0005.

24. de Groot SJ, Arner JW, Smith CN, et al. Arthroscopic SLAP IIb Repair Using Knot-Tying Versus Knotless Suture Anchors: Is There a Difference? Am J Orthop (Belle Mead NJ) 2018;47(12). https://doi.org/10.12788/ajo.2018.0101.

Current Concepts in Assessment and Management of Failed Posterior Labral Repair

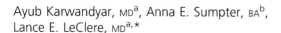

Ayub Karwandyar, MD[a], Anna E. Sumpter, BA[b],
Lance E. LeClere, MD[a],*

KEYWORDS

- Posterior shoulder instability • Failure • Revision

KEY POINTS

- Failed posterior labral repair poses a challenge for both physicians and patients.
- Potential risk factors for failed posterior stabilization include sex, glenoid bone width/glenoid bone loss, concomitant rotator cuff injury, number of anchors used in the index surgery, and patient activity level.
- Bony abnormalities, specifically glenoid dysplasia, bone loss, and significant retroversion, are important to consider in the setting of posterior labral repair, as they have been shown to be associated with increased rates of failure.
- There does not presently exist a standard for assessing and discerning clinical failure of posterior labral repairs.

INTRODUCTION & BACKGROUND

Persistent pain and instability following a posterior labral repair poses a unique challenge for both patients and physicians. Though posterior instability was previously thought to represent just 2% to 12% of all reported instability,[1–3] this estimate has increased to as high as 20% to 24%.[4–6] Furthermore, recurrence rates following surgical intervention as high as 14% have been demonstrated[1,7] with most published posterior instability surgery revision rates falling between 5% and 8%.[1,7] This has important repercussions for the return to pre-operative activity level in the impacted patient population, which is disproportionately composed of athletes and military personnel.[6,7] This is likely due to the increased incidence of traumatic and microtraumatic events that occur

[a] Department of Orthopaedic Surgery, Vanderbilt University Medical Center, Nashville, TN, USA; [b] School of Medicine, Vanderbilt University, Nashville, TN, USA
* Corresponding author. Department of Orthopaedic Surgery, Vanderbilt University Medical Center, 1215 21st Avenue South, MCE South Tower, Suite 4200, Nashville, TN 37232.
E-mail address: l.leclere@vumc.org

Clin Sports Med 43 (2024) 755–767
https://doi.org/10.1016/j.csm.2023.12.003
0278-5919/24/© 2023 Elsevier Inc. All rights reserved.

in these settings, which place a large degree of posteriorly-directed forces on the shoulder, resulting in capsulolabral attenuation and detachment.[6,7]

Existing research has explored a number of risk factors associated with clinical failure of posterior labral repairs, including but not limited to sex, glenoid bone width, concomitant rotator cuff injury, number of anchors used in the index surgery, and patient activity level.[1,7] However, standardization of assessment and failure metrics are currently lacking. As such, further distinction and definition are necessary. This article will review and summarize the current understanding of failed posterior labral repair with respect to incidence and impact, risk factors, clinical and radiographic assessment, and treatment strategies.

INCIDENCE & IMPACT

There is discrepancy regarding the rates of recurrent instability and reoperation among patients who undergo posterior stabilization surgery. Even within a specific patient subpopulation, such as active military personnel, reported incidence varies.[6,8,9] Chan and colleagues found that, of 65 active-duty military service members who underwent primary, isolated arthroscopic posterior labral repair, just 1 individual required a revision arthroscopic repair (1.5%). However, more than 15% of the patients reported activity-limiting shoulder pain, preventing them from making a full return to active duty.[9] Conversely, Scanaliato and colleagues found that less than 5% of active-duty servicemen were unable to return to their pre-operative active-duty status following posterior stabilization. Just 3 of the 75 patients in this study were reported to have recurrent instability (4.11%) and only 1 underwent revision surgery.[8] Provencher and colleagues found much higher rates of clinical failure among US Navy or Marine Corps active-duty personnel, as indicated by either recurrent instability (12.1%) or persistent pain (9%), totaling 7 of 33 patients (21%).

Much of the existing research has also focused on the athlete patient subpopulation, seeking to understand the outcomes of posterior stabilization, including both revision rate and return-to-sport (RTS). Bradley and colleagues explored the incidence of revision surgeries across 297 shoulders that underwent arthroscopic posterior capsulolabral repair, of which 19 were identified (6.4%). Between the revision and non-revision groups, there was an enormous disparity in the return to pre-operative level of sport (64.3% vs 15.4%, respectively). The revision group also demonstrated smaller improvements from pre-to post-op with regard to pain, range of motion, and strength compared to the non-revision group. Similarly, those who underwent revision repair did not achieve significant stability improvement post-operatively, while the primary repair group did.[1]

Another study investigating the incidence of failed posterior stabilization among throwing athletes found that 9 of 105 individuals underwent revision surgery (8.6%) at an average of 2.8 years after the index procedure (Vaswani and colleagues). In contrast to the Bradley and colleagues findings, the revision and non-revision cohorts had similar post-operative outcomes as indicated by American Shoulder and Elbow Score (ASES), Kerlan-Jobe Orthopaedic Clinic Shoulder and Elbow Score (KJOC), pain, stability, and patient satisfaction. However, a lower return-to-sport was noted in the revision group, though this was not statistically significant.[10]

Reddy and colleagues explored differences in return-to-sport and recurrent instability in young athletes, with a particular focus on differences in post-operative return-to-sport testing regimens (criteria-based vs time-based). Recurrent instability in each of the 2 cohorts was 6.7% and 9.0%, respectively, while persistent pain was 23.3% and 25.4%, respectively. Similar to the aforementioned studies, overall RTS rate was roughly 94% for both groups, but return to pre-injury level of sport was between 80% and 84%.[11] Whicker and colleagues studied a similar patient population—the adolescent athlete—in order to discern rates of revision and post-operative outcomes. Ultimately, this study found that 9.3% of the patients required revision surgery, and these patients demonstrated lower ASES scores, and poorer range of motion, among other metrics. Interestingly, however, revision and non-revision groups had comparable rates of return to sport and pre-injury sport level.[12]

RISK FACTORS

There are a number of risk factors that have been identified in posterior labral repair failure. Prior literature has repeatedly demonstrated a higher risk of failure among females compared to males.[1,10,11] Additionally, Bradley and colleagues reported on the association of smaller glenoid bone width (≤26 mm) with the need for revision surgery.[1] These measurements were obtained on axial MRI and were determined to be the distances between the apices of subchondral bone anteriorly and posteriorly. An average width difference of 3 mm was found between the non-revision and revision groups. There were no significant inter-group differences in labral width, nor glenoid labral, chondral, or glenoid version. Conversely, Vaswani and colleagues found no significant differences in any bony or labral widths or version between the revision and non-revision cohorts.[10] The utilization of fewer than 3 suture anchors during the index posterior labral repair surgery has also been proposed as a risk factor, though this has been disputed by other research.[1,9,13] Additionally, Delong and colleagues noted higher rates of failure could result from poor-quality posterior capsular tissue as a consequence of prior surgical intervention.[14] The authors particularly noted that thermal capsulorrhaphy can cause shrinkage of capsular tissue which may weaken the capsule labral complex which can lead to failure.[15–17] Finally, Bradley and colleagues identified concomitant rotator cuff injury as being a risk factor for failure of posterior labral repair.[1]

SPECIAL CONSIDERATIONS

Bony abnormalities, specifically glenoid dysplasia, bone loss, and significant retroversion, are important to consider in the setting of posterior labral repair, as they have been shown to be associated with increased rates of failure.[18,19] Recurrent posterior instability events may produce bony defects, particularly in the posteroinferior quadrant of the glenoid (**Fig. 1**)[20,21] To date, the impact of bone loss on the post-operative outcomes of reverse Bankart repairs has not been extensively researched, though biomechanical models have suggested that pathomechanics such as posterior humeral head translation, unable to be corrected with a reverse Bankart procedure alone, may contribute to increased risk.[20,22] In a study, Wolfe and colleagues found that moderate posterior glenoid bone deficiency (>13.5%) at the time of the index posterior labral repair and glenoid-based capsulorrhaphy was associated with significantly greater retroversion (7°) and higher clinical failure rate compared to minimal bone deficiency (44.4% vs 10.5%, respectively). This highlights the critical need to adequately address recurrent posterior instability, as each instability event has been shown to be associated with a glenoid bone loss as much as 5%.[19]

ASSESSMENT/EVALUATION
Physical Examination

Posterior shoulder instability may be difficult to initially diagnose due to the variation of clinical complaints. Most patients initially will present with pain rather than instability,

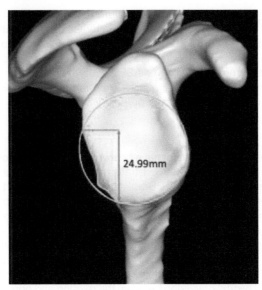

Fig. 1. Superior to inferior measurement of the bony defect by utilizing glenoid en face view with an example of posterior bone loss. (Reused with permission from Ernat et al.[23])

but those presenting with recurrent instability are more likely to fail nonoperative management.[24] Although nonspecific, the most common symptom associated with instability after reconstruction is posterior shoulder pain with decreased athletic activity.[25] Assessment of the shoulder should always be compared to the contralateral shoulder. Assessment should begin with history taking, inspection, palpation, assessment of range of motion, evaluation of scapular kinematics, specific muscle strength tests, and physical examination tests to obtain important diagnostic clues.[26] Specific tests for posterior shoulder instability include the posterior apprehension test, load and shift test, posterior drawer test, Kim test, and Jerk test. A comprehensive review of shoulder instability examinations and their efficacy can be found in articles written by Hippensteel and colleagues in 2019 and Hedgeus and colleagues in 2012.[27,28] The Kim test has a sensitivity of 80%, specificity of 94%, positive predictive value of 73%, and negative predictive value of 96% in detecting posterior inferior labral lesions.[29] The jerk test has a specificity of 85%, sensitivity of 89.7%, positive predictive value of 72.2%, and negative predictive value of 94.4% in diagnosing posterior inferior labral lesions.[30] A comprehensive assessment of the shoulder for instability can help aid in the work-up of failed posterior labral repairs.

Defining Failure

No consensus exists on how to define patients who failed treatment of posterior capsulolabral repair. Provencher and colleagues in their review of military patients who underwent posterior shoulder stabilization procedures defined failure as persistent pain or instability postoperatively.[17] Bradley and colleagues in their study defined failure as patients who required revision surgery, American Shoulder and Elbow Surgeons shoulder score of less than 60 (range 0–100; >80 excellent; <40 poor), or a subjective shoulder stability score of greater than 5 (range 0–10; 0 as completely stable; 10 completely unstable).[1] Similarly, Jewett and colleagues in their systematic review highlighted the inconsistencies for the definition of failure in posterior shoulder instability literature.[31] While no optimal definition exists, continued pain and instability are the most commonly utilized criteria for failure in the literature.

Imaging

Even with adequate physical examination, recurrent or persistent posterior shoulder instability after prior surgery may be challenging to diagnose. Imaging examinations play a key role in identification and management of this condition.

Radiography

Radiographic imaging for the work-up for posterior shoulder instability includes standard 4-view radiographs of the glenohumeral joint. Radiographs should be evaluated for signs of glenoid dysplasia, changes in the size of the acromion, dysplasia of the distal clavicle, hypoplasia of the ribs and flattening of the humeral head, and any post-surgical changes, to include glenohumeral bone loss.[25]

Computed tomography

Computed tomography (CT) scans are helpful for evaluating bony structures and bony pathology and can assess bone loss. Weishaupt and colleagues reviewed CT scans of 15 patients with atraumatic recurrent posterior instability, 93% had some loss of the posterior inferior glenoid rim.[21] Furthermore, those with a deficiency of 12 mm or more in the craniocaudal length were defined as abnormal and sensitivity and specificity for diagnosing recurrent posterior instability were 86.7% and 83.3%, respectively.[21]

MRI and arthrography

MRI and magnetic resonance arthrography (MRA) are helpful in evaluating soft tissues particularly the posterior labrum and the posterior capsule. Liu and colleagues reviewed the diagnostic performance of MRI versus MRA for detecting labral lesions which showed a sensitivity of 77% versus 92% and specificity of 95% versus 98%, respectively.[32] While MRA enhances sensitivity, specificity is only marginally superior. Liu suggests that since MRAs are invasive and associated with adverse reactions related to injections and contrast, MRAs should be reserved for patients with chronic symptoms or pathologic abnormality that may be more subtle to detect on MRI, and therefore may be beneficial in the evaluation of failed prior posterior labral reapir.[32] Imaging for recurrent posterior shoulder instability can reveal glenoid bone loss that shows reverse bony Bankart lesions or fractures, attritional bone loss, or dysplasia.[33]

Measuring glenoid bone loss

Dickens and colleagues reviewed the common method for measuring posterior glenoid bone loss by using sagittal CT or MRI cuts to place a "best fit" circle along the inferior two-third of the glenoid. The width of the posterior osseous defect is measured and divided by the diameter of the "best fit" circle to calculate a percent bone loss.[33] (**Fig. 2**).

Location of glenoid bone loss

Dekker and colleagues studied the location of glenoid defect in recurrent posterior shoulder instability by using a "clock-face" on 3-dimensional (3D) CT reformats. The supraglenoid tubercle defined the 12 o'clock position. Six-o'clock was defined by a vertical line drawn from supraglenoid tubercle to the inferior portion of the glenoid. Regardless of laterality, 9-o'clock was always posterior and 3-o'clock anterior.[20] In Dekker's review of 71 patients, the mean posterior bone loss defect extended from the 6:44 to 9:28 position or in the posteroinferior quadrant.[20] The authors discuss that knowledge of the precise location of glenoid bone loss as well as angle from

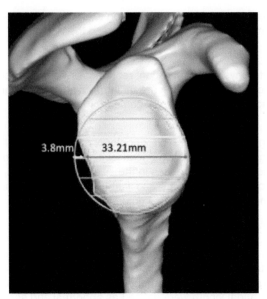

Fig. 2. Anterior to posterior width of the defect measured at 5 different levels on the glenoid en face view. This is calculated by subtracting the remaining glenoid width from the width of the uninjured glenoid (*perfect fit circle*) and then dividing that by the diameter of the perfect fit circle. (Reused with permission from Ernat et al.[23])

the long axis can help improve outcomes in revision surgery by optimizing bone block placements.[20] The significance of glenoid bone loss was investigated by Arner and colleagues The authors defined risk factors for failure of posterior shoulder capsulolabral repair which included patients with overall smaller glenoid bone width and noted a 10 times higher failure rate when glenoid bone loss was greater than 11%.[34] (**Fig. 3**).

Glenoid version
Another measurement of glenoid morphology includes glenoid version. Beaulieu-Jones et al reviewed glenoid version in patients with posterior shoulder instability.[36] The authors measured version using the glenoid vault described by Matsumura and

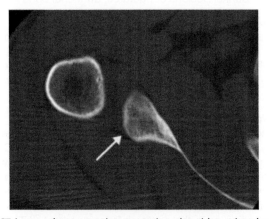

Fig. 3. The axial CT image demonstrating posterior glenoid erosion (*arrow*) and glenoid retroversion. (Reused with permission from Mulcahey et al.[35])

colleagues[37] Glenoid vault is measured using MRI or CT axial sections perpendicular to the glenoid face. The glenoid vault axis is described as a line from the tip of the scapula to the center of the glenoid.[36,37] Glenoid version is then calculated as angle between the glenoid line and the line perpendicular to the glenoid vault axis.[36,37] (**Fig. 4**) This measurement is taken at 5 equal intervals of the inferior two-thirds of the glenoid face.[36,37] A positive number represents retroversion, and a negative number represents anteversion.[36] Owens and colleagues showed that for every 1° of increased retroversion, there was a 17% increased risk in recurrence of posterior shoulder instability.[18] Furthermore, retroversion of greater than 10° in isolation has been associated with posterior instability, and may contribute to failure of primary repairs.[38]

Posterior glenoid slope

Beaulieu-Jones et al describe their novel measurement of the slope of the osseous defect defined as the angle between the glenoid line and a line parallel to the surface of the glenoid defect at 3 equal intervals along the inferior two-thirds of the glenoid face.[36] The mean slope of the posterior defect relative to the glenoid fossa was 26.8° ± 11.5°.[36] Beaulieu-Jones et al study highlighted how patients with posterior shoulder instability have bone loss that is sloped relative the glenoid fossa (**Fig. 5**).

TREATMENT STRATEGIES

Differing treatment strategies exist for failed posterior labral repair. Similar to primary posterior shoulder instability, the majority of patients with recurrent instability after surgery may first attempt nonoperative therapy. Patients who have undergone adequate therapy and continue to have symptomatic and recurrent posterior instability and/or pain with an identifiable anatomic cause should be considered for revision surgery.[25] No formal guidelines exist for treatment of recurrent posterior instability.

Nonoperative Treatment

Initial nonoperative management should focus on preventing instability, strengthening, scapular positioning, proprioception, and modification of sport-specific movements.[33]

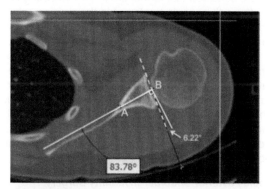

Fig. 4. Measurement of glenoid vault version. The glenoid vault axis (AB) was defined as the line connecting the tip of the scapular vault and the center of the glenoid. Glenoid version was calculated as the angle between the glenoid line (*dashed line*) and the line perpendicular to the glenoid vault axis (*solid white line*) and was measured at 5 intervals, spanning the inferior two-thirds of the face of the glenoid. In this example, glenoid version is 6.22°. (Reused with permission from Beaulieu-Jones et al.[36])

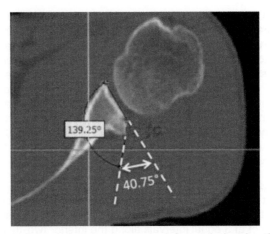

Fig. 5. Measurement of slope of posterior osseous defect. Calculated as the angle between the glenoid line and a line parallel to the surface of the glenoid bone defect. The slope was measured at 3 equal intervals, spanning the inferior two-thirds of the face of the glenoid. C denotes the measured anterior-posterior width of the glenoid defect. In this example, the slope of the posterior defect is 40.75°, relative to the glenoid fossa. (Reused with permission from Beaulieu-Jones et al.[36])

Surgical Interventions

Arthroscopic procedures for posterior capsule and labral repair include suture anchors as well as capsular plication. However, some surgeons have advocated that these procedures should be limited to patients with posterior glenoid bone loss of less than 13.5% as noted by a study from Wolfe and colleagues[39] Additionally, Provencher and colleagues showed an association of a higher failure rate if the bone loss of the glenoid surface area was greater than 11%.[34] The efficacy of revision arthroscopic labral repair and capsulorrhaphy in the setting of minimal or no bone loss is not clear. In a recent systematic review, Jewett and colleagues reviewed outcomes of revision arthroscopic posterior labral repair and cited failure rates of 21% to 75%[7,31,40] The authors conclude that further studies are needed to identify risk factors that lead to failure after arthroscopic treatment in the revision setting.

Surgeries to address glenohumeral bone loss or glenoid dysplasia include glenoid osteotomy, humeral rotational osteotomy, humeral head grafting, or glenoid bone block procedures. Augmentation with a posterior bone block may be indicated in patients with failed primary arthroscopic repair and glenohumeral bone loss. The specific techniques, indications, and outcomes for the most common osseous augmentation procedures are detailed in articles written by Dickens and colleagues and Millet and colleagues[20,33] While these articles highlight the current lack of established guidelines for revision posterior stabilization surgeries due to insufficient literature demonstrating the superiority of one technique over another, clinical algorithms are currently available to guide clinicalz

Revision Arthroscopic Posterior Shoulder Instability Surgery

The outcomes for revision arthroscopic posterior shoulder instability surgery are largely unknown.[31] Jewett and colleagues in their systematic review reported failure rates of 21% to 75%.[31] Furthermore, subjective patient scores, based on whether the surgery was worthwhile, were low, ranging from 15% to 25%[31] Jewett and colleagu systematic review was limited to 3 papers. The authors noted that more knowledge about this procedure is needed to help identify which patients may benefit from arthroscopic surgery alone or who may need open repair.[31] Given the high rate of failure of posterior instability surgery and revision posterior instability surgery, revision arthroscopic repair should be reserved for cases in which there is no appreciable bone loss and quality labral and capsular tissue that is amenable to robust repair.

Glenoid Bone Block Procedures

Posterior bone block procedures or augmentations become an option in the setting of increased glenoid retroversion, failed soft tissue repair or poor soft tissue quality, or posterior bone loss.[33] The augmentations can be done through open or arthroscopic approaches. Arthroscopic posterior bone augmentation has potential advantages which include improved joint visibility, ability to address concomitant pathologies, deltoid sparing, and improved cosmesis.[41]

Posterior bone augmentation graft options include distal tibia allograft, distal clavicle autograft, scapular spine autograft, or tricortical iliac crest graft.[33] Autograft has the benefit of decreased cost and avoidance of immune reactions and donor infection risk, but disadvantages include donor site morbidity and limited available donor sites. Fixation of the graft can be accomplished by screws or suspensory fixation, with no clear superiority demonstrated at this time. Outcomes data for bone block augmentation are limited. Gilat and colleagues found a 10% recurrence rate and 20% revision rate for patients undergoing distal tibia allograft stabilization surgery.[42] Cognetti and colleagues performed a systematic review on posterior glenoid bone block augmentation. The authors found high rates of complications which include large ranges of rates of revision surgery (0% to 67%), symptomatic hardware (0% to 73%), the development of osteoarthritis (0% to 100%), and partial or complete osteolysis (0% to 100%) of the bone block.[43] Cognetti and colleagues concluded posterior bone augmentation did not reliably yield positive outcomes and is associated with high rates of complications.[43] The data were limited to draw conclusions of the superiority of one technique over another.[43] Mojica and colleagues also reviewed bone block procedures for posterior shoulder instability and found a moderate rate of recurrent instability and high complication rate of 14% after bone block transfer.[44] However, Mojica and colleagues found that patient-reported outcomes, most commonly reported by Rowe, Constant, and Walch-Duplay scores, were consistently high.[44] These results are in contrast to Cognetti and colleagues review which found low patient satisfaction scores.[44] Both studies concluded that posterior glenoid bone block augmentation is a rare technique associated with a high likelihood of failure[44]

Humeral Rotational Osteotomy

A humeral rotational osteotomy can be performed when the reverse Hill Sachs lesion is large or medial enough to engage with the glenoid. Typically done with open approach, the humeral osteotomy rotates the impaction fracture to prevent recurrent instability and engagement.[33] Keppler and colleagues reviewed the procedure and noted that the osteotomy is appropriate for patients with less than 40% defect of the articular surface.[45] They recommend defects greater than 40% may be better served with arthroplasty.[45] Outcomes for this procedure are limited. Brooks-Hills et al performed this procedure on 19 patients. There were 25 complications and 9shoulders underwent revision surgery.[46] Because of the limited data and unpredictable outcomes, Dickens and colleagues recommended reserving this treatment as a salvage option.

Glenoid Osteotomy

A glenoid osteotomy is typically reserved for patients with posterior shoulder instability due to significant glenoid retroversion by performing an opening wedge osteotomy. Sardar and colleagues performed a systematic review of this procedure and found 85% satisfaction rates, but complications were frequent at 34% which included glenoid fracture, graft loosening, infection, and nerve injury.[47] Additionally, recurrent instability was seen in 20% of the patients. Sardar and colleagues recommended this procedure be performed with iliac crest graft due to its high fixation strength to minimize the risk of recurrent instability. Waltenspül and colleagues noted in their series of 7 shoulders that despite correction of retroversion, 6 had recurrent instability and 5 patients did not have the humeral head centered on the glenoid after the opening wedge osteotomy.[48] Because of the technical demands of this surgery and poor outcomes, this procedure is rarely performed.[33]

Rehabilitation

Rehabilitation is procedure, patient, and surgeon dependent. In general, most patients will be kept in an abduction sling for 4 to 6 weeks. Codman exercises can be initiated immediately. Progressing from passive to active-assisted range of motion is advanced over 4 weeks. At 4 to 6 weeks, the patient can begin internal rotation progression, with a goal of achieving full range of motion at around 8 weeks. At 3 months, strength training can be initiated. Depending on the sport or work, return to sport or unrestricted activity can usually start around 6 months.

SUMMARY

Recurrent posterior shoulder instability after primary repair is uncommon, but presents a challenging clinical scenario. Most revisions in failed labral repair were associated with glenoid bone morphology related to critical bone loss, retroversion, or dysplasia. A variety of treatment options exist which include revision labral repair with or without capsular plication, glenoid osteotomy, humeral rotational osteotomy, or glenoid bone augmentation. No single technique has been shown to be superior and each technique has strengths and limitations. Therefore, thoughtful evaluation and planning is critical to address each patient's individual pathology to maximize success after revision surgery.

CLINICS CARE POINTS

- The diagnosis and management of revision posterior shoulder stabilization surgery remains challenging.
- No clear definition exists for failure for surgery, but recurrent pain and instability were the most frequently cited in the literature.
- Risk factors for failure include a combination of soft tissue pathology with glenoid bone loss or glenoid retroversion.
- The literature is limited on providing ideal surgical techniques for optimal outcomes in revision posterior shoulder stabilization procedures. In general, revision arthroscopic soft tissue repair should be reserved for rare situations in which there is no appreciate bone loss and good soft tissue quality. Arthroscopic bone augmentation procedures may improve outcomes of revision posterior repairs, especially in the setting of glenoid bone loss. However, there are limited long-term outcomes data at this time.

DISCLOSURE

There are no conflicts of interest to disclose.

REFERENCES

1. Bradley JP, Arner JW, Jayakumar S, et al. Risk Factors and Outcomes of Revision Arthroscopic Posterior Shoulder Capsulolabral Repair. Am J Sports Med 2018; 46(10):2457–65.
2. Antoniou J, Harryman DT. 2nd. Posterior instability. Orthop Clin North Am 2001; 32(3):463–73, ix.
3. Provencher MT, LeClere LE, King S, et al. Posterior instability of the shoulder: diagnosis and management. Am J Sports Med 2011;39(4):874–86.
4. Swan ER, Lynch TB, Sheean AJ, et al. High Incidence of Combined and Posterior Labral Tears in Military Patients With Operative Shoulder Instability. Am J Sports Med 2022;50(6):1529–33.
5. Song DJ, Cook JB, Krul KP, et al. High frequency of posterior and combined shoulder instability in young active patients. J Shoulder Elbow Surg. Feb 2015; 24(2):186–90.
6. Yow BG, Wade SM, Bedrin MD, et al. The Incidence of Posterior and Combined AP Shoulder Instability Treatment with Surgical Stabilization Is Higher in an Active Military Population than in the General Population: Findings from the US Naval Academy. Clin Orthop Relat Res 2021;479(4):704–8.
7. DeLong JM, Jiang K, Bradley JP. Posterior Instability of the Shoulder: A Systematic Review and Meta-analysis of Clinical Outcomes. Am J Sports Med 2015; 43(7):1805–17.
8. Scanaliato JP, Childs BR, Dunn JC, et al. Arthroscopic Posterior Labral Repair in Active-Duty Military Patients: A Reliable Solution for an At-Risk Population, Regardless of Anchor Type. Am J Sports Med 2022;50(11):3036–44.
9. Chan S, O'Brien LK, Waterman BR, et al. Low Risk of Recurrence After Posterior Labral Repair of the Shoulder in a High-Risk United States Military Population. Arthrosc Sports Med Rehabil 2020;2(1):e47–52.
10. Vaswani R, Arner J, Freiman H, et al. Risk Factors for Revision Posterior Shoulder Stabilization in Throwing Athletes. Orthop J Sports Med 2020;8(12). 2325967120967652.
11. Reddy RP, Rai A, Como M, et al. Criteria-based return-to-sport testing helps identify functional deficits in young athletes following posterior labral repair but may not reduce recurrence or increase return to play. JSES Int 2023;7(3):385–92.
12. Whicker EA, Arner JW, Edwards C, et al. Outcomes After Revision Posterior Shoulder Capsulolabral Repair in Adolescent Athletes. Orthop J Sports Med 2023;11(8). 23259671231188390.
13. Boileau P, Villalba M, Héry JY, et al. Risk factors for recurrence of shoulder instability after arthroscopic Bankart repair. J Bone Joint Surg Am 2006;88(8): 1755–63.
14. DeLong JM, Bradley JP. Posterior shoulder instability in the athletic population: Variations in assessment, clinical outcomes, and return to sport. World J Orthop 2015;6(11):927–34.
15. Bradley JP, Baker CL, Kline AJ, et al. Arthroscopic Capsulolabral Reconstruction for Posterior Instability of the Shoulder: A Prospective Study of 100 Shoulders. Am J Sports Med 2006;34(7):1061–71.

16. McIntyre LF, Caspari RB, Savoie FH 3rd. The arthroscopic treatment of multidirectional shoulder instability: two-year results of a multiple suture technique. Arthroscopy 1997;13(4):418–25.

17. Provencher MT, Bell SJ, Menzel KA, et al. Arthroscopic treatment of posterior shoulder instability: results in 33 patients. Am J Sports Med 2005;33(10): 1463–71.

18. Owens BD, Campbell SE, Cameron KL. Risk factors for posterior shoulder instability in young athletes. Am J Sports Med 2013;41(11):2645–9.

19. Bedrin MD, Owens BD, Slaven SE, et al. Prospective Evaluation of Posterior Glenoid Bone Loss After First-time and Recurrent Posterior Glenohumeral Instability Events. Am J Sports Med 2022;50(11):3028–35.

20. Dekker TJ, Peebles LA, Goldenberg BT, et al. Location of the Glenoid Defect in Shoulders With Recurrent Posterior Glenohumeral Instability. Am J Sports Med 2019;47(13):3051–6.

21. Weishaupt D, Zanetti M, Nyffeler RW, et al. Posterior glenoid rim deficiency in recurrent (atraumatic) posterior shoulder instability. Skeletal Radiol 2000;29(4): 204–10.

22. Nacca C, Gil JA, Badida R, et al. Critical Glenoid Bone Loss in Posterior Shoulder Instability. Am J Sports Med 2018;46(5):1058–63.

23. Ernat JJ, Golijanin P, Peebles AM, et al. Anterior and posterior glenoid bone loss in patients receiving surgery for glenohumeral instability is not the same: a comparative 3-dimensional imaging analysis. JSES Int 2022;6(4):581–6.

24. Antosh IJ, Tokish JM, Owens BD. Posterior Shoulder Instability. Sports Health 2016;8(6):520–6.

25. Chalmers PN, Hammond J, Juhan T, et al. Revision posterior shoulder stabilization. J Shoulder Elbow Surg 2013;22(9):1209–20.

26. Yang S, Kim TU, Kim DH, et al. Understanding the physical examination of the shoulder: a narrative review. Ann Palliat Med 2021;10(2):2293–303.

27. Hippensteel KJ, Brophy R, Smith MV, et al. Comprehensive Review of Provocative and Instability Physical Examination Tests of the Shoulder. J Am Acad Orthop Surg 2019;27(11):395–404.

28. Hegedus EJ, Goode AP, Cook CE, et al. Which physical examination tests provide clinicians with the most value when examining the shoulder? Update of a systematic review with meta-analysis of individual tests. Br J Sports Med 2012; 46(14):964–78.

29. Kim SH, Park JS, Jeong WK, et al. The Kim test: a novel test for posteroinferior labral lesion of the shoulder–a comparison to the jerk test. Am J Sports Med 2005;33(8):1188–92.

30. Kim SH, Park JC, Park JS, et al. Painful jerk test: a predictor of success in nonoperative treatment of posteroinferior instability of the shoulder. Am J Sports Med 2004;32(8):1849–55.

31. Jewett CA, Reardon P, Cox C, et al. Outcomes of Revision Arthroscopic Posterior Labral Repair and Capsulorrhaphy: A Systematic Review. Orthop J Sports Med 2023;11(6). https://doi.org/10.1177/23259671231174444. 23259671231174474.

32. Liu F, Cheng X, Dong J, et al. Imaging modality for measuring the presence and extent of the labral lesions of the shoulder: a systematic review and meta-analysis. BMC Muscoskel Disord 2019;20(1).

33. Dickens JF, Hoyt BW, Kilcoyne KG, et al. Posterior Glenoid Bone Loss and Instability: An Evidence-based Approach to Diagnosis and Management. J Am Acad Orthop Surg 2023;31(9):429–39.

34. Arner JW, Ruzbarsky JJ, Midtgaard K, et al. Defining Critical Glenoid Bone Loss in Posterior Shoulder Capsulolabral Repair. Am J Sports Med 2021;49(8):2013–9.
35. Mulcahey MK, Campbell KJ, Golijanan P, et al. Posterior Bone Grafting for Glenoid Defects of the Shoulder. Operat Tech Sports Med 2015;23(1):32–42.
36. Beaulieu-Jones BR, Peebles LA, Golijanin P, et al. Characterization of Posterior Glenoid Bone Loss Morphology in Patients With Posterior Shoulder Instability. Arthroscopy 2019;35(10):2777–84.
37. Matsumura N, Ogawa K, Ikegami H, et al. Computed tomography measurement of glenoid vault version as an alternative measuring method for glenoid version. J Orthop Surg Res 2014;9(1):17.
38. Imhoff FB, Camenzind RS, Obopilwe E, et al. Glenoid retroversion is an important factor for humeral head centration and the biomechanics of posterior shoulder stability. Knee Surg Sports Traumatol Arthrosc 2019;27(12):3952–61.
39. Wolfe JA, Elsenbeck M, Nappo K, et al. Effect of Posterior Glenoid Bone Loss and Retroversion on Arthroscopic Posterior Glenohumeral Stabilization. Am J Sports Med 2020;48(11):2621–7.
40. Bradley JP, Baker CL 3rd, Kline AJ, et al. Arthroscopic capsulolabral reconstruction for posterior instability of the shoulder: a prospective study of 100 shoulders. Am J Sports Med 2006;34(7):1061–71.
41. Zhang AL, Montgomery SR, Ngo SS, et al. Arthroscopic versus open shoulder stabilization: current practice patterns in the United States. Arthroscopy 2014; 30(4):436–43.
42. Gilat R, Haunschild ED, Tauro T, et al. Distal Tibial Allograft Augmentation for Posterior Shoulder Instability Associated With Glenoid Bony Deficiency: A Case Series. Arthrosc Sports Med Rehabil 2020;2(6):e743–52.
43. Cognetti DJ, Hughes JD, Kay J, et al. Bone Block Augmentation of the Posterior Glenoid for Recurrent Posterior Shoulder Instability Is Associated With High Rates of Clinical Failure: A Systematic Review. Arthroscopy 2022;38(2):551–63.e5.
44. Mojica ES, Schwartz LB, Hurley ET, et al. Posterior glenoid bone block transfer for posterior shoulder instability: a systematic review. J Shoulder Elbow Surg 2021; 30(12):2904–9.
45. Keppler P, Holz U, Thielemann FW, et al. Locked posterior dislocation of the shoulder: treatment using rotational osteotomy of the humerus. J Orthop Trauma 1994;8(4):286–92.
46. Brooks-Hill AL, Forster BB, van Wyngaarden C, et al. Weber osteotomy for large Hill-Sachs Defects: clinical and CT assessments. Clin Orthop Relat Res 2013; 471(8):2548–55.
47. Sardar H, Lee S, Horner NS, et al. Indications and outcomes of glenoid osteotomy for posterior shoulder instability: a systematic review. Shoulder Elbow 2023;15(2): 117–31.
48. Waltenspül M, Häller T, Ernstbrunner L, et al. Long-term results after posterior open glenoid wedge osteotomy for posterior shoulder instability associated with excessive glenoid retroversion. J Shoulder Elbow Surg 2022;31(1):81–9.

UNITED STATES POSTAL SERVICE

Statement of Ownership, Management, and Circulation
(All Periodicals Publications Except Requester Publications)

1. Publication Title	**2. Publication Number**	**3. Filing Date**
CLINICS IN SPORTS MEDICINE	000 – 702	9/18/2024

4. Issue Frequency	**5. Number of Issues Published Annually**	**6. Annual Subscription Price**
JAN, APR, JUL, OCT	4	$390.00

7. Complete Mailing Address of Known Office of Publication (Not printer) (Street, city, county, state, and ZIP+4®)

ELSEVIER INC.
230 Park Avenue, Suite 800
New York, NY 10169

Contact Person
Malathi Samayan

Telephone (Include area code)
91-44-4299-4507

8. Complete Mailing Address of Headquarters or General Business Office of Publisher (Not printer)

ELSEVIER INC.
230 Park Avenue, Suite 800
New York, NY 10169

9. Full Names and Complete Mailing Addresses of Publisher, Editor, and Managing Editor (Do not leave blank)

Publisher (Name and complete mailing address)

Dolores Meloni, ELSEVIER INC.
1600 JOHN F KENNEDY BLVD. SUITE 1600
PHILADELPHIA, PA 19103-2899

Editor (Name and complete mailing address)

Megan Ashdown, ELSEVIER INC.
1600 JOHN F KENNEDY BLVD. SUITE 1600
PHILADELPHIA, PA 19103-2899

Managing Editor (Name and complete mailing address)

PATRICK MANLEY, ELSEVIER INC.
1600 JOHN F KENNEDY BLVD. SUITE 1600
PHILADELPHIA, PA 19103-2899

10. Owner (Do not leave blank. If the publication is owned by a corporation, give the name and address of the corporation immediately followed by the names and addresses of all stockholders owning or holding 1 percent or more of the total amount of stock. If not owned by a corporation, give the names and addresses of the individual owners. If owned by a partnership or other unincorporated firm, give its name and address as well as those of each individual owner. If the publication is published by a nonprofit organization, give its name and address.)

Full Name	Complete Mailing Address
WHOLLY OWNED SUBSIDIARY OF REED/ELSEVIER, US HOLDINGS	1600 JOHN F KENNEDY BLVD. SUITE 1600 PHILADELPHIA, PA 19103-2899

11. Known Bondholders, Mortgagees, and Other Security Holders Owning or Holding 1 Percent or More of Total Amount of Bonds, Mortgages, or Other Securities. If none, check box. ► ☐ None

Full Name	Complete Mailing Address
N/A	

12. Tax Status (For completion by nonprofit organizations authorized to mail at nonprofit rates) (Check one)
The purpose, function, and nonprofit status of this organization and the exempt status for federal income tax purposes:
☒ Has Not Changed During Preceding 12 Months
☐ Has Changed During Preceding 12 Months (Publisher must submit explanation of change with this statement)

PS Form **3526**, July 2014 [Page 1 of 4 (see instructions page 4)] PSN: 7530-01-000-9931 PRIVACY NOTICE: See our privacy policy on www.usps.com.

---

13. Publication Title	**14. Issue Date for Circulation Data Below**
CLINICS IN SPORTS MEDICINE	JULY 2024

15. Extent and Nature of Circulation

		Average No. Copies Each Issue During Preceding 12 Months	No. Copies of Single Issue Published Nearest to Filing Date
a. Total Number of Copies (Net press run)		125	121
b. Paid Circulation (By Mail and Outside the Mail)	(1) Mailed Outside-County Paid Subscriptions Stated on PS Form 3541 (Include paid distribution above nominal rate, advertiser's proof copies, and exchange copies)	63	64
	(2) Mailed In-County Paid Subscriptions Stated on PS Form 3541 (Include paid distribution above nominal rate, advertiser's proof copies, and exchange copies)	0	0
	(3) Paid Distribution Outside the Mails Including Sales Through Dealers and Carriers, Street Vendors, Counter Sales, and Other Paid Distribution Outside USPS®	46	44
	(4) Paid Distribution by Other Classes of Mail Through the USPS (e.g., First-Class Mail®)	9	6
c. Total Paid Distribution (Sum of 15b (1), (2), (3), and (4))	►	118	114
d. Free or Nominal Rate Distribution (By Mail and Outside the Mail)	(1) Free or Nominal Rate Outside-County Copies included on PS Form 3541	6	6
	(2) Free or Nominal Rate In-County Copies Included on PS Form 3541	0	0
	(3) Free or Nominal Rate Copies Mailed at Other Classes Through the USPS (e.g., First-Class Mail)	0	0
	(4) Free or Nominal Rate Distribution Outside the Mail (Carriers or other means)	1	1
e. Total Free or Nominal Rate Distribution (Sum of 15d (1), (2), (3) and (4))	►	7	7
f. Total Distribution (Sum of 15c and 15e)	►	125	121
g. Copies not Distributed (See Instructions to Publishers #4 (page #3))	►	0	0
h. Total (Sum of 15f and g)	►	125	121
i. Percent Paid (15c divided by 15f times 100)		94.38%	94.21%

* If you are claiming electronic copies, go to line 16 on page 3. If you are not claiming electronic copies, skip to line 17 on page 3.

16. Electronic Copy Circulation

	Average No. Copies Each Issue During Preceding 12 Months	No. Copies of Single Issue Published Nearest to Filing Date
a. Paid Electronic Copies ►		
b. Total Paid Print Copies (Line 15c) + Paid Electronic Copies (Line 16a) ►		
c. Total Print Distribution (Line 15f) + Paid Electronic Copies (Line 16a) ►		
d. Percent Paid (Both Print & Electronic Copies) (16b divided by 16c × 100) ►		

☒ I certify that 50% of all my distributed copies (electronic and print) are paid above a nominal price.

17. Publication of Statement of Ownership

☒ If the publication is a general publication, publication of this statement is required. Will be printed in the OCTOBER 2024 issue of this publication.   ☐ Publication not required.

18. Signature and Title of Editor, Publisher, Business Manager, or Owner

Malathi Samayan

Malathi Samayan - Distribution Controller

Date: 9/18/2024

I certify that all information furnished on this form is true and complete. I understand that anyone who furnishes false or misleading information on this form or who omits material or information requested on the form may be subject to criminal sanctions (including fines and imprisonment) and/or civil sanctions (including civil penalties).

PS Form **3526**, July 2014 (Page 3 of 4)   PRIVACY NOTICE: See our privacy policy on www.usps.com.

Moving?

Make sure your subscription moves with you!

To notify us of your new address, find your **Clinics Account Number** (located on your mailing label above your name), and contact customer service at:

Email: journalscustomerservice-usa@elsevier.com

800-654-2452 (subscribers in the U.S. & Canada)
314-447-8871 (subscribers outside of the U.S. & Canada)

Fax number: 314-447-8029

Elsevier Health Sciences Division
Subscription Customer Service
3251 Riverport Lane
Maryland Heights, MO 63043

*To ensure uninterrupted delivery of your subscription, please notify us at least 4 weeks in advance of move.

Printed and bound by CPI Group (UK) Ltd, Croydon, CR0 4YY

13/05/2025

01869643-0001